W9-BSA-945

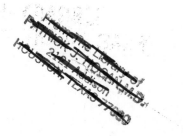

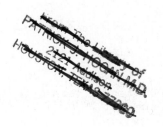

FUNDAMENTALS OF

Clinical
Trials

THIRD EDITION

FUNDAMENTALS OF

Clinical Trials

Lawrence M. Friedman

National Heart, Lung, and Blood Institute,
National Institutes of Health

Curt D. Furberg

Department of Public Health Sciences,
Bowman Gray School of Medicine

David L. DeMets

Biostatistics Department,
University of Wisconsin

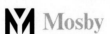

St. Louis Baltimore Boston Carlsbad Chicago Naples New York Philadelphia Portland
London Madrid Mexico City Singapore Sydney Tokyo Toronto Wiesbaden

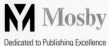
Mosby

Dedicated to Publishing Excellence

A Times Mirror
Company

Publisher: Anne Paterson
Editor: Stephanie Manning
Developmental Editors: Carolyn Malik, Laura Berendson
Project Manager: Mark Spann
Production Editor: Elizabeth Fathman
Editing and Production: A-R Editions
Designer: David Zielinski
Manufacturing Manager: Betty Richmond

THIRD EDITION
Copyright © 1996 by Mosby-Year Book, Inc.

Previous editions copyrighted 1981, 1985

All rights reserved. No part of this publication may be reproduced, stored in a retrieval system, or transmitted, in any form or by any means, electronic, mechanical, photocopying, recording or otherwise, without prior written permission from the publisher.

Permission to photocopy or reproduce solely for internal or personal use is permitted for libraries or other users registered with the Copyright Clearance Center, provided that the base fee of $4.00 per chapter plus $.10 per page is paid directly to the Copyright Clearance Center, 27 Congress Street, Salem, MA 01970. This consent does not extend to other kinds of copying, such as copying for general distribution, for advertising or promotional purposes, for creating new collected works, or for resale.

Printed in the United States of America
Composition by A-R Editions
Printing/binding by R.R. Donnelley

Mosby-Year Book, Inc.
11830 Westline Industrial Drive
St. Louis, Missouri 63146

Library of Congress Cataloging in Publication Data

Friedman, Lawrence M., 1942–
    Fundamentals of clinical trials / Lawrence M. Friedman, Curt D.
Furberg, David L. DeMets. — 3rd ed.
       p.   cm.
    Includes bibliographical references and index.
    ISBN 0-8151-3356-1
    1. Clinical trials.   I. Furberg, Curt.   II. DeMets, David L.,
1944–   .   III. Title.
    [DNLM: 1. Clinical Trials.   2. Research Design.   W 20.5 F911f
1995]
    R853.C55F75   1995
    615.5'072–dc20
    DNLM/DLC
    for Library of Congress   95-41923
                                      CIP

95 96 97 98 99 / 9 8 7 6 5 4 3 2 1

ABOUT THE AUTHORS

Lawrence M. Friedman, M.D., is Director, Division of Epidemiology and Clinical Applications, National Heart, Lung, and Blood Institute, National Institutes of Health. He was formerly Chief of the Clinical Trials Branch of the Institute. He has had major involvement in several large clinical trials and has been a consultant on many others. He has a research interest in clinical trials methodology.

Curt D. Furberg, M.D., Ph.D., is Professor and Chair, Department of Public Health Sciences, Bowman Gray School of Medicine and former Associate Director, Clinical Applications and Prevention Program, National Heart, Lung, and Blood Institute, National Institutes of Health. He has played major scientific and administrative roles in numerous multicenter clinical trials and has served in a consultative or advisory capacity on others. Dr. Furberg's research activities include the areas of clinical trials methodology and cardiovascular epidemiology.

David L. DeMets, Ph.D. in Biostatistics, is Professor of Statistics and Biostatistics, Chair of the Biostatistics Department, University of Wisconsin, and former Chief of the Mathematical and Applied Statistics Branch, National Heart, Lung, and Blood Institute, National Institutes of Health. Since 1970, he has had major roles in the design, monitoring, and analysis of data from several clinical trials, especially in the cardiology and pulmonary disease area. Since 1982, he has been involved in clinical trials of cancer therapy and acquired immunodeficiency syndrome (AIDS). Recent research interests involve monitoring and early stopping procedures in clinical trials.

Preface

The clinical trial is "the most definitive tool for evaluation of the applicability of clinical research." It represents "a key research activity with the potential to improve the quality of health care and control costs through careful comparison of alternative treatments."[10]

While many reported clinical trials are of high quality, a careful reviewer of the medical literature will notice that a significant number have deficiencies in design, conduct, analysis, presentation, or interpretation of results. Although improvements have occurred in clinical studies,[2,13] there is still considerable doubt that major progress has occurred.[2,3,7] Certainly, many studies could have been upgraded if the authors had had a better understanding of the fundamentals. The U.S. Food and Drug Administration (FDA) has issued stricter guidelines for drug approval that are consistent with the principles expressed in this book.[4] Similar guidelines for the approval of devices have also been established by the FDA.

Since the publication of the first (1981) and second (1985) editions of this book, several other texts on clinical trials have appeared.* Few of them, however, discuss general as well as specific issues involved in the development, management, and analysis of clinical trials. The purpose of this third edition is to update areas in which considerable progress has recently been made, and to broaden the scope, in the light of clinical trials in new areas. All chapters have been updated; several have been substantially expanded or cover additional topics.

In this book we hope to assist investigators in academia and industry in improving the quality of clinical trials by discussing fundamental concepts with examples from our experience and the literature. It is intended for investigators with some clinical trial experience as well as for those who plan to conduct a trial for the first time. It is also intended to be used as a textbook in the teaching of clinical trial methodology and to assist members of the scientific and medical community who wish to evaluate and interpret published reports of trials. Although not a technically oriented text, it may be used as a reference for a graduate course on statistical methods in clinical trials.

The first half of the book concerns design and development phases of a trial. These chapters are relevant for all investigators. Chapter 9 reviews recruitment techniques and may be of special interest to investigators not having ready access to participants. Methods for collecting high quality data and some common problems in data collection are included in Chapter 10. Chapters 11 and 12 focus on the important areas of assessment of adverse effects and quality of life. Measures to enhance and monitor participant adherence are presented in Chapter 13. Chapter

---

*References: 1, 5, 6, 8, 9, 10, 12, 14, 15, 16, 17.

14 reviews techniques of survival analysis. Chapter 15 covers data monitoring. Which participants should be included in analyses? We develop this question, posed in Chapter 16, by discussing reasons for not withdrawing participants from analysis. Topics such as subgroup analysis and meta-analysis are also addressed. Chapter 17 deals with phasing out clinical trials, and Chapter 18 with reporting and interpretation of results. Finally, in Chapter 19 the text presents information about multicenter studies, which have features requiring special attention. Several points covered in the final chapter may also be of value to investigators conducting single center studies.

This book is a collaborative effort and is based on knowledge gained during more than 2 decades in developing, conducting, overseeing, and analyzing data from many clinical trials. This experience is chiefly, but not exclusively, in large trials of heart and lung diseases, cancer, and AIDS. As a consequence, many of the examples cited are based on work done in these fields. However, the principles are applicable to clinical trials in general.

The views expressed in this book are those of the authors and do not necessarily represent the views of the organizations with which the authors have been or are affiliated. Use of the singular pronoun is unavoidable but does not necessarily imply the gender of the actor in any example of this book.

A portion of this book was supported in part by NIH grant no. CA 18332 (Statistical Problems in Cancer Research).

REFERENCES

1. Bulpitt CJ. Randomised controlled clinical trials, The Hague, Martinus Nijhoff, 1983.
2. Chalmers TC, Schroeder B: Letter to the editor, *N Engl J Med* 301:1293,1979.
3. Fletcher RH Fletcher SW: Clinical research in general medical journals: a 30-year perspective, *N Engl J Med* 301:180-183, 1979.
4. Guideline for the Format and Content of the Clinical and Statistical Sections of New Drug Applications. Center for Drug Evaluation and Research, Food and Drug Administration, Department of Health and Human Services, July 1988.
5. Iber FL, Riley WA, Murray PJ: Conducting clinical trials, New York, 1987, Plenum.
6. Ingelfinger JA, Mosteller F, Thibodeau LA et al. Biostatistics in clinical medicine, New York, Macmillan, 1983.
7. Juhl E, Christensen E, Tygstrup N: The epidemiology of the gastrointestinal randomized clinical trial, *N Engl J Med* 296:20-22, 1977.
8. Meinert CL: Clinical trials: Design, conduct and analysis, New York, Oxford University Press, 1986.
9. Miké V, Stanley KE (eds): Statistics in medical research: methods and issues, with applications in cancer research, New York, John Wiley & Sons, 1982.
10. NIH inventory of clinical trials: fiscal year 1979, Volume I. National Institutes of Health, Division of Research Grants, Research Analysis and Evaluation Branch, Bethesda, MD.
11. Peace KE (ed): Statistical issues in drug research and development, New York, Marcel Dekker, 1990.
12. Pocock SJ: Clinical trials: a practical approach, New York, John Wiley & Sons, 1983.
13. Ross OB, Jr.: Use of control in medical research, *JAMA* 145:72-75, 1951.
14. Shapiro SH, Louis TA (eds): Clinical trials: issues and approaches, New York, Marcel Dekker, 1983.
15. Spilker B: Guide to clinical trials, New York, Raven Press, 1991.
16. Spriet A, Dupin-Spriet T, Simon P: Methodology of clinical drug trials, ed 2, Basel, 1994, Karger.
17. Tygstrup N, Lachin JM, Juhl E (eds): The randomized clinical trial and therapeutic decisions, New York, Marcel Dekker, 1982.

ACKNOWLEDGMENTS

Most of the ideas and concepts discussed in this book represent what we learned during our years at the National Heart, Lung, and Blood Institute. We are indebted to many colleagues, particularly Dr. William T. Friedewald and the late Dr. Max Halperin, with whom we had numerous hours of discussion concerning theoretical and operational aspects of the design, conduct, and analysis of clinical trials.

Many contributed to the preparation of the first two editions of this book. We are especially grateful for the advice and assistance of Dr. Byron W. Brown, Dr. Max Halperin, Dr. Darwin R. Labarthe, Dr. Graham May, and Dr. Hans Wedel. We appreciate the many constructive comments of others in preparing the third edition, plus the efforts of Dr. Michelle Naughton and Dr. Sally Shumaker in revising the chapter on health-related quality of life. Finally, we want to particularly acknowledge the outstanding secretarial support of Sarah Hutchens, Kathleen O'Brien, and Julie Olson.

Contents

CHAPTER 1

Introduction to Clinical Trials

The evolution of the clinical trial dates from the eighteenth century.[10,55] Lind, in his classical study on board the *Salisbury*, evaluated six treatments for scurvy in 12 patients. One of the two who were given oranges and lemons recovered quickly and was fit for duty after 6 days. The second was the best recovered of the others and was assigned the role of nurse to the remaining 10 patients. Several other comparative studies were also conducted in the eighteenth and nineteenth centuries. The comparison groups comprised literature controls, other historical controls, and concurrent controls.[55]

The concept of randomization was introduced by Fisher and applied in agricultural research in 1926.[8] The first clinical trial that used a form of random assignment of subjects to study groups was reported in 1931 by Amberson et al.[2] After careful matching of 24 patients with pulmonary tuberculosis into comparable groups of 12 each, a flip of a coin determined which group received sanocrysin, a gold compound commonly used at that time. The British Medical Research Council trial of streptomycin in patients with tuberculosis, reported in 1948, was the first to use random numbers in the allocation to experimental and control groups.[42,58]

The principle of blindness was also introduced in the trial by Amberson et al.[2] The patients were not aware of whether they received intravenous injections of sanocrysin or distilled water. In a trial of cold vaccines in 1938, Diehl et al.[26] referred to the saline solution given to the subjects in the control group as a placebo.

It is only in the past few decades that the clinical trial has emerged as the preferred method in the evaluation of medical interventions. Techniques of implementation and special methods of analysis have been developed during this period. Many of the principles have their origins in work by Hill.[27,46,47,48]

Because the authors of this book have all spent formative years at the National Institutes of Health (NIH), it is also pertinent to cite a series of papers that reviews the history of clinical trials development at the NIH.*

The purpose of this chapter is to define clinical trials; review the need for them; and discuss timing, phasing, and ethics of clinical trials.

---

*References 13, 36, 40, 43, 66

FUNDAMENTAL POINT

A properly planned and executed clinical trial is a powerful experimental technique for assessing the effectiveness of an intervention.

WHAT IS A CLINICAL TRIAL?

A *clinical trial* is defined as a prospective study comparing the effect and value of intervention(s) against a control in human beings. Note that a clinical trial is prospective, rather than retrospective. Study participants must be followed forward in time. They need not all be followed from an identical calendar date. In fact, this will occur only rarely. Each participant, however, must be followed from a well-defined point, which becomes time zero or baseline for the study. This contrasts with a case-control study, a type of retrospective study in which participants are selected on the basis of presence or absence of an event or condition of interest. By definition, such a study is not a clinical trial. People can also be identified from hospital records or other data sources and subsequent records can be assessed for evidence of new events. This is not considered to be a clinical trial since the participants are not directly observed from the moment of initiation of the study and at least some of the follow-up data are retrospective.

A clinical trial must employ one or more *intervention* techniques. These may be "prophylactic, diagnostic or therapeutic agents, devices, regimens, procedures, etc."[62] Intervention techniques should be applied to participants in a standard fashion in an effort to change some aspect of the participants. Follow-up of people over time without active intervention may measure the natural history of a disease process, but it does not constitute a clinical trial. Without active intervention the study is observational because no experiment is being performed.

A clinical trial must contain a *control* group against which the intervention group is compared. At baseline, the control group must be sufficiently similar in relevant respects to the intervention group so that differences in outcome may reasonably be attributed to the action of the intervention. Methods for obtaining an appropriate control group are discussed in Chapter 4. Most often a new intervention is compared with best current standard therapy. If no such standard exists, the people in the intervention group may be compared with people who are on no active intervention. "No active intervention" means that the participant may receive either a placebo or no intervention at all. Obviously, participants in all groups may be on a variety of additional therapies and regimens, so-called concomitant interventions, which may be either self-administered or prescribed by others (e.g., private physicians).

For purposes of this book, only studies on human beings will be considered as clinical trials. Certainly, animals (or plants) may be studied using similar techniques.

However, this book focuses on trials in people, and each clinical trial must therefore incorporate participant safety considerations into its basic design. Equally important is the need for, and responsibility of, the investigator to fully inform potential participants about the trials.[60, 63]

Unlike animal studies, in clinical trials the investigator cannot dictate what an individual participant should do. He can only strongly encourage participants to avoid certain medications or procedures that might interfere with the trial. Since it may be impossible to have "pure" intervention and control groups, an investigator may not be able to compare interventions, but only intervention strategies. Strategies refer to attempts at getting all participants to comply to the best of their ability with their originally assigned intervention. When planning a trial, the investigator should recognize the difficulties inherent in studies with human subjects and attempt to estimate the magnitude of participants' failure to comply strictly with the protocol.

As discussed in Chapters 5 and 6, the ideal clinical trial is one that is randomized and double-blinded. Deviation from this standard has potential drawbacks that will be discussed in the relevant chapters. In some clinical trials compromise is unavoidable, but often deficiencies can be prevented by adhering to fundamental features of design, conduct, and analysis.

Several people distinguish between demonstrating efficacy of an intervention and effectiveness of an intervention. The former refers to what the intervention accomplishes in an ideal setting; the latter to what it accomplishes in actual practice, taking into account incomplete compliance to protocol. As discussed in Chapter 16 and elsewhere, our preferred analytic approach emphasizes the importance of the concept of effectiveness. Only in special circumstances, will the focus of the clinical trial described in this book be on efficacy.

CLINICAL TRIAL PHASES

While we focus on the design and analysis of randomized trials comparing the effectiveness of one or more interventions with a control, several steps or phases of clinical research must occur before this comparison can be implemented.

Phase I studies

Although useful preclinical information may be obtained from in vitro studies or animal models, early data must be obtained in humans. The first step, or phase in developing a drug or a biologic is to understand how well it can be tolerated in a small number of individuals. Although it does not meet our definition of a clinical trial, this phase is commonly called a phase I trial. People who participate in phase I trials have typically already tried and failed to improve on the existing standard interventions. Most phase I designs are relatively simple. One of the first steps in evaluating drugs is to estimate how large a dose can be given before unacceptable toxicity is experienced by patients.* This dose is usually referred to as the maximally tolerated dose, or MTD. Much of the literature has discussed how to extrapolate animal model data to the starting dose in humans[74] or how to step-up the dose levels to achieve the MTD. As Storer and DeMets describe,[83] there is a sparsity of phase I design literature; somewhat surprising since the goals are not dissimilar from those of bioassay methods for which a large literature exists.

In estimating the MTD in cancer drug development, the investigator usually starts with a very low dose and escalates the dose until a prespecified level of toxicity in patients is obtained. Typically, a small number of patients, usually three, are entered sequentially at a particular dose. If no specified level of toxicity is observed, the next predefined higher dose level is used. If unacceptable toxicity is observed in any of the three patients, an additional number of patients, usually three, are treated at the same dose. If no further toxicity is seen, the dose is escalated to the next higher dose. If additional unacceptable toxicity is observed, then the dose escalation is terminated and that dose, or perhaps the previous dose, is declared to be the MTD. This particular design assumes that the MTD occurs when approximately one third of the patients experience unacceptable toxicity. Variations of this design exist, but most are similar.

Some investigators[64,65,82] have recently proposed more sophisticated designs that specify a sampling scheme for dose escalation and a statistical model for the estimate of the MTD and its standard error. The sampling scheme must be conservative in dose escalation so as not to overshoot the MTD by very much, but at the same time be efficient in the number of patients studied. Many of the proposed schemes use a step-up/step-down approach; the simplest being to step-up with a single patient until toxicity is first observed. Further increase or decrease in the dose level depends on whether or not toxicity is observed at a given dose. Dose escalation stops when the process seems to have converged around a particular dose level. Once the data are generated, a dose response model is fit to the data and estimates of the MTD can be obtained as a function of the specified probability of a toxic response.[82]

Phase II studies

Once the MTD is established, the next goal is to evaluate whether the drug has any biologic activity or effect and to estimate the rate of adverse events. If the design of the phase I trial has not been adequate, the investigator may evaluate the drug for activity at too low or high a dose. Thus, the phase II design depends on the quality and adequacy of the phase I study. The results of the phase II trial will, in turn, be used to design the comparative phase III trial. The statistical literature for phase II trials is also quite limited.**

---

*References 3, 16, 38, 82, 83, 96
**References 23, 29, 35, 37, 45, 78, 94

One of the most commonly used phase II designs in cancer is based on the work of Gehan,[35] which is a version of a two-stage design. In the first stage the investigator attempts to rule out drugs that have no or little biologic activity. For example, he may specify that a drug must have some minimal level of activity, say, in 20% of patients. If the estimated activity level is less than 20%, he chooses not to consider this drug further, at least not at that MTD. If the estimated activity level exceeds 20%, he will add more patients to get a better estimate of the response rate. A typical study for ruling out a 20% or lower response rate enters 14 patients. If no response is observed in the first 14 patients, the drug is considered not likely to have a 20% or higher activity level. That is, failure 14 times in a row would happen 5% or less if the drug were truly effective 20% or more of the time. The number of additional patients added depends on the degree of precision desired, but ranges from 10 to 20. Thus a typical cancer phase II trial might include fewer than 30 patients to estimate the response rate. As is discussed in Chapter 7, the precision of the estimated response rate is important in the design of the comparative trial. In general, phase II trials are smaller than they ought to be.

Others[29,52,82] have proposed phase II designs that have more stages or a sequential aspect. Some[73,94] have considered hybrids of phases II and III designs to enhance efficiency. While these designs have desirable statistical properties, the most vulnerable aspect of phase II, as well as phase I studies, is the type of patients enrolled. Usually, patients entered in phase II trials have more exclusion criteria than those who will be considered in the phase III comparative trials. Furthermore, the outcome in the phase II trial (e.g., tumor response) may be different from that used in the definitive comparative trial (e.g., survival).

Phase III/IV trials

The phase III trial is the clinical trial defined above. It is generally designed to assess the effectiveness of the new intervention and thereby, its role in clinical practice. As noted, the intervention need not be a drug, but the term phase III trial is still commonly applied. The focus of this text is on phase III trials. However, many design assumptions for phase III trials depend on a series of phase I and II studies.

Phase III trials of chronic conditions or diseases often have a short follow-up period for evaluation, relative to the time the intervention might be used in clinical practice. In addition, they focus on effectiveness, but knowledge of safety is also necessary to evaluate fully the proper role of an intervention. A procedure or device may fail after a few years and have adverse sequelae for the patient. Thus long-term surveillance of an intervention believed to be effective in phase III trials is necessary. Such long-term studies, which do not involve control groups, are referred to as phase IV trials.

WHY ARE CLINICAL TRIALS NEEDED?

A clinical trial is the clearest method of determining whether an intervention has the postulated effect. Only seldom is a disease or condition so completely characterized that people fully understand its natural history and can say, from a knowledge of pertinent variables, what the subsequent course of a group of patients will be. Even more rarely can a clinician predict with certainty the outcome in individual patients. By outcome is meant not simply that an individual will die, but when, and under what circumstances; not simply that he will recover from a disease, but what complications of that disease he will suffer; not simply that some biologic variable has changed, but to what extent the change has occurred. Given the uncertain knowledge about disease course and the usual large variations in biologic measures, it is often difficult to say on the basis of uncontrolled clinical observation whether a new treatment has made a difference to outcome, and if it has, what the magnitude is. A clinical trial offers the possibility of such judgment because there exists a control group—which, ideally, is comparable to the intervention group in every way except for the intervention being studied.

The consequences of not conducting appropriate clinical trials at the proper time can be serious or costly. An example is the continued uncertainty as to the efficacy and safety of digitalis in congestive heart failure. Only recently, after the drug has been used for more than 200 years, has a large clinical trial evaluating the effect of digitalis on mortality been mounted.[87] Intermittent positive pressure breathing became an established therapy for chronic obstructive pulmonary disease without good evidence of benefits. Much later, one trial suggested no major benefit from this very expensive procedure.[89] Similarly, high concentration of oxygen was used for therapy in premature infants until a clinical trial demonstrated its harm.[77] A clinical trial can determine the incidence of adverse effects of complications of the intervention. Few interventions, if any, are entirely free of undesirable effects. However, drug toxicity might go unnoticed without the systematic follow-up measurements obtained in a clinical trial of sufficient size. The Cardiac Arrhythmia Suppression Trial documented that commonly used antiarrhythmic drugs were harmful in patients who had had a myocardial infarction and raised questions about routine use of an entire class of antiarrhythmic agents.[28]

In the final evaluation, an investigator must compare the benefit of an intervention with its other, possibly unwanted effects to decide whether, and under what circumstances, its use should be recommended. The cost implications of an intervention, particularly if there is limited benefit, must also be considered. Thrombolytic therapy has been repeatedly shown to be beneficial in acute myocardial infarction. The cost of different thrombolytic agents, however, varies several-fold. Are the added benefits of the most expensive agents[88] worth the extra cost? Such assessments are not statistical. They must rely on the judgment of the investigator and the physician.

It has been argued, most commonly and most forcefully by those suffering from and interested in the acquired immunodeficiency syndrome (AIDS), that traditional clinical trials are not the sole legitimate way of determining whether interventions are useful.[14,53,79] This is undeniably true, and clinical trial researchers need to be willing to modify, when necessary, aspects of study design or management. If the patient community is unwilling to participate in clinical trials conducted along traditional lines, or in ways that are scientifically pure, trials are not feasible and no information will be forthcoming. Investigators need to involve the relevant communities or populations at risk, even though this could lead to some compromises in design and scientific purity. Investigators need to decide when such compromises so invalidate the results that the study is not worth conducting. It should be noted that the rapidity with which trial results are demanded, the extent of community involvement, and the consequent effect on study design can change as knowledge of the disease increases, as at least partially effective therapy becomes available, and as understanding of the need for valid research designs, including clinical trials, develops. This has happened to some extent with AIDS trials.

Clinical trials are conducted because it is expected that they will influence practice.* It is undoubtedly true that the influence depends on numerous factors, including direction of the findings, means of dissemination of the results, and existence of evidence from other relevant research. However, well-designed clinical trials can certainly have pronounced effects on clinical practice.[51]

There is no such thing as a perfect study. A well thought-out, well-designed, appropriately conducted and analyzed clinical trial, however, is an effective tool. While even well-designed clinical trials are not infallible, they can provide a sounder rationale for intervention than is obtainable by other methods of investigation. On the other hand, poorly designed and conducted trials can be misleading. Also, without supporting evidence, no single study ought to be definitive. When interpreting the results of a trial, consistency with data from laboratory, animal, epidemiologic, and other clinical research must be considered.

PROBLEMS IN THE TIMING OF A TRIAL

Once drugs and procedures of unproved clinical benefit have become part of general medical practice, performing an adequate clinical trial becomes difficult ethically and logistically. Some people advocate instituting clinical trials as early as possible in the evaluation of new therapies.[20,81] The trials, however, must be feasible. Assessing feasibility takes into account several factors. Before conducting a trial, an investigator needs to have the necessary knowledge and tools. He must know something about

---

*References 4, 5, 33, 34, 51, 69, 75

the safety of the intervention and what outcomes to assess and have the techniques to do so. Well-run clinical trials of adequate magnitude are costly and should be done only when preliminary evidence of the efficacy of an intervention looks promising enough to warrant the effort and expenses involved.

Another aspect of timing is consideration of the relative stability of the intervention. If active research will be likely to make the intended intervention outmoded in a short time, studying such an intervention may be inappropriate. This is particularly true in long-term clinical trials or studies that take many months to develop. One of the criticisms of trials of surgical interventions has been that surgical methods are constantly being improved. Evaluating an operative technique of several years past, when a study was initiated, may not reflect the current status of surgery.[7,70,90]

These issues were raised in connection with the Veterans Administration study of coronary artery bypass surgery.[59] The trial showed that surgery was beneficial in subgroups of patients with left main coronary artery disease and three vessel disease, but not overall.[25,59,85] Critics of the trial argued that when the trial was started, the surgical techniques were still evolving. Therefore, surgical mortality in the study did not reflect what occurred in actual practice at the end of the long-term trial. In addition, there were wide differences in surgical mortality between the cooperating clinics,[68] which may have been related to the experience of the surgeons. Defenders of the study maintained that the surgical mortality in the Veterans Administration hospitals was not very different from the national experience at the time.[22] In the Coronary Artery Surgery Study,[17] surgical mortality was lower than in the Veterans Administration trial, reflecting better technique. The control group mortality, however, was also lower.

Review articles show that surgical trials have been successfully undertaken.[11,84] While the best approach would be to postpone a trial until a procedure has reached a plateau and is unlikely to change greatly, such a postponement will probably mean waiting until the procedure has been widely accepted as efficacious for some indication, thus making it impossible to conduct the trial. However, as noted by Chalmers and Sacks,[21] allowing for improvements in operative techniques in a clinical trial is possible. As in all aspects of conducting a clinical trial, judgment must be used in determining the proper time to evaluate an intervention.

ETHICS OF CLINICAL TRIALS

People have debated the ethics of clinical trials for as long as they have been done. The arguments have changed over the years and perhaps become more sophisticated, but in general, they center around the issues of the physician's obligations to his patient vs. societal good, informed consent, randomization, and the use of placebo.* Studies that require ongoing intervention or studies that continue to

---

*References 6, 9, 12, 15, 44, 49, 57, 67, 71, 72, 76, 80, 92, 93, 95

enroll participants after trends in the data have appeared have raised some of the controversy.[32,57,91] The indicated references argue a number of these issues.

We take the view that properly designed and conducted clinical trials are ethical. A well-designed trial can answer important public health questions without impairing the welfare of individuals. There may, at times, be conflicts between a physician's perception of what is good for his patient, and the needs of the trial. In such instances, the needs of the participants must predominate.

Proper informed consent is essential. The requirements of the U.S. Department of Health and Human Services are reasonable ones.[63] Also pertinent are the International Ethical Guidelines for Biomedical Research Involving Human Subjects.[24,54] Several investigators have shown that simply adhering to legal requirements does not ensure informed consent.[19,41] In many clinical trial settings, though, true informed consent can be obtained.[50] Sometimes, during a trial, important information derives from either other studies or the trial being conducted, which is relevant to the informed consent. In such cases, the investigator is obligated to update the consent form and notify current participants in an appropriate manner. A trial of antioxidants in Finnish male smokers indicated that beta carotene and vitamin E may have been harmful with respect to cancer or cardiovascular disease, rather than beneficial.[86] Because of those findings, investigators of other ongoing trials of antioxidants informed the participants of the results and the possible risks. Not only is it an ethical stance, but a well-informed participant is usually a better trial participant. The situations where participant enrollment must be done immediately, in comatose patients, or in highly stressful circumstances and where the prospective participants are minors or not fully competent to understand the study are more complicated and may not have optimal solutions.

The use of finders fees, that is, payment to physicians for referring participants to a clinical trial investigator, is inappropriate in that it might lead to undue pressure on a prospective participant.[56] This differs from the common and accepted practice of paying investigators a certain amount for the effort of recruiting each enrolled participant. Even this practice becomes questionable if the amount of the payment is so great as to induce the investigator to enroll inappropriate participants.

Randomization has generally been more of a problem for physicians and investigators than for participants.[18] The objection to random assignment should only apply if the investigator believes that a preferred therapy exists. If that is the case, he should not participate in the trial. On the other hand, if he truly cannot say that one treatment is better than another, there should be no ethical problem with randomization. Such judgments regarding efficacy obviously vary among investigators. Because it may be unreasonable to expect that an individual investigator have no preference, not only at the start of a trial but during its conduct, the concept of "clinical equipoise" has been proposed.[30] In this concept, the presence of uncertainty as to the benefits or harm from an intervention among the expert medical community rather than in the investigator, is justification for a clinical trial. Similarly, the use of a placebo is acceptable if there is no known best therapy and in other special circumstances (e.g., the commonly used therapy is poorly tolerated).[31] Of course, all participants must be told that there is a specified probability, for example, 50%, of their receiving placebo. The use of a placebo also does not imply that control group participants will receive no treatment. In many trials, the objective is to see whether a new intervention plus standard care is better or worse than a placebo plus standard care. In all trials, there is the ethical obligation to allow the best standard care to be used.

The issue of how to handle accumulating data from an ongoing trial is a difficult one, and is discussed in Chapter 15. With advance understanding by both participants and investigators that they will not be told interim results, and that there is a responsible data monitoring group, ethical concerns should be lessened, if not totally alleviated.

There has been concern about falsification of data and entry of ineligible, or even phantom participants in clinical trials.[1,61] We condemn all such data fabrication. It is important to emphasize that confidence in the integrity of the trial and its results is essential to every trial. If, through intentional or inadvertent actions, that confidence is impaired, not only have the participants and potentially others in the community been harmed, the trial loses its rationale and ability to influence science and medical practice. Chapter 10 covers issues of data quality assurance.

STUDY PROTOCOL

Every well-designed clinical trial requires a protocol. The study protocol can be viewed as a written agreement between the investigator, the participant, and the scientific community. The contents provide the background, specify the objectives, and describe the design and organization of the trial. Every detail explaining how the trial is carried out does not need to be included, provided that a comprehensive manual of procedures contains such information. The protocol serves as a document to assist communication among those working in the trial. It should also be made available to others on request.

The protocol should be developed before the beginning of participant enrollment and should remain essentially unchanged except perhaps for minor updates. Careful thought and justification should go into any changes. Major revisions that alter the direction of the trial should be rare. If they occur, the rationale behind such changes needs to be clearly descried. An example is the Cardiac Arrhythmia Suppression Trial, which, on the basis of important study findings, changed intervention, participant eligibility criteria, and sample size.[39]

An outline of a typical protocol is given below:

A. Background of the study
B. Objectives
    1. Primary question and response variable
    2. Secondary questions and response variables
    3. Subgroup hypotheses
    4. Adverse effects
C. Design of the study
    1. Study population
        a. Inclusion criteria
        b. Exclusion criteria
    2. Sample size assumptions and estimates
    3. Enrollment of participants
        a. Informed consent
        b. Assessment of eligibility
        c. Baseline examination
        d. Intervention allocation (e.g., randomization method)
    4. Intervention
        a. Description and schedule
        b. Measures of compliance
    5. Follow-up visit description and schedule
    6. Ascertainment of response variables
        a. Training
        b. Data collection
        c. Quality control
    7. Data analysis
        a. Interim monitoring
        b. Final analysis
    8. Termination policy
D. Organization
    1. Participating investigators
        a. Statistical unit or data coordinating center
        b. Laboratories and other special units
        c. Clinical center(s)
    2. Study administration
        a. Steering committees and subcommittees
        b. Data monitoring committee
        c. Funding organization
Appendix
    Definitions of eligibility criteria
    Definitions of response variables

REFERENCES

1. Altman LK: Probe into flawed cancer study prompts federal reforms, *The New York Times,* B6, Tuesday, April 26, 1994.
2. Amberson JB, Jr, McMahon BT, Pinner M: A clinical trial of sanocrysin in pulmonary tuberculosis, *Am Rev Tuberc* 24:401-435, 1931.
3. Anbar D: Stochastic approximation methods and their use in bioassay and Phase I clinical trials, *Comm Stat* Ser A 13:2451-2467, 1984.
4. Ayanian JZ, Hauptman PJ, Guadagnoli E, et al: Knowledge and practices of generalist and specialist physicians regarding drug therapy for acute myocardial infarction, *N Engl J Med* 331:1136-1142, 1994.
5. Boissel JP: Impact of randomized clinical trials on medical practices, *Controlled Clin Trials* 10:Suppl:120S-134S, 1989.
6. Bok S: The ethics of giving placebos, *Sci Am* 231:17-23, November 1974.
7. Boncheck LI: Are randomized trials appropriate for evaluating new operations? *N Engl J Med* 301:44-45, 1979.
8. Box JF: R.A. Fisher and the design of experiments, 1922-1926. *Am Stat* 34:1-7, 1980.
9. Brewin TB: Consent to randomised treatment, *Lancet* ii:919-921, 1982.
10. Bull JP: The historical development of clinical therapeutic trials, *J Chronic Dis* 10:218-248, 1959.
11. Bunker JP, Hinkley D, McDermott WV: Surgical innovation and its evaluation, *Science* 200: 937-941, 1978.
12. Burkhardt R, Kienle G: Controlled clinical trials and medical ethics, *Lancet* ii:1356-1359, 1978.
13. Byar DP: Discussion of papers on "historical and methodological developments in clinical trials at the National Institutes of Health," *Stat Med* 9:903-906, 1990.
14. Byar DP, Schoenfeld DA, Green SB et al.: Design considerations for AIDS trials, *N Engl J Med* 323: 1343-1348, 1990.
15. Cancer Research Campaign Working Party in Breast Conservation: Informed consent: ethical, legal, and medical implications for doctors and patients who participate in randomized clinical trials, *Br Med J* 286:1117-1121, 1983.
16. Carbone PP, Krant MJ, Miller SP, et al: The feasibility of using randomization schemes early in the clinical trials of new chemotherapeutic agents: hydroxyurea (NSC-32065), *Clin Pharmacol Thera* 6: 17-24, 1965.
17. CASS Principal Investigators and their Associates: Myocardial infarction and mortality in the Coronary Artery Surgery Study (CASS) randomized trial, *N Engl J Med* 310:750-758, 1984.
18. Cassileth BR, Lusk EJ, Miller DS et al: Attitudes toward clinical trials among patients and the public, *JAMA* 248:968-970, 1982.
19. Cassileth BR, Zupkis RV, Sutton-Smith K et al: Informed consent—why are its goals imperfectly realized? *N Engl J Med* 301:896-900, 1980.
20. Chalmers TC: Randomization of the first patient, *Med Clin North Am* 59:1035-1038, 1975.
21. Chalmers TC, Sacks H: Letter to the editor, *N Engl J Med* 301:1182, 1979.
22. Chalmers TC, Smith H, Jr, Ambroz A et al: In defense of the VA randomized control trial of coronary artery surgery, *Clin Res* 26:230-235, 1978.
23. Chang MN, Therneau TM, Wieand, HS, Cha SS: Designs for group sequential phase II clinical trials, *Biometrics* 43:865-874, 1987.
24. CIOMS/WHO: International Ethical Guidelines for Biomedical Research Involving Human Subjects, Geneva:CIOMS, 1993.
25. Detre K, Peduzzi P, Murphy M et al: Effect by bypass surgery on survival in patients in low- and high-risk subgroups delineated by the use of simple clinical variables, *Circulation* 63:1329-1338, 1981.
26. Diehl HS, Baker AB, Cowan DW: Cold vaccines; an evaluation based on a controlled study, *JAMA* 111:1168-1173, 1938.
27. Doll R: Clinical trials: retrospect and prospect, *Stat Med* 1:337-344, 1982.
28. Echt DS, Liebson PR, Mitchell LB, et al: Mortality and morbidity in patients receiving encainide, flecainaide, or placebo. The Cardiac Arrhythmia Suppression Trial, *N Engl J Med* 324:781-788, 1991.
29. Fleming TR: One-sample multiple testing procedure for phase II clinical trials, *Biometrics* 38: 143-151, 1982.

30. Freedman B: Equipose and the ethics of clinical research, *N Engl J Med* 317:141-145, 1987.

31. Freedman B.: Placebo-controlled trials and the logic of clinical purpose, *IRB* 12:1-6, 1990 (Nov–Dec).

32. Friedman L, DeMets D: The data monitoring committee: How it operates and why, *IRB* 3:6-8, 1981.

33. Friedman L., Wenger NK, Knatterud GL: Impact of the Coronary Drug Project findings on clinical practice, *Controlled Clin Trials* 4:513-522, 1983.

34. Furberg CD: The impact of clinical trials on clinical practice, *Arzneim-Forsch/Drug Res* 39:986-988, 1989.

35. Gehan EA: The determination of the number of patients required in a preliminary and a follow-up trial of a new chemotherapeutic agent, *J Chron Dis* 13:346-353, 1961.

36. Gehan EA, Schneiderman MA: Historical and methodological developments in clinical trials at the National Cancer Institute, *Stat Med* 9:871-880, 1990.

37. Geller NL: Design of phase I and II clinical trials in cancer: a statisticians's view, *Cancer Invest* 2:483-491, 1984.

38. Gordon NH, Willson JKV: Using toxicity grades in the design and analysis of cancer phase I clinical trials, *Stat Med* 11:2063-2075, 1992.

39. Greene HL, Roden DM, Katz RJ, et al: The Cardiac Arrhythmia Suppression Trial: first CAST...then CAST-II, *J Am Coll Cardiol* 19:894-898, 1992.

40. Greenhouse SW: Some historical and methodological developments in early clinical trials at the National Institutes of Health, *Stat Med* 9:893-901, 1990.

41. Grunder TM: On the readability of surgical consent forms, *N Engl J Med* 302:900-902, 1980.

42. Hart PD'A: Randomised controlled clinical trials, Letter to the editor *Br Med J* 302:1271-1272, 1991.

43. Halperin M, DeMets DL, Ware JH: Early methodological developments for clinical trials at the National Heart, Lung, and Blood Institute, *Stat Med* 9:881-892, 1990.

44. Hellman S, Hellman DS: Of mice but not men: problems of the randomized clinical trial, *N Engl J Med* 324:1585-1589, 1991.

45. Herson J: Predictive probability early termination plans for phase II clinical trials, *Biometrics* 35:775-783, 1979.

46. Hill AB: The clinical trial, *Br Med Bull* 7:278-282, 1951.

47. Hill AB: The clinical trial, *N Engl J Med* 247:113-119, 1952.

48. Hill AB: *Statistical methods of clinical and preventive medicine,* New York, Oxford University Press, 1962.

49. Howard J, Friedman L: Protecting the scientific integrity of a clinical trial: some ethical dilemmas, *Clin Pharmacol Ther* 29:561-569, 1981.

50. Howard JM, DeMets D, the BHAT Research Group: How informed is informed consent? The BHAT experience, *Controlled Clin Trials* 2:287-303,1981.

51. Lamas GA, Pfeffer MA, Hamm P, et al: Do the results of randomized clinical trials of cardiovascular drugs influence medical practice? *N Engl J Med* 327:241-247, 1992.

52. Lee YJ, Staquet M, Simon R et al: Two-stage plans for patient accrual in phase II cancer clinical trials, *Cancer Treat Rep* 63:1721-1726, 1979.

53. Levine C, Dubler NN, Levine RJ: Building a new consensus: ethical principles and policies for clinical research on HIV/AIDS, *IRB* 13:1-17, 1991 (Jan–Apr).

54. Levine RJ: New international ethical guidelines for research involving human subjects, *Ann Intern Med* 119:339-341, 1993.

55. Lilienfeld AM: Ceteris paribus: the evolution of the clinical trial, *Bull History Medicine* 56:1-18, 1982.

56. Lind SE: Finder's fees for research subjects, *N Engl J Med* 323:192-195, 1990.

57. Marquis D: Leaving therapy to chance, *The Hastings Center Rep* 13:40-47, August 1983.

58. Medical Research Council: Streptomycin treatment of pulmonary tuberculosis, *Br Med J* 2: 769-782, 1948.

59. Murphy ML, Hultgren HN, Detre K, et al: Treatment of chronic stable angina—a preliminary report of survival data for the randomized Veterans Administration cooperative study, *N Engl J Med* 297: 621-627, 1977.

60. National Commission for the Protection of Human Subjects of Biomedical and Behavioral Research: The Belmont Report: ethical principles and guidelines for the protection of human subjects of research, *Fed Regist* 44:23192-23197, 1979.

61. Neaton JD, Bartsch GE, Broste SK, et al: A case of data alteration in the Multiple Risk Factor Intervention Trial (MRFIT), *Controlled Clin Trials* 12:731-740, 1991.
62. NIH Inventory of Clinical Trials: Fiscal Year 1979, vol I, National Institutes of Health, Division of Research Grants, Research Analysis and Evaluation Branch, Bethesda, MD.
63. OPRR Reports: Code of Federal Regulations: (45 CFT 46) Protection of Human Subjects. National Institutes of Health, Department of Health and Human Services, Revised June 18, 1991. Reprinted March, 1994.
64. O'Quigley J, Chevret S: Methods for dose finding studies in cancer clinical trials: a review and results of a Monte Carlo Study, *Stat Med* 10:1647-1664, 1991.
65. O'Quigley J, Pepe M, Fisher L: Continual reassessment method: a practical design for phase I clinical trials in cancer, *Biometrics* 46:33-48, 1990.
66. Organization, review, and administration of cooperative studies (Greenberg Report): A report from the Heart Special Project Committee to the National Advisory Heart Council, May 1967, *Controlled Clin Trials* 9:137-148, 1988.
67. Passamani E: Clinical trials—are they ethical? *N Engl J Med* 324:1589-1592, 1991.
68. Proudfit WL: Criticisms of the VA randomized study of coronary bypass surgery, *Clin Res* 26:236-240, 1978.
69. Rosenberg Y, Schron E, Parker A: How clinical trial results are disseminated: use and influence of different sources of information in a survey of US physicians, *Controlled Clin Trials* 15:(suppl): 46S, 1994.
70. Rudicel S, Esdail J: The randomized clinical trial in orthopaedics: obligation or option? *J Bone Joint Surg* 67A:1284-1293, 1985.
71. Rutstein DD: The ethical design of human experiments. In Freund PA, ed: *Experimentation with human subjects,* New York, George Braziller, 1970.
72. Schafer A: The ethics of the randomized clinical trial, *N Engl J Med* 307:719-724, 1982.
73. Schaid DJ, Ingle JN, Wieand S, Ahmann DL: A design for phase II testing of anticancer agents within a phase III clinical trial, *Controlled Clin Trials* 9:107-118, 1988.
74. Schneiderman MA: Mouse to man: statistical problems in bringing a drug to clinical trial, *Proceedings of the Fifth Berkeley Symposium on Mathematical Statistics and Probability, Univ of California* 4:855-866, 1967.
75. Schron E, Rosenberg Y, Parker A, Stylianou M: Awareness of clinical trials results and influence on prescription behavior: a survey of US physicians, *Controlled Clin Trials* 15 (suppl):108S, 1994.
76. Shaw LW, Chalmers TC: Ethics in cooperative clinical trials, *Ann NY Acad Sci* 169:487-495, 1970.
77. Silverman WA: The lesson of retrolental fibroplasia, *Sci Am* 236:100-107, June 1977.
78. Simon R, Wittes RE, Ellenberg SS: Randomized phase II clinical trials, *Cancer Treat Rep* 69: 1375-1381, 1985.
79. Spiers HR: Community consultation and AIDS clinical trials, Part I. *IRB* 13:7-10, 1991, (May–June).
80. Spodick DH: The randomized controlled clinical trial: scientific and ethical basis, *Am J Med* 73: 420-425, 1982.
81. Spodick DH: Randomize the first patient: scientific, ethical, and behavioral bases, *Am J Cardiol* 51: 916-917, 1983.
82. Storer BE: Design and analysis of phase I clinical trials, *Biometrics* 45:925-937, 1989.
83. Storer B, DeMets D: Current phase I/II designs: are they adequate? *J Clin Res Drug Devel* 1: 121-130, 1987.
84. Strachan CJL, Oates GD: Surgical trials. In Johnson FN, Johnson S, eds: *Clinical trials,* Oxford, 1977, Blackwell Scientific.
85. Takaro T, Hultgren HN, Lipton MJ et al: The VA cooperative study of surgery for coronary arterial occlusive disease. 11. Subgroup with significant left main lesions, *Circulation* 54 (suppl III):III-107 to III-117, 1976.
86. The Alpha-Tocopherol, Beta Carotene Cancer Prevention Study Group: The effect of vitamin E and beta carotene on the incidence of lung cancer and other cancers in male smokers, *N Engl J Med* 330:1029-1035, 1994.

87. The Digitalis Investigation Group: Rationale, design, implementation and baseline characteristics of patients in the DIG trial: a large, simple trial to evaluate the effect of digitalis on mortality in heart failure, *Controlled Clin Trials* (in press).
88. The GUSTO Investigators: An international randomized trial comparing four thrombolytic strategies for acute myocardial infarction, *N Engl J Med* 329:673-682, 1993.
89. The Intermittent Positive Pressure Breathing Trial Group: Intermittent positive pressure breathing therapy of chronic obstructive pulmonary disease—a clinical trial, *Ann Intern Med* 99:612-620, 1983.
90. Van der Linden W: Pitfalls in randomized surgical trials, *Surgery* 87:258-262, 1980.
91. Veatch RM: Longitudinal studies, sequential design, and grant renewals: What to do with preliminary data, *IRB* 1:1-3, 1979.
92. Vere D: Controlled clinical trials: the current ethical debate, *JR Soc Med* 74:85-88, 1981 (editorial).
93. Vere DW: Ethics of clinical trials. In Good CS, ed: *The principles and practice of clinical trials,* Edinburgh, Churchill Livingstone, 1976.
94. Whitehead J: Sample sizes for phase II and phase III clinical trials: an integrated approach, *Stat Med* 5:459-464, 1986.
95. Wilhelmsen L: Ethics of clinical trials—the use of placebo, *Eur J Clin Pharmacol* 16:295-297, 1979 (editorial).
96. Williams DA: Interval estimation of the median lethal dose, *Biometrics* 42:641-645, 1986.

CHAPTER 2

What Is the Question?

The planning of a clinical trial depends on the question that the investigator is addressing. The general objective is usually obvious, but the specific question to be answered by the trial is often not stated well. Stating the question clearly and in advance encourages proper design. It also enhances the credibility of the findings. One would like answers to several questions, but the study should be designed with only one major question in mind. This chapter will discuss the selection of this primary question and appropriate ways of answering it. In addition, types of subsidiary questions will be reviewed.

FUNDAMENTAL POINT

Each clinical trial must have a primary question. The primary question, as well as any secondary or subsidiary questions, should be carefully selected, clearly defined, and stated in advance.

SELECTION OF THE QUESTIONS
Primary question

The primary question should be the one the investigators are most interested in answering and one that is capable of being adequately answered. It is the question on which the sample size of the study is based and that must be emphasized in the reporting of the trial results. The primary question may be framed in the form of testing a hypothesis,[9] because most of the time an intervention is postulated to have a particular outcome that, on the average, will be different from the outcome in a control group. The outcome may be a beneficial action such as saving a life, ameliorating an illness, reducing symptoms, or improving quality of life, or the modification of an intermediate or surrogate characteristic such as blood pressure.

In some instances, however, the investigator may be interested in demonstrating no difference in outcome between intervention and control or between two interventions. For example, are people equally as well off if treated at home for a myocardial infarction as they are if hospitalized? This particular question was addressed some time ago.[15] Proving that responses to different interventions are the same on the average is not straightforward and is not the same as failing to demonstrate that a difference exists between the groups. Such proof requires special attention to statistical power (sensitivity); that is, the ability to show a difference had one truly been present.

Secondary questions

There may also be a variety of subsidiary, or secondary questions related to the primary question. The study may be designed to help address these, or data collected for the purpose of answering the primary question may also elucidate the secondary questions. They can be of two types. In the first, the response variable is different from that in the primary question. For example, the primary question might ask whether mortality from any cause is altered by the intervention. Secondary questions might relate to incidence of cause-specific death (such as coronary heart disease mortality), incidence of nonfatal myocardial infarction, incidence of stroke, or reduction in a risk factor.

The second type of secondary question relates to subgroup hypotheses. For example, in a study of cancer therapy, the investigator may want to look specifically at people by stage of disease at entry into the trial. Such subsets of people in the intervention group can be compared with similar people in the control group. Subgroup hypotheses should be: (1) specified before data collection begins, (2) based on reasonable expectations, and (3) limited in number. In any event, the number of participants in any subgroup is usually too small to prove or disprove a subgroup hypothesis.

Recently, there has been recognition that certain subgroups of people have not been adequately represented in clinical research, including clinical trials.[3] In the United States, this has led to requirements that women and minority populations be included in appropriate numbers in trials.[19] The issue is whether the number of participants of each sex and racial/ethnic group must be adequate to answer the key questions that the trial addresses, or whether there must merely be adequate diversity of people. As has been noted,[14,22] the design of the trial should be driven by reasonable expectations that the intervention will or will not operate materially differently among the various subsets of participants. If so, then it is appropriate to design the trial to detect those differences. If not, adequate diversity with the opportunity to examine subgroup responses at the end of the trial is more appropriate.

Both types of secondary questions raise several methodologic issues; for example, if enough statistical tests are done, a few will be significant by chance alone when there is no true intervention effect. An example is provided by the Second International Study of Infarct Survival, a factorial-design trial of aspirin and streptokinase on vascular and total mortality in patients with acute myocardial infarction.[16] Participants born under the Gemini or Libra astrological birth signs did somewhat worse on aspirin than on no aspirin, whereas for all other signs, and overall, there was an impressive and highly significant benefit from aspirin. The investigators of that trial note the erroneous conclusions drawn from such subgroup analyses.

Therefore, when a number of tests are carried out, results should be interpreted cautiously. Shedding light or raising new hypotheses is a more proper outcome of these analyses than are conclusive answers. See Chapter 16 for further discussion of subgroup analysis.

Both primary and secondary questions should be important and relevant scientifically, medically, or for public health purposes. Participant safety and well-being must always be considered in evaluating importance. As reviewed in Chapter 1, potential benefit and risk of harm should be looked at by the investigator, as well as by local Institutional Review Boards (Human Experimentation Committees), and, often, data monitoring committees.

Adverse effects

Important questions can be answered by clinical trials concerning adverse or side reactions to therapy (Chapter 11). Here, unlike the primary or secondary questions, it is not always possible to specify in advance the question to be answered. What adverse reactions might occur, and their severity, may be unpredictable. Furthermore, rigorous, convincing demonstration of serious toxicity is usually not achieved because it is generally thought unethical to continue a study to the point at which a drug has been conclusively shown to be more harmful than beneficial.[6,30,31] Investigators traditionally monitor a variety of laboratory and clinical measurements, look for possible adverse effects, and compare these in the intervention and control groups. Statistical significance and the previously mentioned problem of multiple response variables become secondary to clinical judgment and participant safety. While this will lead to the conclusion that some purely chance findings are labeled as adverse effects, moral responsibility to the participants requires a conservative attitude toward safety monitoring, particularly if an alternative therapy is available.

Ancillary questions, substudies

Often a clinical trial can be used to answer questions that do not bear directly on the intervention being tested, but are nevertheless of interest. The structure of the trial and the ready access of participants may make it the ideal vehicle for such investigations. Weinblatt, Ruberman, et al.[40] reported that low level of education among survivors of a myocardial infarction was a marker of poor risk of future survival. The authors[27] subsequently evaluated whether the educational level was an indicator of psychosocial stress. To further investigate these findings, they performed a study ancillary to the Beta-Blocker Heart Attack Trial,[4] a trial that evaluated whether the regular administration of propranolol could reduce 3-year mortality in people with acute myocardial infarctions. Interviews assessing factors such as social interaction, attitudes, and personality were conducted in more than 2300 men in the ancillary study.[28] Inability to cope with high life stress and social isolation were found to be significantly and independently associated with mortality. Effects of low education were accounted for by these two factors. By enabling the investigators to perform this study, the Beta-Blocker Heart Attack Trial provided an opportunity to examine an important issue in a large sample, even though it was peripheral to the main question.

In the Studies of Left Ventricular Dysfunction (SOLVD),[33] the investigators evaluated whether an angiotensin-converting enzyme inhibitor would reduce mortality in symptomatic and asymptomatic people with reduced left ventricular ejection fraction. In selected participants, special studies were done with the objective of getting a better understanding of the disease process and of the mechanisms of action of the intervention. These substudies did not require the large sample size of the main studies (more than 6000 participants). Therefore, most participants had a relatively simple and short evaluation and did not undergo the expensive and time-consuming procedures of interviews demanded by the substudies. This combination of a rather limited assessment in many participants, designed to address an easily monitored response variable, and detailed measurement in subsets of participants, can be extremely effective.

Natural history

Though it is not intervention-related, an often valuable use of the collected data, especially in long-term trials, is a natural history study in the control group.[29] If the control group is receiving either a placebo or no systematic treatment, various baseline factors may be studied for their relation to specific outcomes. Assessment of the prognostic importance of these factors can lead to better understanding of the disease under study and development of new hypotheses. Of course, generally only predictive association—and not necessarily causation—may properly be inferred from such data. The study participants may be a highly selected group, and natural history findings must be interpreted in that light.

Since they are not study hypotheses, specific natural history questions need not be specified in advance. Properly designed baseline forms, however, require some advance consideration of which factors might be related to outcome. After the study has started, going back to ascertain missing baseline information to answer natural history questions is generally a fruitless pursuit. At the same time, collecting large amounts of baseline data on the slight chance that they might provide useful information costs money, consumes valuable time, and may lead to less careful collection of important data. It is better to restrict data collection to those baseline factors that are known, or seriously thought, to be related to prognosis.

Large, simple clinical trials

As discussed in more detail in Chapter 4, the concept of large, simple clinical trials has become popular.[42] The general idea is that for common conditions and important outcomes, such as total mortality, even modest benefits of intervention, particularly an intervention that is easily implemented in a large population, are worthwhile. Because an intervention is likely to have similar effects in different sorts of participants, careful characterization of people at entry is unnecessary. The study must have unbiased allocation of participants to intervention or control and unbiased assessment of outcome. Sufficiently large numbers of participants are more important in providing the power necessary to answer the question than careful attention to quality of data. This model depends on a relatively easily administered intervention, brief forms, an easily ascertained outcome, such as a fatal or nonfatal clinical event, and, typically, a relatively short follow-up time.

INTERVENTION

When the question is conceived, investigators, at the very least, have in mind a class or type of intervention. More commonly, they know the precise drug, procedure, or lifestyle modification they wish to study. In reaching such a decision, they need to consider several aspects. First, the potential benefit of the intervention must be maximized, while possible toxicity is kept to a minimum. Thus, dose of drug or intensity of rehabilitation and frequency of administration are key factors that need to be determined. Can the intervention be standardized and remain reasonably stable over the duration of the trial? Investigators must also decide whether to use a single drug or device, fixed or adjustable doses of drugs, sequential drugs, or drug or device combinations. The composition of the control group regimen is an additional factor.

Second, the availability of the drug or device for testing needs to be determined. If it is not yet licensed, special approval from the regulatory agency and cooperation or support by the manufacturer are required.

Third, investigators must take into account design aspects, such as time of initiation and duration of the intervention, need for special tests or laboratory facilities, and the logistics of blinding in the case of drug studies.

RESPONSE VARIABLES

Response variables are outcomes measured during the course of the trial, and they define and answer the questions. A response variable may be total mortality, death from a specific cause, incidence of a disease, a complication or specific adverse effect of disease, symptomatic relief, a clinical finding, a laboratory measurement, or the cost and ease of administering the intervention. If the primary question concerns total mortality, the occurrence of deaths in the trial clearly answers the question. If the primary question involves severity of arthritis, on the other hand, extent of mobility or a measure of freedom from pain may be reasonably good indicators. In other circumstances, a specific response variable may only partially reflect the overall question. As seen from the above examples, the response variable may show a change from one discrete state (living) to another (dead), from one discrete state to any of several other states (changing from one stage of disease to another), or from one level of a continuous variable to another. If the question can be appropriately defined using a continuous variable, the required sample size may be reduced (see Chapter 7). However, the investigators need to be careful that this variable and any observed differences are clinically meaningful and relevant and that the use of a continuous variable is not simply a device to reduce sample size.

In general, a single response variable should be identified to answer the primary question. If more than one are used, the probability of getting a nominally significant result by chance alone is increased (see Chapter 16). In addition, if several response variables give inconsistent results, interpretation becomes difficult. The investigators would then need to consider which outcome is most important and explain why the others gave conflicting results. Unless they have made the determination of relative importance prior to data collection, their explanations are likely to be unconvincing.

Although the practice is not advocated, there may be circumstances when more than one primary response variable needs to be looked at. This may be the case when investigators truly cannot state which of several response variables relates most closely to the primary question. Ideally, the trial would be postponed until this decision can be made. However, overriding concerns, such as increasing use of the intervention in general medical practice, may compel them to conduct the study earlier. In these circumstances, rather than arbitrarily selecting one response variable that may, in retrospect, be inappropriate, investigators prefer to list several primary outcomes.[38] For instance, in the Urokinase Pulmonary Embolism Trial[38] lung scan, arteriogram and hemodynamic measures were given as the primary response variables in assessing the effectiveness of the agents urokinase and streptokinase. Chapter 7 discusses the calculation of sample size when a study with several primary response variables is designed.

Combining events to make up a response variable might be useful if any one event occurs too infrequently for the investigator reasonably to expect a significant difference without using a large number of participants. It must be emphasized, however, that the combined events should be capable of meaningful interpretation such as being related through a common underlying condition. In answering a question where the response variable involves a combination of events, only *one event per participant* should be counted. That is, the analysis is by participant, not by event.

One kind of combination response variable involves two kinds of events. In a study of heart disease, combined events might be death from coronary heart disease plus nonfatal myocardial infarction. This is clinically meaningful since death from coronary heart disease and nonfatal myocardial infarction might together represent a measure of coronary heart disease. Difficulties in interpretation can arise if the results of each of the components in such a response variable are inconsistent. In the Physicians' Health Study report of aspirin to prevent cardiovascular disease, there was no difference between intervention and control groups in mortality, a large reduction in myocardial infarction in the aspirin-treated group, and an increase in stroke, primarily hemorrhagic.[32] In this case, cardiovascular mortality was the primary response variable, rather than a combination. If it had been a combination, the interpretation of the results would have been even more difficult than it was.[10] When a combination response variable is used, and more than one event may occur in an individual, the rules for establishing a hierarchy of events should be established in advance. Thus a fatal event would take precedence over a nonfatal event, and only the fatal event would be counted, or, in the case of two nonfatal events, the first to occur would be counted.

Another kind of combination response variable involves multiple events of the same sort. Rather than simply asking whether an event has occurred, the investigator can look at the frequency with which it occurs. This may be a more meaningful way of looking at the question than seeking a yes–no outcome. For example, frequency of recurrent transient ischemic attacks or epileptic seizures within a specific follow-up period might constitute the primary response variable of interest. Simply adding up the number of recurrent episodes and dividing by the number of participants in each group to arrive at an average is improper. Multiple events in an individual are not independent, and averaging gives undue weight to those participants with more than one episode. One approach is to compare the number of participants with none, one, two, or more episodes; that is, the distribution, by individual, of the number of episodes.

Regardless of whether investigators are measuring a primary or secondary response variable, certain rules apply. First, they should define and write the questions in advance, being as specific as possible. They should not simply ask, "Is A better than B?" Rather, they should ask "In population W is drug A at daily dose X more efficacious in reducing Z over a period of time T than drug B at daily dose Y?" Implicit here is the magnitude of the difference that the investigators are interested in detecting. Stating the questions and response variables in advance is essential for planning of study design and calculation of sample size. As shown in Chapter 7, sample size calculation requires specification of the response variables as well as estimates of the effect of intervention. In addition, the investigators are forced to consider what they mean by a successful intervention. For example, does the intervention need to reduce mortality by 10% or 25% before a recommendation for its general use is made? Since such recommendations also depend on the frequency and severity of adverse effects, a successful result cannot be completely defined beforehand. However, if a 10% reduction in mortality is clinically important, that should be stated, since it has sample size implications. Specifying response variables and anticipated benefit in advance also eliminates the possibility of the legitimate criticism that can be made if the investigators looked at the data until they found a statistically significant result and then decided that *that* response variable was what they really had in mind the entire time.

Second, the primary response variable must be capable of being assessed in all participants. Selecting one response variable to answer the primary question in some participants and another response variable to answer the same primary question in other participants is not a legitimate practice. It implies that each response variable answers the question of interest with the same precision and accuracy; that each measures exactly the same thing. Such agreement is unlikely. Similarly, response variables should be measured in the same way for all participants. Measuring a given variable by different instruments or techniques implies that the instruments or techniques yield precisely the same information. This rarely, if ever, occurs. If response variables can be measured only one way in some participants and another way in other participants, two separate studies are actually being performed, each of which is likely to be too small.

Third, unless there is a combination primary response variable in which the participant remains at risk of having additional events, participation generally ends when the primary response variable occurs. *Generally* is used here because, unless death is the primary response variable, the investigator may well be interested in certain events subsequent to the occurrence of the primary response variable. These events will not change the analysis of the primary response variable but may affect the interpretation of results. For example, deaths occurring after a nonfatal primary response variable, but before the official end of the trial as a whole, may be of interest. On the other hand, if a secondary response variable occurs, the participant should remain in the study (unless, of course, it is a fatal secondary response variable). He must continue to be followed because he is still at risk of developing the primary response variable. A study of heart disease may have, as its primary question, death from coronary heart disease and, as a secondary question, incidence of nonfatal myocardial infarction. If a participant suffers a nonfatal myocardial infarction, this counts toward the secondary response variable. However, he ought to remain in the study for analytic purposes and be at risk of dying (the primary response variable). This is true whether or not he is continued on the intervention regimen. If he does not remain in the study for purposes of analysis of the primary response variable, bias may result. (See Chapter 16 for more discussion of participant withdrawal).

Fourth, response variables should be capable of unbiased assessment. Truly double-blind studies have a distinct advantage over other studies in this regard. If a trial is not double-blinded (Chapter 6), then, whenever possible, response variable assessment should be done by people who are not involved in participant follow-up and who are blinded to the identity of the study group. Independent reviewers are often helpful. Of course, the use of blinded or independent reviewers does not entirely solve the problem of bias. Unblinded investigators sometimes fill out forms, and the participants may be influenced by the investigators. This may be the case during an exercise performance test, where the impact of the person administering the test on the results may be considerable. Some studies arrange to have the intervention administered by one investigator and response variables evaluated by another. Unless the participant is blinded (or otherwise unable to communicate), this procedure is also vulnerable to bias. One solution to this dilemma is to use only "hard," or objective, response variables (which are unambiguous and not open to interpretation). This assumes complete and honest ascertainment of outcome. Double-blind studies have the advantage of allowing the use of softer response variables, since the risk of assessment bias is minimized.

Fifth, it is important to have response variables that can be ascertained as completely as possible. A hazard of long-term studies is that participants may fail to return for follow-up appointments. If the response variable is one that depends on an interview or an examination and participants fail to return for follow-up appointments, information will be lost. Not only will it be lost, but it may be differentially lost in the intervention and control groups. Death or hospitalization are useful response variables because the investigator can usually ascertain vital status or occurrence of a hospital admission, even if the participant is no longer active in a study. However, only in a minority of clinical trials are they appropriate.

All clinical trials are compromises between the ideal and the practical. This is true in the selection of primary response variables. The most objective or those most easily measured may occur too infrequently, may fail to define adequately the primary question, or may be too costly. To select a response variable that can be reasonably and reliably assessed and yet that can provide an answer to the primary question requires judgment. If such a response variable cannot be found, the wisdom of conducting the trial should be reevaluated.

Surrogate response variables

A common criticism of clinical trials is that they are expensive and of long duration. This is particularly true for trials that use the occurrence of clinical events as the primary response variable. It has been suggested that response variables that are intermediate or continuous in nature might substitute for the clinical outcomes. Thus, instead of monitoring cardiovascular mortality or myocardial infarction an investigator could examine progress of atherosclerosis by means of angiography, ultrasound imaging, or change in cardiac arrhythmia by means of ambulatory electrocardiograms. In the cancer field, change in tumor size might replace mortality. In AIDS trials, change in CD-4 lymphocyte level has been used as a response to treatment instead of incidence of AIDS or mortality in HIV-positive patients. Osteoporosis has been used as a surrogate for bone fractures.

An argument for use of these surrogate response variables is that since the variables are continuous, the sample size can be smaller and the study less expensive than otherwise. Also, changes in the variables are likely to occur before the clinical event, shortening the time required for the trial.

It has been argued that in the case of truly life-threatening diseases (e.g., AIDS and certain cancers), formal clinical trials should not be necessary to license a drug or other intervention. Given the severity of the condition, lesser standards of proof should be required. If clinical trials are done, surrogate response variables ought to be acceptable, since speed in determining possible benefit is crucial. Potential errors in declaring an intervention useful may not be as important as early discovery of a truly effective treatment.

Even in such instances, however, one should not uncritically use surrogate endpoints.[11,13] It has been known for years that the presence of ventricular arrhythmias correlated with increased likelihood of sudden death and total mortality in people with heart disease,[5] as it was presumably one mechanism for the increased mortality. Therefore, it has been common practice to administer antiarrhythmic drugs with the aim of reducing the incidence of sudden cardiac death.[18,39] The Cardiac Arrhythmia Suppression Trial demonstrated, however, that drugs that effectively treated ventricular arrhythmias were not only ineffective in reducing sudden cardiac death, but actually caused increased mortality.[35,36]

A second example concerns the use of inotropic agents in people with heart failure. These drugs have been shown to improve exercise tolerance and symptomatic manifestations of heart failure.[20] It was expected that mortality would also be reduced. Unfortunately, clinical trials subsequently showed that mortality was worsened.[21,37]

It was noted that the level of CD-4 lymphocytes in the blood is associated with severity of AIDS. Therefore, despite some concerns,[8] several clinical trials used change in CD-4 lymphocyte concentration as an indicator of disease status. If the level rose, the drug was considered to be beneficial. Lin et al.,[17] however, argued that CD-4 lymphocyte count accounts for only part of the relationship between treatment with zidovudine and outcome. Choi et al.[7] came to similar conclusions. In a trial comparing zidovudine with zalcitabine, zalcitabine was found to lead to a slower decline in CD-4 lymphocytes but had no effect on the death rate.[12] Also troubling were the results of a large trial which, although showing an early rise in CD-4 lymphocytes, did not demonstrate any long-term benefit from zidovudine.[1] Whether zidovudine or another treatment is, or is not, truly beneficial is not the issue. The main point is that the effect of a drug on a surrogate endpoint (CD-4 lymphocytes) is not necessarily a good indicator of clinical outcome. This is summarized by Fleming, who notes that the CD-4 lymphocyte count showed positive results in seven out of eight trials where clinical outcomes were also positive. The CD-4 count, however, was also positive in six out of eight trials in which the clinical outcomes were not favorably affected by the intervention.[13]

Similar seemingly contradictory results have been seen with cancer clinical trials. In trials of 5-fluorouracil plus leucovorin compared with 5-fluorouracil alone, the combination led to significantly better tumor response, but no difference in survival.[2] Fleming[13] cites other cancer examples as well. Sodium fluoride, because of its stimulation of bone formation, was widely used in the treatment of osteoporosis. Despite this, it was found in a trial in women with postmenopausal osteoporosis to increase skeletal fragility.[26]

These examples do not mean that surrogate response variables should never be used in clinical trials. Nevertheless, they do point out that they should only be used after considering the advantages and disadvantages, recognizing that erroneous conclusions about interventions might occasionally be reached.

When are surrogate response variables useful? They are certainly useful in the early stages of development of a new intervention; i.e., in phase I or phase II studies. Before using surrogate response variables in a phase III trial or any trial that seeks to clearly address a clinical question, however, an investigator needs to consider several issues. First, does the variable truly reflect the clinical outcome? Have changes in the surrogate variable been shown to be highly correlated with changes in the clinical variable? Even if there is a strong correlation, it is not necessarily true that the surrogate variable is a cause of the clinical variable. Second, can the surrogate variable be assessed accurately and reliably? Is there so much measurement error that, in fact, the sample size increases or the results are questioned? Third, will the evaluation be so unacceptable to the participant that the study will become infeasible? If it requires invasive techniques, participants may refuse to join the trial, or worse, discontinue participation before the end. Fourth, measurement can require expensive equipment and highly trained staff, which may, in the end, make the trial more costly than if clinical events are monitored. Fifth, the small sample size of surrogate response variable trials may mean that important data on safety are not obtained.[24] The intervention may have various adverse effects. It may even cause the anticipated clinical outcomes to go in the wrong direction through some unanticipated mechanism of action. Finally, will the conclusions of the trial be accepted by the scientific and medical communities? If there is insufficient acceptance that the surrogate variable reflects clinical outcome, in spite of the investigator's conviction, there is little point in using such variables. Wittes et al.[41] discuss examples of savings in sample size by the use of surrogate response variables.

Prentice has summarized several key criteria that must be met if a surrogate response variable is to be useful.[23] He proposes that the surrogate response variable "'capture' any relationship between the treatment and the true endpoint." Temple[34] has reviewed a variety of circumstances in which supposed surrogate response variables did not turn out to be valid. He cites, however, the U.S. Food and Drug Administration use of surrogate response variables as part of its "accelerated approval" process for proposed treatments of serious illnesses as appropriate. Further clinical studies, though, might be required afterward. In all decisions, the issues of biologic plausibility, risk, benefits, and history of success must be considered.

GENERAL COMMENTS

Although this text attempts to provide straightforward concepts concerning the selection of study response variables, things are rarely as simple as one would like them to be. Investigators often encounter problems related to design, data monitoring, and ethical issues and interpretation of study results.

In long-term studies of participants at high risk, where total mortality is not the primary response variable, many may nevertheless die. They are, therefore, removed from the population at risk of developing the response variable of interest. Even in relatively short studies, if the participants are seriously ill, death may occur. In designing studies, therefore, if the primary response variable is a continuous measurement, a nonfatal event, or cause-specific mortality, the investigator needs to consider the impact of total mortality for two reasons. First, it will reduce the effective sample size. One would like to allow for this reduction by estimating the overall mortality and increasing sample size accordingly. However, a methodology for estimating mortality and increasing sample size is not yet well defined. Second, if mortality is related to the intervention, either favorably or unfavorably, excluding from study analysis those who die may bias results for the primary response variable.

One solution, whenever the risk of mortality is high, is to choose total mortality as the primary response variable. Alternatively, the investigator can combine total mortality with a pertinent nonfatal event as a combined primary response variable. Neither of these solutions may be appropriate and, in that case, the investigator should monitor total mortality and the primary response variable. Evaluation of the primary response variable will then need to consider those who died during the study, or else the censoring may bias the comparison.

Whether or not it is the primary response variable, total mortality, and any other adverse occurrence, needs to be monitored during a study (see Chapter 15). The ethics of continuing a study that, despite a favorable trend for the primary response variable, shows equivocal or even negative results for important secondary response variables, or the presence of major adverse effects, are questionable. Deciding what to do is difficult if an intervention is giving promising results with regard to death from a specific cause, which may be the primary response variable, yet total mortality is unchanged or increased. This issue arose in a study of clofibrate in people with elevated serum cholesterol.[25]

Finally, conclusions from data are not always clear-cut. Issues such as alterations in quality of life or annoying long-term side effects may cloud results that are clear with regard to primary response variables such as increased survival. In such circumstances, the investigator must offer her best assessment of the results but should report sufficient detail about the study to permit others to reach their own conclusions (see Chapter 18).

REFERENCES

 1. Aboulker J-P, Swart AM: Preliminary analysis of the Concorde trial, *Lancet* 341:889-890, 1993.
 2. Advanced Colorectal Cancer Meta-Analysis Project: Modulation of fluorouracil by leucovorin in patients with advanced colorectal cancer. Evidence in terms of response rate, *J Clin Oncol* 10:896-903, 1992.
 3. Angell M: Caring for women's health—what is the problem? *N Engl J Med* 329:271-272, 1993.
 4. Beta-Blocker Heart Attack Trial Research Group: A randomized trial of propranolol in patients with acute myocardial infarction. 1. Mortality results, *JAMA* 247:1707-1714, 1982.
 5. Bigger JT Jr, Fleiss JL, Kleiger R et al: The relationships among ventricular arrhythmias, left ventricular dysfunction, and mortality in the 2 years after myocardial infarction, *Circulation* 69:250-258, 1984.
 6. Chalmers TC: Invited remarks: National conference on clinical trials methodology, *Clin Pharmacol Ther* 25:649-650, 1979.
 7. Choi S, Lagakos SW, Schooley RT, Volberding PA: CD4$^+$ lymphocytes are an incomplete surrogate marker for clinical progression in persons with asymptomatic HIV infection taking zidovudine, *Ann Intern Med* 118:674-680, 1993.
 8. Cohen J: Searching for markers on the AIDS trail, *Science* 258:388-390, 1992.
 9. Cutler SJ, Greenhouse SW, Cornfield J, Schneiderman MA: The role of hypothesis testing in clinical trials: biometrics seminar, *J Chronic Dis* 19:857-882, 1966.
10. Data Monitoring Board of the Physicians' Health Study: Cairns J, Cohen L, Colton T, et al: Issues in the early termination of the aspirin component of the Physicians' Health Study, *Ann Epidemiol* 1:395-405, 1991.
11. DeMets DL, Fleming T: The role of surrogates in clinical trials (submitted for publication).
12. Fischl MA, Olson RM, Follansbee SE, et al: Zalcitabine compared with zidovudine in patients with advanced HIV-1 infection who received previous zidovudine therapy, *Ann Intern Med* 118:762-769, 1993.
13. Fleming TR: Surrogate markers in AIDS and cancer trials, *Stat Med* 13:1423-1435, 1995.
14. Freedman LS, Simon R, Foulkes MA, et al: Inclusion of women and minorities in clinical trials and the NIH Revitalization Act of 1993—the perspective of NIH clinical trialists, *Controlled Clin Trials* 16:277-285, 1995.
15. Hill JD, Hampton JR, Mitchell JRA: A randomised trial of home-versus-hospital management for patients with suspected myocardial infarction, *Lancet* i:837-841, 1978.
16. ISIS-2 (Second International Study of Infarct Survival) Collaborative Group: Randomised trial of intravenous streptokinase, oral aspirin, both, or neither among 17 187 cases of suspected acute myocardial infarction: ISIS-2, *Lancet* ii:349-360, 1988.
17. Lin DY, Fischl MA, Schoenfeld DA: Evaluating the role of CD-4 lymphocyte counts as surrogate endpoints in human immunodeficiency virus clinical trials, *Stat Med* 12:835-842, 1993.
18. Morganroth J, Bigger JT Jr, Anderson JL: Treatment of ventricular arrhythmias by United States cardiologists: a survey before the Cardiac Arrhythmia Suppression Trial (CAST) results were available, *Am J Cardiol* 65:40-48, 1990.
19. NIH Revitalization Act of 1993, Public Law 103-43.
20. Packer M: Vasodilator and inotropic drugs for the treatment of chronic heart failure: distinguishing hype from hope, *J Am Coll Cardiol,* 12:1299-1317, 1988.
21. Packer M, Carver JR, Rodeheffer RJ et al: Effect of oral milrinone on mortality in severe chronic heart failure, *N Engl J Med* 325:1468-1475, 1991.
22. Piantadosi S, Wittes J: Letter to the editor, *Controlled Clin Trials* 14:562-567, 1993.
23. Prentice RL: Surrogate endpoints in clinical trials: definition and operational criteria, *Stat Med* 8:431-440, 1989.
24. Ray WA, Griffin MR, Avorn J: Evaluating drugs after their approval for clinical use, *N Engl J Med* 329:2029-2032, 1993.
25. Report from the Committee of Principal Investigators: A cooperative trial in the primary prevention of ischaemic heart disease using clofibrate, *Br Heart J* 40:1069-1118, 1978.
26. Riggs BL, Hodgson SF, O'Fallon WM, et al: Effect of fluoride treatment on the fracture rate in post-menopausal women with osteoporosis, *N Engl J Med* 322:802-809, 1990.

27. Ruberman W, Weinblatt E, Goldberg JD et al: Education, psychosocial stress, and sudden cardiac death, *J Chronic Dis* 36:151-160, 1983.
28. Ruberman W, Weinblatt E, Goldberg JD, et al: Psychosocial influences on mortality after myocardial infarction, *N Engl J Med* 311:552-559, 1984.
29. Schlant RC, Forman S, Stamler J, Canner PL: The natural history of coronary heart disease: prognostic factors after recovery from myocardial infarction in 2789 men. The 5-year findings of the Coronary Drug Project, *Circulation* 66:401-414, 1982.
30. Shimkin MB: The problem of experimentation on human beings. I. The research worker's point of view, *Science* 117:205-207, 1953.
31. Stamler J: Invited Remarks: National Conference on Clinical Trials Methodology, *Clin Pharmacol Ther* 25:651-654, 1979.
32. Steering Committee of the Physicians' Health Study Research Group: Final report on the aspirin component of the ongoing Physicians' Health Study, *N Engl J Med* 321:129-135, 1989.
33. Studies of Left Ventricular Dysfunction: Protocol, National Heart, Lung, and Blood Institute, Division of Epidemiology and Clinical Applications, Clinical Trials Branch, Bethesda, MD.
34. Temple RJ: A regulatory authority's opinion about surrogate endpoints, In Nimmo WS, Tucker GT, eds: *Clinical Measurement in Drug Evaluation,* New York, 1995, John Wiley & Sons.
35. The Cardiac Arrhythmia Suppression Trial (CAST) Investigators: Preliminary report: effect of encainide and flecainide on mortality in a randomized trial of arrhythmia suppression after myocardial infarction, *N Engl J Med* 321:406-412, 1989.
36. The Cardiac Arrhythmia Suppression Trial II Investigators: Effect of the antiarrhythmic agent moricizine on survival after myocardial infarction, *N Engl J Med* 327:227-233, 1992.
37. The Xamoterol in Severe Heart Failure Study Group: Xamoterol in severe heart failure, *Lancet* 336:1-6, 1990.
38. Urokinase Pulmonary Embolism Trial Study Group: Urokinase Pulmonary Embolism Trial: phase I results, *JAMA* 214:2163-2172, 1970.
39. Vlay SC: How the university cardiologist treats ventricular premature beats: a nationwide survey of 65 university medical centers, *Am Heart J* 110:904-912, 1985.
40. Weinblatt E, Ruberman W, Goldberg JD et al: Relation of education to sudden death after myocardial infarction, *N Engl J Med* 299:60-65, 1978.
41. Wittes J, Lakatos E, Probstfield J: Surrogate endpoints in clinical trials: cardiovascular diseases. *Stat Med* 8:415-425, 1989.
42. Yusuf S, Collins R, Peto R: Why do we need some large, simple randomized trials? *Stat Med* 3:409-420, 1984.

CHAPTER 3

Study Population

Defining the study population is an integral part of posing the primary question. It is not enough to claim that an intervention is or is not effective without describing the type of participant on which the intervention was tested. The description requires specification of criteria for subject eligibility. This chapter focuses on how to define the study population. In addition, it considers two questions. First, to what extent will the results of the trial be generalizable to a broader population? Second, what impact does selection of eligibility criteria have on participant recruitment, or, more generally, study feasibility? This issue is also discussed in Chapter 9.

FUNDAMENTAL POINT

The study population should be defined in advance, stating unambiguous inclusion (eligibility) criteria. The impact that these criteria will have on study design, ability to generalize, and participant recruitment must be considered.

DEFINITION OF STUDY POPULATION

The study population is the subset of the population with the condition or characteristics of interest defined by the eligibility criteria. The group of participants actually studied in the trial is selected from the study population (Fig. 3-1).

In reporting the study, the investigator needs to say what people were studied and how they were selected. The reasons for this are several. First, if an intervention is shown to be successful or unsuccessful, the medical and scientific communities must know to what kinds of people the findings apply.

Second, knowledge of the study population helps other investigators assess the study's merit and appropriateness. For example, an antianginal drug may be found to be ineffective. Close examination of the description of the study population, however, could reveal that the participants represented a variety of ill-defined conditions characterized by chest pain. Thus the study may not have been properly designed to evaluate the antianginal effects of the agent. Since many literature reports contain inadequate characterization of the study participants, readers are often unable to assess fully the merit of the studies. Third, in order for other investi-

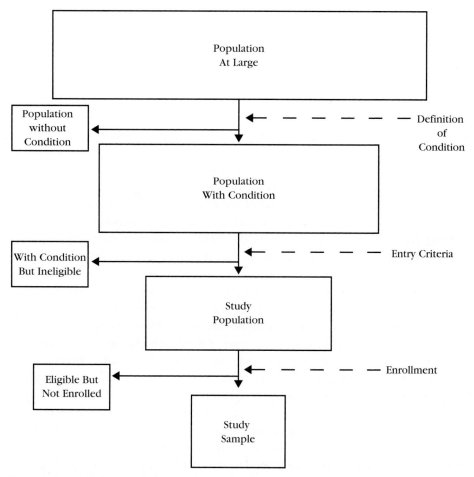

Fig. 3-1 Relationship of study sample to study population and population at large (those with and those without the condition under study).

gators to be able to replicate the study, they need data descriptive of the partici-pants enrolled. A similar issue is sometimes found in laboratory research. Because of incomplete discussion of details of the methods, procedures, and preparation of materials, other investigators find it impossible to replicate an experiment. Before most research findings are widely accepted, they need to be confirmed by indepen-dent scientists. Only small trials are likely to be repeated, but these are the ones, in general, that most need confirmation.

Inclusion criteria and reasons for their selection should be stated in advance. Ideally, all eligibility criteria should be precisely specified, but this is often impractical. Therefore those criteria central to the study should be the most carefully defined. For example, in a study of survivors of a myocardial infarction, the investigator may be interested in excluding people with severe hypertension. He will require an explicit definition of myocardial infarction; but with regard to hypertension, it may be sufficient to state that people with a diastolic blood pressure above a specified level will be excluded. Note that even here, the definition of severe hypertension, though arbitrary, is fairly specific. In a study of antihypertensive agents, however, the above definition of severe hypertension is inadequate. An investigator who wants to include only people with diastolic blood pressure over 105 mm Hg, should specify how often it is to be determined, when, with what instrument, by whom, and in what circumstances. If the etiology of the blood pressure is also important (e.g., only people with hypertension secondary to pheochromocytoma), the investigator needs to specify the etiology and how it is to be determined. For any study of antihypertensive agents, the criterion of hypertension is central; a detailed definition of myocardial infarction, on the other hand, may be less important.

If age is a restriction, the investigator should ideally specify not only that a participant must be less than 70, for example, but *when* he must be less than 70. If a prospective participant is 69 at the time of a prebaseline screening examination, but 70 at baseline, is he eligible? This should be clearly indicated. If diabetes mellitus is an exclusion criterion, is this only insulin-dependent diabetes, only juvenile-onset diabetes, or all diabetes? Does elevated glucose warrant exclusion? How is diabetes mellitus defined? Often there are no correct ways of defining inclusion and exclusion criteria and arbitrary decisions must be made. Regardless, they need to be as clear as possible, with appropriate specifications of the technique and laboratory methods.

As discussed in Chapter 4, many recent clinical trials are of the large, simple model. In such trials, not only are the interventions relatively easy to implement, and the baseline and outcome variables limited, so too are the eligibility criteria. Definitions of eligibility criteria may not require repeated visits or special procedures. They may rely on previously measured variables that are part of a diagnostic evaluation, or on variables that are measured using any of several techniques, or on investigator judgment. For example, a detailed definition of myocardial infarction or hypertension may be replaced with, "Does the investigator believe a myocardial infarction has occurred?" or "Is hypertension present?" The advantage of this kind of criterion is its simplicity. The disadvantage is the possible difficulty that a reader of the results of the trial will have in deciding if the results are applicable to specific patients under her care. It should be noted, however, that even with the large simple trial model, the criteria are selected and specified in advance.

In general, eligibility criteria relate to participant safety and anticipated effect of the intervention. The following categories outline the framework on which to develop individual criteria:

1. Participants who have the potential to benefit from the intervention are obviously candidates for enrollment into the study. The investigators select

participants on the basis of their scientific knowledge and the expectation that the intervention will work in a specific way on a certain kind of participant. For example, participants with a genito-urinary coliform infection are appropriate to enroll in a study of a new antibiotic agent known to be effective in vivo and thought to penetrate to the site of the infection in sufficient concentration. It should be evident from this example that selection of the participant depends on knowledge of the mechanism of action of the intervention. Knowing the mechanism of action may enable the investigator to identify a well-defined group of participants likely to respond to the intervention. Thus people with similar characteristics with respect to the relevant variable, that is, a homogeneous population, can be studied. In the above example, participants are homogeneous with regard to the type and strain of bacteria, and to the site of infection. If age or renal or liver function are also critical, these too might be considered, creating an even more highly selected group.

Even if the mechanism of action of the intervention is known, however, it may not be feasible to identify a homogeneous population because the technology to do so may not be available. For instance, the causes of a headache are numerous and, with few exceptions, not easily or objectively determined. If a potential therapy were developed for one kind of headache, it would be difficult to identify precisely the people who might benefit.

If the mechanism of action of the intervention is unclear, or if there is uncertainty at which stage of a disease a treatment might be most beneficial, a specific group of participants likely to respond cannot easily be selected. The Diabetic Retinopathy Study[7] evaluated the effects of photocoagulation. In this trial, each participant had one eye treated while the other eye served as the control. Participants were subgrouped on the basis of existence, location, and severity of vessel proliferation. Before the trial was scheduled to end, it became apparent that treatment was dramatically effective in the four most severe of the 10 subgroups. To have initially selected for study only those four subgroups who benefited was not possible given existing knowledge.

Some interventions may have more than one potentially beneficial mechanism of action. For example, if exercise reduces mortality or morbidity, is it because of its effect on cardiac performance, its weight-reducing effect, its effect on the person's sense of well being, some combination of these effects, or some as yet unknown effect? The investigator could select study participants who have poor cardiac performance, or who are obese or who, in general, do not feel well. If he chose incorrectly, his study would not yield a positive result. If he chose participants with all three characteristics and then showed benefit from exercise, he would never know which of the three aspects was important.

One could, of course, choose a study population where the members differ in one or more identifiable aspects of the condition being evaluated, or a heterogeneous group. These aspects could include stage or severity of a disease, etiology, or demographic factors. In the previous exercise example, studying a heterogeneous population may be preferable. By comparing outcome with presence or absence of initial obesity or sense of well being, the investigator may discover the relevant characteristics and gain insight into the mechanism of action. Also, when the study group is too restricted, there is no opportunity to discover whether an intervention is effective in a subgroup not initially considered. The broadness of the Diabetic Retinopathy Study[8] was responsible for showing that the remaining six subgroups also benefited from therapy. If knowledge had been more advanced, only the four subgroups with the most dramatic improvement might have been studied. Obviously, after publication of the results of these four subgroups, another trial might have been initiated. However, valuable time would have been wasted. Extrapolation of conclusions to milder retinopathy might even have made a second study impossible. Of course, the effect of the intervention on a heterogeneous group may be diluted, and the ability to detect a benefit may be reduced. That is the price to be paid for incomplete knowledge about mechanism of action.

Large, simple trials are, by nature, more heterogeneous in their study populations than other sorts of trials. It is assumed, in the design, that the intervention affects a diverse group, and that despite such diversity, the effect of the intervention is more similar among the various kinds of participants than not.

Homogeneity and heterogeneity are matters of degree and knowledge. As scientific knowledge advances, ability to classify is improved. Today's homogeneous group may be considered heterogeneous tomorrow. The discovery of Legionnaires' Disease[9] as a separate entity caused by a specific organism improved possibilities for categorizing respiratory disease. Presumably, until that discovery, people with Legionnaires' Disease were simply lumped together with people having other respiratory ailments.

2. In selecting participants to be studied, not only does the investigator require people in whom the intervention might work; he also wants to choose people in whom there is a high likelihood that he can detect the hypothesized results of the intervention. Careful choice will enable investigators to detect results in reasonable time, given a reasonable number of participants and finite amount of money.

For example, in a trial of an antianginal agent, an investigator would not wish to enroll a person who, in the past 2 years, has had only one brief angina pectoris episode (assuming such a person could be identified). The likelihood of finding an effect of the drug on this person is limited since his likelihood of having many angina episodes during the expected duration of the trial is minimal. Persons with frequent episodes would be more appropriate. Similarly, many people accept the hypothesis that low density lipoprotein (LDL) cholesterol is a continuous variable in its impact on the risk of developing cardiovascular disease. That is, there is no specific level below which the serum LDL cholesterol concentration is good with respect to coronary heart disease. Theoretically, an investigator could take any population with moderate or low LDL cholesterol, attempt to lower its cholesterol, and see if occurrence of cardiovascular disease is reduced. However, this trial would require studying an impossibly large number of people since the calculation of sample size (see Chapter 7) considers expected frequency of the primary response variables. When the expected frequency in the control group is low, as it would likely be in people who do not have elevated serum cholesterol, the number of people studied must be correspondingly high. From a sample size point of view it is, therefore, desirable to begin studying people with a high expected event rate. If results from a first trial are positive, the investigator can then go to groups with lower levels. The initial Veterans Administration study[20] of hypertension treatment involved people with diastolic blood pressure from 115 through 129 mm Hg. After therapy was shown to be beneficial in that group, a second trial was undertaken using people with diastolic blood pressures from 90 through 114 mm Hg.[21] The latter study suggested that treatment should be instituted for people with diastolic blood pressure over 104 mm Hg. Results were less clear for people with lower blood pressure. Subsequently, the Hypertension Detection and Follow-up Program[12,13] demonstrated benefit from treatment for people with diastolic blood pressure of 90 mm Hg or above.

Generally, if the primary response is continuous (e.g., blood pressure, blood sugar, and body weight), change is easier to detect when the initial level is extreme. In a study to see whether a new drug is antihypertensive, one might expect a more pronounced drop of blood pressure in a participant with diastolic pressure of 130 mm Hg than in one with diastolic pressure of 102 mm Hg. There are exceptions to this rule, especially if a condition has multiple causes. The relative frequency of each cause might be different across the spectrum of values. For example, genetic disorders might be heavily represented among people with extremely high cholesterol. These lipid disorders may require alternative therapies or may even be resistant to usual methods of reducing cholesterol. In addition, use of participants with lower levels of a variable such as cholesterol might be less costly.[18] This is because of lower screening costs. Therefore, while in general use of higher risk participants is preferable, other considerations can modify this.

3. Most interventions are likely to have adverse effects. The investigator needs to weight these effects against possible benefit when he evaluates the feasibility of the study. However, any participant for whom the intervention is known to be harmful should not be admitted to the trial. Pregnant women often have been excluded from drug trials (unless, of course, the primary question concerns pregnancy). The amount of additional data obtained may not justify the risk of possibly teratogenicity. Some have recently questioned, however, if pregnancy is a valid exclusion criterion.[4] Investigators would probably exclude from a study of almost any of the antiinflammatory drugs people with a history of gastric bleeding. Gastric bleeding is a fairly straightforward and absolute contraindication for enrollment.

Yet, an exclusion criterion such as "history of major gastric bleed," leaves much to the judgment of the investigator. The word "major" implies that gastric hemorrhaging is not an absolute contraindication, but a relative one that depends upon clinical judgment. The phrase also recognizes the question of anticipated risk vs. benefit, because it does not clearly prohibit people with a mild bleeding episode in the distant past from being placed on an anti-inflammatory drug. It may very well be that such people take aspirin or similar agents, possibly for a good reason, and studying such people may prove more beneficial than hazardous.

Note that these exclusions apply only before enrollment into the trial. During a trial participants may develop symptoms or conditions that would have excluded them had any of these conditions been present earlier. In these circumstances, the participant may be removed from the intervention regimen, but should be kept in the trial for purposes of analysis. (See Chapter 16.)

4. The issue of competing risk is generally of greater interest in long-term studies. Participants at high risk of developing conditions that preclude the ascertainment of the event of interest should be excluded from enrollment. The intervention may or may not be efficacious in such participants, but the necessity for excluding them from enrollment relates to design considerations. In many studies of people with heart disease, those who have cancer or severe kidney or liver disorders are excluded because these diseases might cause the participant to die or withdraw from the study before the primary response variable can be observed. Even in short-term studies, however, the competing risk issue needs to be considered. For example, an investigator may be studying a new intervention for a specific congenital heart defect in infants. Such infants are also likely to have other life-threatening defects. The investigator would not want to enroll infants if one of these other conditions was likely to lead to the death of the infant before the investigator had an opportunity to evaluate the effect of the intervention. (This matter is similar to the one raised in Chapter 2 that presented the problem of the impact of high expected total mortality on a study in which the primary response variable is morbidity or cause-specific mortality.) When there is competing risk, the ability to assess the true impact of the intervention is, at best, lessened. At worst, if the intervention somehow has either a beneficial or harmful effect on the coexisting condition, biased results for the primary question can be obtained.

5. Investigators prefer, ordinarily, to enroll only participants who are likely to adhere to the study protocol. Participants are expected to take their assigned intervention (usually a drug) and return for scheduled follow-up appointments regardless of the intervention assignment. In unblinded studies, participants are asked to accept the random assignment, even after knowing its identity, and abide by the protocol. Moreover, participants should not receive the study intervention from sources outside the trial during the course of the study. Participants should also refrain from using other interventions that may compete with the study intervention. Nonadher-

ence by participants reduces the opportunity to observe the true effect of the intervention. Unfortunately, there are no failsafe ways of selecting perfect participants. Traditional guidelines have led to disappointing results. See Chapter 13 for a further discussion of adherence.

GENERALIZATION

Study samples or participants are usually nonrandomly chosen from the study population, which in turn is defined by the eligibility criteria (Fig. 3-1). As long as selection of participants into a trial occurs, they must be regarded as special. Therefore investigators have the problem of generalizing from participants actually in the trial to the study population and then to the population with the condition. Defined medical conditions and quantifiable or discrete variables such as age, sex, or elevated blood sugar can be clearly stated and measured. For these characteristics, specifying in what way the study participants and study population are different from the population with the condition is relatively easy. Judgments about the appropriateness of generalizing study results can, therefore, be made. Other factors of the study participants are less easily characterized. Obviously, investigators study only those participants available to them. If they live in Florida, they will not be studying people living in Maine. Even within a geographical area, most investigators are hospital based. Except in rare instances, participants are not drawn from the community at large. Furthermore, many hospitals are referral centers. Only certain types of participants come to the attention of investigators at these institutions. It may be impossible to decide whether these factors are relevant when generalizing to other geographical areas or patient care settings.

It is often forgotten that participants must agree to enroll in a study. What sort of person volunteers for a study? Why do some agree to participate while others do not? The requirement that study participants sign informed consent or return for periodic examinations is sufficient to make certain people unwilling to participate. The reasons are not often obvious. What is known, however, is that volunteers can be different from nonvolunteers.[11,17,22] They are usually in better health, and they are more likely to adhere to the study protocol. However, the reverse could also be true. People might be more motivated if they have disease symptoms. In the absence of knowing what motivates the particular study participants, appropriate compensatory adjustments cannot be made. Because specifying how volunteers differ from others is difficult, an investigator cannot confidently identify those segments of the study or general populations that these study participants supposedly represent. One approach to answering the question of representativeness is to maintain a log or registry that lists prospective participants identified, but not enrolled, and the reasons for excluding them. This log can provide an estimate of the proportion of all potentially eligible people who meet study entrance requirements and can also indicate how many otherwise eligible people refused enrollment. In an effort to further assess the issue of representativeness, response variables in those excluded have also been monitored. In the Norwegian Multicenter Study[14] on timolol, people excluded because of contraindication to the study drug or competing risks had a mortality rate twice that of enrolled participants.

The Coronary Artery Surgery Study[3] included a randomized trial that compared coronary artery bypass surgery against medical therapy and a registry of people eligible for the trial but who refused to participate. The enrolled and not enrolled groups were alike in most identifiable respects. Survival in the participants randomly assigned to medical care was the same as those receiving medical care but not in the trial. The findings for those undergoing surgery were similar. Therefore, in this particular case, the trial participants appeared to be representative of the study population.

Since the investigator can describe only to a limited extent the kinds of participants in whom an intervention was evaluated, a leap of faith is always required when applying any study findings to the population with the condition. In taking this jump, one must always strike a balance between making unjustifiably broad generalizations and being too conservative in one's claims. Some extrapolations are reasonable and justifiable from a clinical point of view, especially in light of subsequent information. The Coronary Drug Project,[5] a trial of lipid-lowering drugs, studied men between the ages of 30 and 64 who had had at least one myocardial infarction. Conclusions from that trial about the hazards of certain methods of lipid lowering and the inefficacy of other methods with respect to reducing mortality might reasonably have been extended to men below 30 and above age 64, since conclusions about younger men in the trial were similar to conclusions about older men.[6] Here too, though, caution needed to be exercised; causes of myocardial infarctions in young men might be different from causes in older men. One might have been tempted to claim that the findings could be extrapolated to women, as men were chosen mainly for statistical reasons (greater incidence of events related to coronary heart disease). An extrapolation from men to women, however could have been hazardous because there was no information at all on women. Several later trials convincingly showed that at least for secondary prevention, lipid lowering is beneficial.[10] Unfortunately, many other lipid-lowering trials also excluded women. Thus, even though epidemiologic data and the small numbers of women in lipid-lowering trials suggest that benefits are likely, definitive proof is lacking that mortality can be reduced. The Scandinavian Simvastatin Survival Study (4S)[16] did, however, demonstrate that major coronary events could be reduced by lipid lowering in women, as well as men, who had known coronary heart disease.

The Physicians' Health Study[19] concluded that aspirin reduced myocardial infarction in men without previously documented heart disease. Although it is reasonable to expect that a similar reduction would occur in women, it is as yet unproven. Importantly, aspirin was shown in the Physicians' Health Study and elsewhere[15] to increase hemorrhagic stroke. Given the lower risk of heart disease in premenopausal women, whether the trade-off between adverse effects and benefit is favorable is far from certain. An ongoing trial is seeking to address that issue.[2] Whether proof in women, separate from men, is necessary, is a matter of clinical judgment.

RECRUITMENT

The impact of eligibility criteria on recruitment of participants should be considered when deciding on these criteria. Using excessive restrictions in an effort to obtain a pure (or homogeneous) sample can lead to extreme difficulty in getting sufficient participants. Age and sex are two criteria that have obvious bearing on the ease of enrolling participants. The Coronary Primary Prevention Trial undertaken by the Lipid Research Clinics was a collaborative trial evaluating a lipid-lowering drug in men between the ages of 35 and 59 with severe hypercholesterolemia. One of the Lipid Research Clinics[1] noted that approximately 35,000 people were screened and only 257 participants enrolled. Exclusion criteria, all of which were perfectly reasonable and scientifically sound, coupled with the number of people who refused to enter the study, brought the overall trial yield down to less than 1%. As discussed in Chapter 9, this example of greater than expected numbers being screened and unanticipated problems in reaching potential participants is common to most clinical trials.

If entrance criteria are properly determined in the beginning of a study, there should be no need to change them. As discussed earlier in this chapter, eligibility criteria are appropriate if they exclude those who might be harmed by the intervention, are not likely to be benefited by the intervention, or are not likely to comply with the study protocol. The reasons for each criterion should be carefully examined during the planning phase of the study. If they do not fall into one of the above categories, they should be reassessed. Whenever investigators consider changing criteria, they need to look at the effect of changes on participant safety and study design. It may be that, in opening the gates to accommodate more participants, they increase the required sample size, because the participants admitted may have lower probability of developing the primary response variable. They can thus lose the benefits of added recruitment. In summary, capacity to recruit participants and carry out the trial effectively could greatly depend on the eligibility criteria that are set. As a consequence, careful thought should go into establishing them.

REFERENCES

1. Benedict GW: LRC Coronary Prevention Trial: Baltimore, *Clin Pharmacol Ther* 25:685-687, 1979.
2. Buring JE, Hennekens CH, for the Women's Health Study Research Group: The Women's Health Study: rationale and background, *J Myocardial Ischemia* 4:30-40, 1992.

3. CASS Principal Investigators et al: Coronary artery surgery study (CASS): a randomized trial of coronary artery bypass surgery. Comparability of entry characteristics and survival in randomized patients and non-randomized patients meeting randomization criteria, *JACC* 3:114-128, 1984.

4. Committee on the Ethical Issues Relating to the Inclusion of Women in Clinical Studies, Institute of Medicine: *Women and Health Research: Ethical and Legal Issues of Including Women in Clinical Studies,* Mastroianni AC, Faden R, Federman D, eds. Washington, D.C. National Academy Press, 1994.

5. Coronary Drug Project Research Group: The Coronary Drug Project: design, methods, and baseline results, *Circulation* 47 (suppl I):I-1–I-50, 1973.

6. Coronary Drug Project Research Group: Clofibrate and niacin in coronary heart disease, *JAMA* 231:360-381, 1975.

7. Diabetic Retinopathy Study Research Group: Preliminary report on effects of photocoagulation therapy, *Am J Ophthalmol* 81:383-396, 1976.

8. Diabetic Retinopathy Study Research Group: Photocoagulation treatment of proliferative diabetic retinopathy: the second report of diabetic retinopathy study findings, *Ophthalmol* (formerly *Trans Am Acad Ophthalmol Otolaryngol*) 85:82-105, 1978.

9. Fraser DW, Tsai TR, Orenstein W et al: Legionnaires' Disease: description of an epidemic of pneumonia, *N Engl J Med* 297:1189-1197, 1977.

10. Gordon DJ: Cholesterol lowering and total mortality. In Rifkind BM, ed: *Lowering cholesterol in high-risk individuals and populations,* New York, 1995, Marcel Dekker.

11. Horwitz D, Wilbeck E: Effect of tuberculosis infection on mortality risk, *Am Rev Respir Dis* 104: 643-655, 1971.

12. Hypertension Detection and Follow-up Program Cooperative Group: The Hypertension Detection and Follow-up Program, *Prev Med* 5:207-215, 1976.

13. Hypertension Detection and Follow-up Program Cooperative Group: Five-year findings of the Hypertension Detection and Follow-up Program. 1. Reduction in mortality of persons with high blood pressure, including mild hypertension, *JAMA* 242:2562-2571, 1979.

14. Pedersen TR: The Norwegian Multicenter Study of timolol after myocardial infarction, *Circulation* 67 (suppl I):I-49–I-53, 1983.

15. Peto R, Gray R, Collins R et al: A randomized trial of the effects of prophylactic daily aspirin among male British doctors, *Br Med J* 296:320-331, 1988.

16. Scandinavian Simvastatin Survival Study Group: Randomised trial of cholesterol lowering in 4444 patients with coronary heart disease: the Scandinavian Simvastatin Survival Study (4S), *Lancet* 344:1383-1389, 1994.

17. Smith P, Arnesen H: Mortality in non-consenters in a post-myocardial infarction trial, *J Intern Med* 228:253-256, 1990.

18. Sondik EJ, Brown BW Jr, Silvers A: High risk subjects and the cost of large field trials, *J Chron Dis* 27:177-187, 1974.

19. Steering Committee of the Physicians' Health Study Research Group: Final report on the aspirin component of the ongoing Physician's Health Study, *N Engl J Med* 321:129-135, 1989.

20. Veterans Administration Cooperative Study Group on Antihypertensive Agents: Effects of treatment on morbidity in hypertension: results in patients with diastolic blood pressures averaging 115 through 129 mm Hg, *JAMA* 202:1028-1034, 1967.

21 Veterans Administration Cooperative Study Group on Antihypertensive Agents: Effects of treatment on morbidity in hypertension: II. Results in patients with diastolic blood pressures averaging 90 through 114 mm Hg, *JAMA* 213:1143-1152, 1970.

22. Wilhelmsen L, Ljungberg S, Wedel H, Werko L: A comparison between participants and non-participants in a primary preventive trial, *J Chron Dis* 29:331-339, 1976.

CHAPTER 4

Basic Study Design

The foundations for the design of controlled experiments were established for agricultural application. They are described in several classical statistics text-books.[22,26,34,35] From these sources evolved the basic design of controlled clinical studies.

Although the history of clinical experimentation contains several instances in which the need for control groups has been recognized,[13,30] this need was not widely accepted until the 1950s.[49] In the past, when a new intervention was first investigated, it was likely to be given to only a small number of patients, and the outcome compared, if at all, to that in patients previously treated in a different manner. The comparison was informal and frequently based on memory alone. Patients were evaluated initially and then reexamined after an intervention had been introduced. In such studies, the changes from the initial state were used as the measure of success or failure of the new intervention. What could not be known was whether the patient would have responded in the same manner if there had been no intervention at all. However, then, and unfortunately sometimes even today, this kind of observation has formed the basis for the widespread use of new interventions.

Of course, some results are so highly dramatic that no comparison group is needed. Successful results of this magnitude, however, are rare. One example is the effectiveness of penicillin in pneumococcal pneumonia. Another example origi-nated with Pasteur, who in 1884 was able to demonstrate that a series of vaccine injections protected dogs from rabies.[63] He suggested that because of the long incu-bation time prompt vaccination of a human being after infection might prevent the fatal disease. The first patient was a 9-year-old boy who had been bitten 3 days ear-lier by a rabid dog. The treatment was completely effective. The confirmation came from another boy who was treated within 6 days of having been bitten. During the next few years, hundreds of patients were given the antirabies vaccine. It was almost always effective if given within certain time limits.

Gocke[42] reported on a similar, uncontrolled study of patients with acute fulmi-nant viral hepatitis. Nine consecutive cases had recently been observed, all of whom had a fatal outcome. The next diagnosed case, a young staff nurse in hepatic coma, was given immunotherapy in addition to standard treatment. The patient survived, as did four others among eight given the antiserum. The author initially thought that this uncontrolled study was conclusive. However, in considering other explanations for the encouraging findings, he could not eliminate the possibility that a tendency to treat patients earlier in the course and more intensive care might be responsible for the observed outcome. Thus he joined a double-blind, randomized trial comparing hyperimmune antiAustralia globulin with normal human serum globulin in patients with severe acute hepatitis. Nineteen of 28 patients (67.9%) randomized to control treatment died, compared with 16 of 25 patients (64%) randomized to treatment with exogenous antibody, a statistically nonsignificant difference.[1]

Several medical conditions are either of short duration or episodic. Therapy evaluation in these cases can be difficult in the absence of controlled studies. Snow and Kimmelman[85] reviewed various uncontrolled studies of surgical procedures for Ménière's disease. They found that about 75% of patients improved, but noted that this is similar to the 70% remission rate occurring without treatment.

Given the wide spectrum of the natural history of almost any disease and variability of an individual patient's response to an intervention, most investigators recognize the need for a defined control or comparison group.

FUNDAMENTAL POINT

Sound scientific clinical investigation almost always demands that a control group be used against which the new intervention can be compared. Randomization is the preferred way of assigning participants to control and intervention groups.

Statistics and epidemiology textbooks and papers* cover various study designs in some detail. Green and Byar[45] also present a "hierarchy of strength of evidence concerning efficacy of treatment." In their scheme, anecdotal case reports are weakest and confirmed randomized clinical trials are strongest, with various observational and retrospective designs in between. This chapter will discuss several major clinical trial designs: randomized, nonrandomized concurrent, historical, cross-over, withdrawal, factorial, and group allocation. The randomized and nonrandomized concurrent control studies both assign participants to either the intervention or control group, but only the former makes the assignment by using a randomized procedure. Historical control studies compare a group of participants on a new therapy or intervention with a previous group of participants on standard or control therapy. The cross-over design uses each participant twice, once as a member of the control group and once as a member of the intervention group.

Questions have been raised concerning the method of selection of the control group, but the major controversy has revolved around the use of historical vs. randomized control.[17,40,95] With regard to drug evaluation, this controversy is less intense

---

*References 4, 10, 11, 12, 15, 33, 48, 60, 64, 71, 74, 86.

than in the past. It is still being hotly contested, however, in the evaluation of new devices or procedures.[80] Each of the designs has advantages and disadvantages, but a randomized control design is the standard by which other studies should be judged. A discussion of sequential designs is postponed until Chapter 15 because the basic feature involves interim analyses.

For each of the designs it is assumed, for the simplicity of discussion, that a single control group and a single intervention group are being considered. These designs can be extended to more than one intervention group and more than one control group.

RANDOMIZED CONTROL STUDIES

Randomized control studies are comparative studies with an intervention group and a control group; the assignment of the participant to a group is determined by the formal procedure of randomization. Randomization, in the simplest case, is a process by which all participants are equally likely to be assigned to either the intervention or control group. The features of this technique are discussed in Chapter 5. There are three advantages of the randomized design over other methods for selecting controls.[17]

First, randomization removes the potential of bias in the allocation of participants to the intervention group or control group. Such allocation bias could easily occur, and cannot be necessarily prevented, in the nonrandomized concurrent or historical control study because the investigator or the participant may influence the choice of intervention. This influence can be conscious or subconscious and can be because of numerous factors, including the prognosis of the participant. The direction of the allocation bias may go either way and can easily invalidate the comparison.

The second advantage, somewhat related to the first, is that randomization tends to produce comparable groups; that is, the measured and unknown prognostic factors and other characteristics of the participants at the time of randomization will be, on the average, evenly balanced between the intervention and control group. This does not mean that in any single experiment all such characteristics, sometimes called baseline variables or covariates, will be perfectly balanced between the two groups. However, it does mean that for independent covariates, whatever the detected or undetected differences that exist between the groups, the overall magnitude and direction of the differences will tend to be equally divided between the two groups. Of course, many covariates are strongly associated; thus any imbalance in one would tend to produce imbalances in the others. As discussed in chapters 5 and 16, stratified randomization and stratified analysis are methods commonly used to guard against and adjust for imbalanced randomizations.

The third advantage of randomization is that the validity of statistical tests of significance is guaranteed. As has been stated,[17] "although groups compared are never perfectly balanced for important covariates in any single experiment, the process of randomization makes it possible to ascribe a probability distribution to the difference in outcome between treatment groups receiving equally effective treatments and thus to assign significance levels to observed differences." How valid the statistical tests of significance are does not depend on the balance of the prognostic factors between the two groups. The chi-square test for 2-by-2 tables and Student's t-test for comparing two means can be justified on the basis of randomization alone without making further assumptions concerning the distribution of baseline variables. If randomization is not used, further assumptions concerning the comparability of the groups and appropriateness of the statistical models must be made before the comparisons will be valid. Establishing the validity of these assumptions may be difficult.

Randomized and nonrandomized trials of the use of anticoagulant therapy in patients with acute myocardial infarctions have been reviewed by Chalmers et al.[21] and the conclusions compared. Of 32 studies, 18 used historical controls and involved a total of 900 patients, 8 used nonrandomized concurrent controls and involved more than 3000 patients, and 6 were randomized trials with a total of more than 3800 patients. The authors reported that 15 of the 18 historical control trials and 5 of the 8 nonrandomized concurrent control trials showed statistically significant results favoring the anticoagulation therapy. Only one of the six randomized control trials showed significant results in support of this therapy. Pooling the results of these six randomized trials yielded a statistically significant 20% reduction in total mortality. Pooling the results of the nonrandomized control studies showed a reduction of about 50% in total mortality in the intervention groups, more than twice the decrease seen in the randomized trials. Peto[70] has assumed that this difference in reduction is because of bias. He suggests that since the presumed bias in the nonrandomized trials was of the same order of magnitude as the presumed true effect, the nonrandomized trials could have yielded positive answers even if the therapy had been of no benefit. Of course, pooling results of several studies can be subject to criticism. As Goldman and Feinstein pointed out,[43] not all randomized trials of anticoagulants study the same kind of participants, use precisely the same intervention, or measure the same response variables. And, of course, not all randomized trials are done equally well. The principles of pooled analysis, or meta-analysis, are covered are Chapter 16.

Grace, Muench, and Chalmers[44] reviewed studies involving portacaval shunt operations for patients with portal hypertension from cirrhosis. In their review, 34 of 47 nonrandomized studies strongly supported the shunt procedure, while only 1 of the 4 randomized control trials indicated support for the operation. The authors concluded that the operation should not be endorsed.

Sacks et al.[78] have expanded the work by Chalmers et al. referenced previously to five other interventions. They concluded that selection biases led historical control studies to favor inappropriately the new interventions. It was also noted that many randomized control trials were of inadequate size, and therefore may have failed to find benefits that truly existed.[79] Chalmers et al.[20] also examined 145 reports of studies of treatment after myocardial infarction. Of the 57 studies that used a blinded randomization process, 14% had at least one significant ($p < 0.05$) maldistribution of baseline variables, with 3.4% of all of the baseline variables being significantly different between study groups. Of these 57 studies, 9% found significant outcome differences between groups. This contrasted with 58% having baseline variable differences among the 43 reports where the control groups were selected by means of a nonrandom process, with 34% of all of the baseline variables being significantly different between groups. The outcome between groups was significantly different 58% of the time. For the 45 studies that used a randomized but unblinded process to select the control groups, the results were in between; 28% had baseline imbalances, 7% of the baseline variables were significantly different, and 24% showed significant outcome differences. It should be noted that in using a $p < 0.05$ to declare a significant difference, such a difference would be seen 5% of the time by chance alone.

The most frequent objections to the use of the randomized control clinical trial are stated by Ingelfinger[54] to be "emotional and ethical." Many clinicians feel that they must not deprive a patient from receiving a new therapy or intervention which they, or someone else, believe to be beneficial, regardless of the validity of the evidence for that claim. The argument aimed at randomization is that in the typical trial it deprives about one half the participants from receiving the new and presumed better intervention.

The ethical aspects of randomization have been discussed by several authors.[17,19,81] What is meant by ethical behavior? Most would agree that it means treating the patient with the intervention believed to be best. Of course, what is ethical behavior for one well-informed investigator might not be ethical for another. Similarly, there are considerable differences among geographic locations (within and between countries) and cultures. Presumably, the reason that a clinical trial is being considered at all is that there is uncertainty about the potential benefits of a new intervention. An investigator who believes, for whatever reason, that the new intervention is more beneficial or harmful than the old, should not participate in the trial. On the other hand, an investigator who has sufficient doubt about which intervention is better is ethically justified in participating in a randomized clinical trial to settle the question. Shaw and Chalmers[81] argue that under these circumstances, randomization is a more ethical way of practicing medicine than the routine prescribing of medication or therapy that has never been proven to be beneficial by standard scientific methods and could possibly be harmful.

A classic example of ethics and randomized clinical trials was presented by Silverman[83] and Meier.[66] Administering high concentrations of oxygen to premature babies was, at one time, routinely practiced to prevent brain damage because of oxygen deficiency. The suspicion that this procedure might cause retrolental fibro-plasia and subsequent blindness led to a clinical trial in which premature babies were randomized to either the accepted high or a lower concentration of oxygen. Trial results indicated that the practice of administering high concentrations of oxygen caused blindness.[58] What was once considered to be unethical behavior in withholding high oxygen concentration was later felt to be ethically correct. How-ever, because of possible harm to other organs caused by withholding high con-centrations of oxygen, questions regarding the overall benefit or harm remained unanswered.[83]

The lesson from the retrolental fibroplasia study was helpful in justifying a clinical trial involving respiratory distress syndrome in premature babies.[23] This study involved randomization of mothers in premature labor to corticosteroid or placebo therapy. The assumption was that the corticosteroid would hasten the lung matura-tion process and protect against respiratory distress syndrome. Pediatricians and obstetricians recalled the oxygen experience and felt ethically able to participate in such a randomized clinical trial before recommending steroid therapy for general use.

Not all clinical studies can use randomized controls. Occasionally, the preva-lence of the disease is so rare that a large enough population cannot be readily obtained. In such an instance, only case-control studies might be possible. Such studies, which are not clinical trials according to the definition in this book, are dis-cussed in standard epidemiology textbooks.[48,60,64]

Zelen[98] has proposed to modify the standard randomized control study. He argued that investigators are often reluctant to recruit prospective trial participants not knowing to which group the participant will be assigned. Expressing ignorance of optimal therapy compromises the traditional doctor-patient relationship. Zelen there-fore suggested randomizing eligible participants before informing them about the trial. Only those assigned to active intervention would be asked if they wish to partic-ipate. The control participants would simply be followed and their outcome moni-tored. Obviously, such a design could not be blinded. Another major criticism of this controversial design centers on the ethical concern of not informing participants that they are enrolled in a trial. The efficiency of the design has also been evaluated.[2] It depends on the proportion of participants consenting to adhere to the assigned inter-vention. To compensate for this possible inefficiency, one needs to increase the sam-ple size. (See Chapter 7.) The Zelen approach has been tried with varying degrees of success.[31,99] Despite its having been proposed in 1979, there is insufficient experience to evaluate it fully. This may indicate its lack of general acceptance.

NONRANDOMIZED CONCURRENT CONTROL STUDIES

Controls in a nonrandomized concurrent control study are participants treated without the new intervention at approximately the same time as the intervention group is treated. Participants are allocated to one of the two groups, but by definition this is not a random process. An example of a nonrandomized concurrent control study would be a comparison of survival results of patients treated at two institutions, one institution using a new surgical procedure and the other using more traditional medical care.

To some investigators, the nonrandomized concurrent control design has advantages over the randomized control design. Those who object to the idea of ceding to chance the responsibility for selecting a person's treatment may favor this design. It is also difficult for some investigators to convince potential participants of the need for randomization. They find it easier to select a group of people to receive the intervention and would prefer to select the control group by means of matching key characteristics.

The major weakness of the nonrandomized concurrent control study is the potential that intervention and control groups are not strictly comparable. It is difficult to prove comparability because investigators must assume that they have information on all the important prognostic factors. Selecting a control group by matching on more than a few factors is impractical, and the comparability of a variety of other characteristics would still need to be evaluated. In small studies, an investigator is unlikely to find real differences that may exist between groups before the initiation of intervention since there is poor sensitivity to detect such differences. Even for large studies that could detect most differences of real clinical importance, the uncertainty about the unknown or unmeasured factors is still a concern.

Is there, for example, some unknown and unmeasurable process that results in one type of participant's being recruited into one group and not into the other? If all participants come from one institution, physicians may select participants into one group based on subtle and intangible factors. In addition, there exists the possibility for subconscious bias in allocating participants to either the intervention or control group. One group might come from a different socioeconomic class than the other group. All of these uncertainties may decrease the credibility of the concurrent but nonrandomized control study. For any particular question, the advantages of reduced cost, relative simplicity, and investigator and participant acceptance must be carefully weighed against the potential biases before a decision is made to use a nonrandomized concurrent control study. We believe this will occur rarely.

HISTORICAL CONTROLS/DATA BASES

In historical control studies, a new intervention is used in a series of participants and the results are compared to the outcome in a previous series of comparable participants. Historical controls are, by this definition, nonrandomized and nonconcurrent.

The argument for using a historical control design is that all new participants can receive the new intervention. As Gehan and Freireich[40] argued, many clinicians believe that no patient should be deprived of the possibility of receiving a new therapy or intervention. Some require less supportive evidence than others to accept a new intervention as being beneficial. Investigators who are already of the opinion that the new intervention is beneficial would most likely consider any restriction on its use unethical. Therefore they would favor a historical control study. In addition, participants may be more willing to enroll in a study if they can be assured of receiving a particular therapy or intervention. Finally, since all new participants will be on the new intervention, the time required to complete recruitment of participants for the trial will be cut approximately in half. This allows investigators to obtain results more quickly or do more studies with given resources.

Gehan[41] has emphasized the ethical advantages of historical control studies and pointed out that they have contributed to medical knowledge. Lasagna has argued that medical practitioners have traditionally relied on historical controls when making therapeutic judgments. He maintains that, while sometimes faulty, these judgments are often correct and useful.[59]

Typically, historical control data can be obtained from two sources. First, control group data may be available in the literature. These data are often undesirable because it is difficult, and perhaps impossible, to establish whether the control and intervention groups are comparable in key characteristics at the onset. Even if such characteristics were measured in the same way, the information may not be published and for all practical purposes it will be lost. Second, data may not have been published but may be available on computer files or in medical charts. Such data on control participants, for example, might be found in a large center that has several ongoing clinical investigations. When one study is finished, the participants in that study may be used as a control group for some future study. Centers doing successive studies, as in cancer research, will usually have a system for storing and retrieving the data from past studies for use at some future time.

Despite the time and cost benefits, and the ethical considerations, historical control studies have potential limitations that should be kept in mind. They are particularly vulnerable to bias. Moertel[67] cites several examples of treatments for cancer that have been claimed beneficial on the basis of historical control studies. Many treatments were declared breakthroughs on the basis of control data as old as 30 years. Pocock[73] identified 19 instances of the same intervention's having been used in two consecutive trials employing similar participants at the same institution. Theoretically, the mortality in the two groups using the same treatment should be similar. Pocock noted that the difference in mortality rates between such groups ranged from –46% to +24%. Four of the 19 comparisons showed differences significant at the 5% level.

An improvement in outcome for a given disease may be attributed to a new intervention when, in fact, the improvement may stem from a change in the patient population or patient management. Shifts in patient population can be subtle and perhaps undetectable. In a Veterans Administration Urological Research Group[93] study of prostate cancer, 2313 patients were randomized to placebo and estrogen treatment groups over 7 years. During the last 2 to 3 years of the study, no differences were found between the placebo and estrogen groups. However, placebo patients entering in the first 2 to 3 years had a shorter survival time than estrogen patients entering in the last 2 to 3 years of the study. The reason for the apparent difference is probably that the patients randomized earlier were older than the later group and thus were at higher risk of death during observation.[17] The results would have been misleading had this been a historical control study and a concurrent randomized comparison group not been available.

On a broader scale, for reasons that are not entirely clear, in many countries, including the United States,[75] coronary heart disease has been on the decline in the general population for more than 20 years. Therefore any clinical trial in the cardiovascular area involving long-term therapy using historical controls would need to separate the treatment effect from the recent trend, an almost impossible task.

The method by which participants are selected for a particular study can have a large impact on their comparability with earlier participant groups or general population statistics. In the Coronary Drug Project,[25] an annual total mortality rate of 6% was anticipated in the control group based on rates from a fairly unselected group of myocardial infarction patients. In fact, a control group mortality rate of about 4% was observed, and no significant differences were seen between the intervention groups and the control group. Using the historical control approach, a 33% reduction in mortality might have been claimed for the treatments. One explanation for the discrepancy between anticipated and observed mortality is that entry criteria typically excluded those most seriously ill.

Shifts in diagnostic criteria for a given disease because of improved technology can cause major changes in the recorded frequency of the disease and in the perceived prognosis of the subjects with the disease. International coding systems and names of diseases change periodically and, unless one is aware of the modifications, prevalence of certain conditions can appear to change abruptly. For example, when the Eighth Revision of the International Classification of Diseases came out in 1968, almost 15% more deaths were assigned to ischemic heart disease than had been assigned in the Seventh Revision.[77] When the Ninth Revision appeared in 1979, there was a correction downward of a similar magnitude.[69]

People identified as having hypertension today may be quite different from those identified 30 years ago. Today, through education, publicity campaigns, and screening programs, people are encouraged to have their blood pressure checked. Many people may be asymptomatic and yet be noted as having hypertension. Several years ago, it was likely that primarily people with symptoms would have chosen to see a physician. As result, those classed as hypertensive in the past might have been at a different risk level than those currently labeled as hypertensive.

A common concern about historical control designs is the accuracy and completeness with which control group data are collected. With the possible exception of special centers that have many ongoing studies, data are generally collected in a nonuniform manner by numerous people with diverse interests in the information. Lack of uniform collection methods can easily lead to incomplete and erroneous records. Data on some important prognostic factors may not have been collected at all. Because of limitations of data collected historically from medical charts, records from a center that conducts several studies and has a computerized data management system may provide the most reliable historical control data.

The historical control study has a place in scientific investigation despite its limitations. As a rapid, relatively inexpensive method of obtaining initial impressions regarding a new therapy, such studies can be important. This is particularly so if investigators understand the potential biases and are willing to miss effective new therapies if bias works in the wrong direction. Bailar et al.[6] have identified several features that can strengthen the conclusions to be drawn from historical control studies. These include an a priori identification of a reasonable hypothesis and advance planning for analysis.

In some special cases where disease diagnosis is clearly established and the prognosis is well known or the disease is highly fatal, a historical control study may be the only reasonable design. The results of penicillin in treatment of pneumococcal pneumonia were so dramatic in contrast to previous experience that no further evidence was really required. Similarly, the benefits of treatment of malignant hypertension became readily apparent from comparisons with previous, untreated populations.[7,8,29]

The use of prospective registries to characterize patients and evaluate effects of therapy has been advocated.[51,52,89] Supporters say that a systematic approach to data collection and follow-up can provide information about the local patient population and can aid in clinical decision making. They argue that clinical trial populations may not be representative of the patients actually seen by a physician. Moon et al.[68] have described the use of data bases derived from clinical trials to evaluate therapy. They stress that the high-quality data obtained through these sources can reduce the problems of the typical historical control study. The use of data bases has expanded in recent years. This so-called outcomes research has burgeoned because of the relative ease of accessing huge computerized medical data bases.[3] Such analyses are faster and cheaper than conducting clinical trials.

Others[14,27,45,82] have emphasized limitations of registry studies such as potential bias in treatment assignment, inappropriate conclusions from multiple comparisons, lack of standardization in collecting and reporting data, and missing data. Another weakness of prospective data-base registries is that they rely heavily on the validity of the model employed to analyze the data.[65]

Undoubtedly, analyses of large data bases can provide important descriptive information about disease occurrence and outcome, and suggestions that certain therapies are preferable. Currently, however, it is no substitute for a randomized clinical trial in evaluating whether one intervention is truly better than another.

CROSS-OVER DESIGNS

The cross-over design is a special case of a randomized control trial and has some appeal to medical researchers. The cross-over design allows each participant to serve as his own control. In the simplest case, namely the two-period cross-over design, each participant will receive either intervention or control (A or B) in the first period and the alternative in the succeeding period. The order in which A and B are given to each participant is randomized. Thus approximately half of the participants receive the intervention in the sequence AB and the other half in the sequence BA. This is so that any trend from first period to second period can be eliminated in the estimate of group differences in response.

James et al. describe 59 cross-over studies of analgesic agents. They conclude that if the studies had been designed using parallel or non–cross-over designs, 2.4 times as many participants would have been needed.[56] Carriere has shown that a three-period cross-over design is even more efficient than a two-period cross-over design.[18] A cross-over study need not have only two groups. A cross-over design for two active interventions and one control has been described.[57]

The advantages and disadvantages of the two-period cross-over design have been reviewed.* The appeal of the cross-over design to investigators is that it allows assessment of whether each participant does better on A or B. Since each participant is used twice, variability is reduced because the measured effect of the intervention is the difference in an individual participant's response to intervention and control. This reduction in variability enables investigators to use smaller sample sizes to detect a specific difference in response.

To use the cross-over design, however, a fairly strict assumption must be made; the effects of the intervention during the first period must not carry over into the second period. This assumption should be independent of which intervention was assigned during the first period and the participant response. In many clinical trials, such an assumption is clearly inappropriate. If, for example, the intervention during the first period cures the disease, then the participant obviously cannot return to

---

*References 10, 11, 36, 57, 61, 97.

the initial state. In other clinical trials, the cross-over design appears more reasonable. If a drug's effect is to lower blood pressure or heart rate, then a drug-vs.-placebo cross-over design might be considered if the drug has no carryover effect once the participant is taken off medication. Obviously, a fatal event cannot serve as the primary response variable in a cross-over trial.

Although the statistical method for checking the assumption of no period-treatment interaction has been described by Grizzle,[46] the test is not as powerful as one would like. What decreases the power of the test is that the mean response of the *AB* group is compared with the mean response of the *BA* group. However, participant variability is introduced in this comparison, which inflates the error term in the statistical test. Thus the ability to test the assumption of no period-intervention interaction is not sensitive enough to detect important violations of the assumption unless many participants are used. The basic appeal of this design is to avoid between-participant variation in estimating the intervention effect, thereby requiring a smaller sample size. Yet the ability to justify the use of the design still depends on a test for carryover that includes between-participant variability. This weakens the main rationale for the cross-over design. Because of this insensitivity, the cross-over design is not as attractive as it as first appears. Fleiss et al.[37] note that even adjusting for baseline variables may not be sufficient if inadequate time has been allowed to return to baseline at the start of the second period. Brown[10,11] and Hills and Armitage[50] discourage the use of the cross-over design in general. Only if there is substantial evidence that the therapy has no carryover effects, and the scientific community is convinced by that evidence, should a cross-over design be considered.

WITHDRAWAL STUDIES

Several studies have been conducted in which the participants on a particular treatment for a chronic disease are taken off therapy or have the dosage reduced. The objective is to assess response to the discontinuation or reduction. This design may be validly used to evaluate the duration of benefit of an intervention already known to be useful. For example, subsequent to the Hypertension Detection and Follow-up Program[53] that demonstrated the benefits of treating mild and moderate hypertension, several investigators withdrew a sample of participants with controlled blood pressure from antihypertensive therapy.[87] One aim was to see if life-long therapy was necessary.

Withdrawal studies have also been used to assess the efficacy of an intervention that has never conclusively been shown to be beneficial. An example is the Sixty Plus Reinfarction Study.[76] Patients doing well on oral anticoagulant therapy since their myocardial infarction, an average of 6 years earlier, were randomly assigned to continue on anticoagulants or assigned to placebo. Those who stayed on the intervention had lower mortality (not statistically significant) and a clear reduction in nonfatal reinfarction. One serious limitation of this type of study is that a highly selected sample is evaluated. Only those participants who physicians thought were benefiting from the intervention were likely to have been on it for several years. Anyone who had major adverse effects from the drug would have been taken off and therefore not been eligible for the withdrawal study. Thus this design can overestimate benefit and underestimate toxicity. Another drawback is that both patients and disease states change over time. In the previous example, it cannot validly be claimed that anticoagulants were shown to be beneficial if administered immediately after an infarction.

If withdrawal studies are conducted, the same standards used with other designs should be followed. Randomization, blinding where feasible, unbiased assessment, and proper data analysis are as important here as in other settings.

FACTORIAL DESIGN

In the simple case, the factorial design attempts to evaluate two interventions compared with control in a single experiment (Table 4–1).[22,26,35] Given the cost and effort in recruiting participants and conducting clinical trials, getting two experiments done at once is appealing. Examples of factorial designs are the Canadian transient ischemic attack study, where aspirin and sulfinpyrazone were compared with placebo,[90] ISIS-3,[55] the Physicians' Health Study,[88] and the Women's Health Initiative.[96] Some factorial design studies are more complex than the 2-by-2 design, employing a third or even a fourth level. It is also possible to leave some of the cells empty, that is use an incomplete factorial design.[16] This would be done if it is inappropriate, infeasible, or unethical to address every possible treatment combination. It is also possible to use a factorial design in a cross-over study.[38]

The appeal of the factorial design might suggest that there really is a free lunch. However, every design has strengths and weaknesses. A concern with the factorial design is the possibility of the existence of interaction and its impact on the sample size. *Interaction* means that the effect of intervention X differs depending on the

Table 4–1 Factorial design

	Intervention X	Control
Intervention Y	a	b
Control	c	d

Cell	Intervention
a	$X + Y$
b	Y + control
c	X + control
d	control + control

presence or absence of intervention Y, or vice versa. It is more likely to occur when the two interventions are expected to have related mechanisms of action.

If one could safely assume there were no interactions, one could show that with a modest increase in sample size two experiments could be conducted in one; one that is considerably smaller than the sum of two independent trials under the same design specifications. However, if one cannot reasonably rule out interaction, one should statistically test for its presence because it may affect the analysis. As is true for the crossover design, the power for testing for interaction is less than the power for testing for the main effects of interventions (cells a + c vs. b + d or cells a + b vs. c + d). Thus, to obtain satisfactory power to detect interaction, the total sample size must be increased. If an interaction is detected, or perhaps only suggested, the comparison of intervention X would have to be done individually for intervention Y and its control (cell a vs. b and cell c vs. d). The power for these comparisons is obviously less than for the main effects comparisons.

As noted, in studies where the various interventions act either on the same response variable or possibly through the same mechanism of action, as with the Canadian transient ischemic attack study,[90] interaction can be more of a concern. Furthermore, there may be a limited amount of reduction in the response variable that can be reasonably expected, restricting the joint effect of the interventions.

In trials such as the Physicians' Health Study,[88] the two interventions, aspirin and beta carotene, were expected to act on two separate outcomes, cardiovascular disease and cancer. Thus interaction was much less likely. It turns out, however, that beta carotene, an antioxidant, may affect both conditions, as may aspirin. Similarly, in the Women's Health Initiative,[96] dietary and hormonal interventions may impact on more than one disease process.

In circumstances where there are two separate outcomes, for example, heart disease and cancer, but one of the interventions may have an effect on both, data monitoring may become complicated. If, during the course of monitoring response variables, it is determined that an intervention has a significant or important effect on one of the outcomes in a factorial design study, it may be difficult or even impossible to continue the trial to fully assess the effect on the other outcome. Chapter 15 reviews data monitoring in more detail.

The factorial design has some distinct advantages. If the interaction of two interventions is important to determine, or if there is little chance of interaction, then such a design with appropriate sample size can be very informative and efficient. However, the added complexity, impact on recruitment and compliance, and potential adverse effect of polypharmacy must be considered. Brittain and Wittes[9] discuss several settings in which factorial designs might be useful or not, and raise several cautions. In addition to the issue of interaction, they note that less-than-full adherence to the intervention can exacerbate problems in a factorial design trial.

GROUP ALLOCATION DESIGNS

In group allocation or cluster randomization designs, a group of individuals, a clinic, or a community is randomized to a particular intervention or control.[5,18,24,84] In the Child and Adolescent Trial for Cardiovascular Health, schools were randomized to different interventions.[100] A trial of vitamin A vs. placebo on morbidity and mortality in children in India randomized villages.[94] Communities have been compared in other trials.[32,39] These designs have been used in cancer trials where a clinic or physician may have difficulty approaching people about the idea of randomization. Giving all participants a specific intervention, however, may be quite acceptable. In this design, the basic sampling units and the units of analysis are groups, not individual participants. This means that the effective sample does not consist of the total number of participants, and the design may not be as efficient as the traditional one. If the response rates vary across clinics or groups, efficiency is further decreased. Chapter 7 contains further discussion of this design.

HYBRID DESIGNS

Pocock[72] has argued that if a substantial amount of data is available from historical controls, then a hybrid, or combination, design could be considered. Rather than a 50:50 allocation of participants, a smaller proportion could be randomized to control, permitting most to be assigned to the new intervention. Several criteria must be met to combine the historical and randomized controls. These include the same entry criteria and evaluation factors, and participant recruitment by the same clinic or investigator. The data from the historical control participants must also be fairly recent. This approach requires fewer participants to be entered into a trial. Machin,[62] however, cautions that if biases introduced from the nonrandomized participants (historical controls) are substantial, more participants might have to be randomized to compensate than would be the case in a corresponding fully randomized trial.

STUDIES OF EQUIVALENCY

In studies of equivalency, or trials with positive controls, the objective is to test whether a new intervention is as good as an established one. Sample size issues for this kind of trial are discussed in Chapter 7. Several design aspects also need to be considered. The control or standard treatment must have been shown to be effective; that is, truly better than placebo or no therapy. The circumstances under which the control was found to be useful ought to be reasonably close to those of the planned trial. Similarity of populations, concomitant therapy, and dosage are important. These requirements also mean that the trials that demonstrated efficacy of the standard should be recent and properly designed and conducted.

As emphasized in Chapter 7, the investigator must specify what is meant by equivalence. It cannot be statistically shown that two therapies are identical, as an infinite sample size would be required. Therefore, if the intervention falls sufficiently close to the standard as defined by reasonable boundaries, the two are claimed to be the same. In this situation, outcomes other than the primary response variable become important factors. A judgment regarding use of similar treatments can depend on frequency and severity of adverse effects, changes in quality of life, ease of applying the intervention, and cost. Thus, the study must be designed to allow for proper evaluation of these factors. (See Chapters 11 and 12.)

LARGE SIMPLE CLINICAL TRIALS

In recent years, the concept of large, simple clinical trials has been promoted. The advocates of this idea maintain that for common pathological conditions, it is important to uncover even modest benefits of intervention, particularly short-term interventions that are easily implemented in a large population. They also argue than an intervention is unlikely to have very different effects in different sorts of participants. Therefore careful characterization of people at entry, or of interim response variables, is unnecessary. The important criteria for a valid study are unbiased (i.e., randomized) allocation of participants to intervention or control and unbiased assessment of outcome. Sufficiently large numbers of participants are more important than modest improvement in data quality. The simplification of the study design and management allows for sufficiently large trials at reasonable cost. Examples of successful large, simple trials are ISIS,[55] GISSI,[47] GUSTO,[92] and a study of digitalis.[91] It should be noted that with the exception of the digitalis trial, these studies were relatively short term.

As indicated, this model depends on a relatively easily administered intervention and an easily ascertained outcome. If the intervention is complex, requiring either special expertise or effort, particularly where adherence to protocol must be maintained over a long time, this kind of study is less likely to be successful. Similarly, if the response variable is a measure of morbidity that requires careful measurement by highly trained investigators, a large simple trial is not feasible.

It has also been pointed out that measurement of baseline characteristics may be useful, not only for natural history studies but for subgroup analysis. The issue of subgroup analysis is discussed more fully in Chapter 16. Although in general, it is likely that the effect of an intervention is qualitatively the same across subgroups, that is, in the same direction, exceptions may exist. In addition, important quantitative differences, or magnitudes of effect, may occur. When there is reasonable expectation of such differences, appropriate baseline variables need to be measured. Variables such as age, gender, past history of a particular condition, or type of medication currently being taken can be assessed in a simple trial. On the other hand, if an invasive laboratory test or a measurement that requires special training is necessary at baseline, such characterization may make a simple trial unfeasible.

The investigator also needs to consider that the results of the trial must be persuasive to others. If other researchers or clinicians seriously question the validity of the trial because of inadequate information about participants or inadequate documentation of quality control, then the study has not achieved its purpose.

Undoubtedly many clinical trials are too expensive and cumbersome, especially multicenter ones. The advent of the large, simple trial is an important step in enabling many meaningful medical questions to be addressed in an efficient manner. In other instances, however, the use of large numbers of participants may not compensate for reduced data collection and quality control. As always, the primary question being asked dictates the optimal design of the trial.

REFERENCES

1. Acute Hepatic Failure Study Group: Failure of specific immunotherapy in fulminant type B hepatitis, *Ann Intern Med* 86:272-277, 1977.
2. Anbar D: The relative efficiency of Zelen's prerandomization design for clinical trials, *Biometrics* 39: 711-718, 1983.
3. Anderson C: Measuring what works in health care, *Science* 263:1080-1082, 1994.
4. Armitage P: *Statistical methods in medical research,* New York, 1971, John Wiley & Sons.
5. Armitage P: The role of randomization in clinical trials, *Stat Med* 1:345-352, 1982.
6. Bailar JC III, Louis TA, Lavori PW, et al: Studies without internal controls, *N Engl J Med* 311:156-162, 1984.
7. Bjork S, Sannerstedt R, Angervall G, Hood B: Treatment and prognosis in malignant hypertension: clinical follow-up study of 93 patients on modern medical treatment, *Acta Med Scand* 166:175-187, 1960.
8. Bjork S, Sannerstedt R, Falkheden T, Hood B: The effect of active drug treatment in severe hypertensive disease: an analysis of survival rates in 381 cases on combined treatment with various hypotensive agents, *Acta Med Scand* 169:673-689, 1961.
9. Brittain E, Wittes J: Factorial designs in clinical trials: the effects of non-compliance and subadditivity, *Stat Med* 8:161-171, 1989.
10. Brown BW: The crossover experiment for clinical trials, *Biometrics* 36:69-80, 1980.
11. Brown BW Jr.: Statistical controversies in the design of clinical trials—some personal views, *Controlled Clin Trials* 1:13-27, 1980.
12. Brown BW, Hollander M: *Statistics: a biomedical introduction,* New York, 1977, John Wiley & Sons.
13. Bull JP: The historical development of clinical therapeutic trials, *J Chronic Dis* 10:218-248, 1959.
14. Byar DP: Why databases should not replace randomized clinical trials, *Biometrics* 36:337-342, 1980.
15. Byar DP: Some statistical considerations for design of cancer prevention trials, *Prev Med* 18: 688-699, 1989.
16. Byar DP, Herzberg AM, Tan W-Y: Incomplete factorial designs for randomized clinical trials, *Stat Med* 12:1629-1641, 1993.
17. Byar DP, Simon RM, Friedewald WT et al: Randomized clinical trials: perspectives on some recent ideas, *N Engl J Med* 295:74-80, 1976.
18. Carriere KC: Crossover designs for clinical trials, *Stat Med* 13:1063-1069, 1994.
19. Chalmers TC, Black JB, Lee S: Controlled studies in clinical cancer research, *N Engl J Med* 287:75-78, 1972.
20. Chalmers TC, Celano P, Sacks HS, Smith HJ Jr: Bias in treatment assignment in controlled clinical trials, *N Engl J Med* 309:1358-1361, 1983.
21. Chalmers TC, Matta RJ, Smith H, Kunzler AM: Evidence favoring the use of anticoagulants in the hospital phase of acute myocardial infarction, *N Engl J Med* 297:1091-1096, 1977.
22. Cochran WG, Cox GM: *Experimental designs,* ed 2, New York, 1957, John Wiley & Sons.

23. Collaborative Group on Antenatal Steroid Therapy: Effect of antenatal dexamethasone administration on the prevention of respiratory distress syndrome, *Am J Obstet Gynecol* 141:276-287, 1981.

24. Cornfield J: Randomization by group: a formal analysis, *Am J Epidemiol* 108:100-102, 1978.

25. Coronary Drug Project Research Group: Clofibrate and niacin in coronary heart disease, *JAMA* 231: 360-381, 1975.

26. Cox DR: *Planning of experiments,* New York, 1958, John Wiley & Sons.

27. Dambrosia JM, Ellenberg JH: Statistical considerations for a medical database, *Biometrics* 36:323-332, 1980.

28. Donner A, Birkett N, Buck C: Randomization by cluster: sample size requirements and analysis, *Am J Epidemiol* 114:906-914, 1981.

29. Dustan HP, Schneckloth RE, Corcoran AC, Page IH: The effectiveness of long-term treatment of malignant hypertension, *Circulation* 18:644-651, 1958.

30. Eliot MM: The control of rickets: preliminary discussion of the demonstration in New Haven, *JAMA* 85:656-663, 1925.

31. Ellenberg SS: Randomization designs in comparative clinical trials, *N Engl J Med* 310:1404-1408, 1984.

32. Farquhar JW, Fortmann SP, Flora JA, et al: Effects of communitywide education on cardiovascular disease risk factors. The Stanford Five-City Project, *JAMA* 264:359-365, 1990.

33. Feinstein AR: *Clinical biostatistics,* St Louis, 1977, CV Mosby.

34. Fisher RA: *Statistical methods for research workers,* Edinburgh, 1925, Oliver & Boyd.

35. Fisher RA: *The design of experiments,* Edinburgh, 1935, Oliver & Boyd.

36. Fleiss JL: A critique of recent research on the two treatment crossover design, *Controlled Clin Trials* 10:237-243, 1989.

37. Fleiss JL, Wallenstein S, Rosenfeld R: Adjusting for baseline measurements in the two-period crossover study: a cautionary note, *Controlled Clin Trials* 6:192-197, 1985.

38. Fletcher DJ, Lewis SM, Matthews JNS: Factorial designs for crossover clinical trials, *Stat Med* 9:1121-1129, 1990.

39. Gail MH, Byar DP, Pechacek TF, Corle DK, for COMMIT Study Group: Aspects of statistical design for the Community Intervention Trial for Smoking Cessation, *Controlled Clin Trials* 13:6-21, 1992.

40. Gehan EA, Freireich EJ: Non-randomized controls in cancer clinical trials, *N Engl J Med* 290:198-203, 1974.

41. Gehan EA: The evaluation of therapies: historical control studies, *Stat Med* 3:315-324, 1984.

42. Gocke DJ: Fulminant hepatitis treated with serum containing antibody to Australia antigen, *N Engl J Med* 284:919, 1971.

43. Goldman L, Feinstein AR: Anticoagulants and myocardial infarction: the problems of pooling, drowning, and floating, *Ann Intern Med* 90:92-94, 1979.

44. Grace ND, Muench H, Chalmers TC: The present status of shunts for portal hypertension in cirrhosis, *Gastroenterology* 50:684-691, 1966.

45. Green SB, Byar DP: Using observational data from registries to compare treatments: the fallacy of omnimetrics, *Stat Med* 3:361-370, 1984.

46. Grizzle JE: The two period change-over design and its use in clinical trials, *Biometrics* 21:467-480, 1965.

47. Gruppo Italiano per lo Studio della Streptochinasi nell' Infarto Miocardico (GISSI): Effectiveness of intravenous thrombolytic treatment in acute myocardial infarction, *Lancet* i:397-402, 1986.

48. Hennekens CH, Buring JE: *Epidemiology in medicine,* Mayrent SL, ed, Boston, 1987, Little, Brown.

49. Hill AB: Observation and experiment, *N Engl J Med* 248:995-1001, 1953.

50. Hills M, Armitage P: The two-period cross-over clinical trial, *Br J Clin Pharmacol* 8:7-20, 1979.

51. Hlatky MA, Califf RM, Harrell FE Jr, et al: Clinical judgment and therapeutic decision making, *J Am Coll Cardiol* 15:1-14, 1990.

52. Hlatky MA, Lee KL, Harrell FE Jr, et al: Tying clinical research to patient care by use of an observational database, *Stat Med* 3:375-384, 1984.

53. Hypertension Detection and Follow-up Program Cooperative Group: Five-year findings of the Hypertension Detection and Follow-Up Program. 1. Reduction in mortality of persons with high blood pressure, including mild hypertension, *JAMA* 242:2562-2571, 1979.

54. Ingelfinger FJ: The randomized clinical trial, *N Engl J Med* 287:100-101, 1972 (editorial).
55. ISIS-3 (Third International Study of Infarct Survival) Collaborative Group: ISIS-3: a randomised comparison of streptokinase vs tissue plasminogen activator vs anistreplase and of aspirin plus heparin vs aspirin alone among 41 299 cases of suspected acute myocardial infarction, *Lancet* 339:753-770, 1992.
56. James KE, Forrest WH Jr, Rose RL: Crossover and noncrossover designs in four-point parallel line analgesic assays, *Clin Pharmacol Ther* 37:242-252, 1985.
57. Koch GG, Amara IA, Brown BW Jr, et al: A two-period crossover design for the comparison of two active treatments and placebo, *Stat Med* 8:487-504, 1989.
58. Lanman JT, Guy LP, Dancis J: Retrolental fibroplasia and oxygen therapy, *JAMA* 155:223-226, 1954.
59. Lasagna L: Historical controls: the practitioner's clinical trials, *N Engl J Med* 307:1339-1340, 1982.
60. Lilienfeld AM: *Foundations of epidemiology*, New York, 1976, Oxford University Press.
61. Louis TA, Lavori PW, Bailar JC III, Polansky M: Crossover and self-controlled designs in clinical research, *N Engl J Med* 310:24-31, 1984.
62. Machin D: On the possibility of incorporating patients from nonrandomising centres into a randomised clinical trial, *J Chron Dis* 32:347-353, 1979.
63. Macfarlane G: *Howard Florey: the making of a great scientist*, Oxford, 1979, Oxford University Press.
64. MacMahon B, Pugh TF: *Epidemiology: principles and methods*, Boston, 1970, Little, Brown.
65. Mantel N: Cautions on the use of medical databases, *Stat Med* 2:355-362, 1983.
66. Meier P: Terminating a trial—the ethical problem, *Clin Pharmacol Ther* 25:633-640, 1979.
67. Moertel CG: Improving the efficiency of clinical trials: a medical perspective, *Stat Med* 3:455-465, 1984.
68. Moon TE, Jones SE, Bonadonna G et al: Using a database of protocol studies to evaluate therapy: a breast cancer example, *Stat Med* 3:333-339, 1984.
69. Morbidity and mortality chartbook on cardiovascular, lung and blood diseases: National Heart, Lung, and Blood Inst, US Department of Health and Human Services, Public Health Service, May, 1994.
70. Peto R: Clinical trial methodology, *Biomedicine* (special issue) 28:24-36, 1978.
71. Peto R, Pike MC, Armitage P, et al: Design and analysis of randomized clinical trials requiring prolonged observation of each patient. 1. Introduction and design, *Br J Cancer* 34:585-612, 1976.
72. Pocock SJ: The combination of randomized and historical controls in clinical trials, *J Chron Dis* 29: 175-188, 1976.
73. Pocock SJ: Letter to the editor, *Br Med J* 1:1661, 1977.
74. Pocock SJ: Allocation of patients to treatment in clinical trials, *Biometrics* 35:183-197, 1979.
75. *Proceedings of the Conference on the Decline in Coronary Heart Disease Mortality*: Havlik RJ, Feinleib M, ed: Washington, DC, NIH Pub. 79-1610, 1979.
76. Report of the Sixty Plus Reinfarction Study Research Group: A double blind trial to assess long-term oral anticoagulant therapy in elderly patients after myocardial infarction, *Lancet* ii:989-994, 1980.
77. Rosenberg HM, Klebba AJ: Trends in cardiovascular mortality with a focus on ischemic heart disease: United States, 1950-1976. In Havlik R, Feinleib M, ed: *Proceedings of the Conference on the Decline in Coronary Heart Disease Mortality*, Washington DC, 1979, NIH Publ 79-1610.
78. Sacks H, Chalmers TC, Smith H Jr: Randomized versus historical controls for clinical trials, *Am J Med* 72:233-240, 1982.
79. Sacks H, Chalmers TC, Smith H Jr: Sensitivity and specificity of clinical trials: randomized *v* historical controls, *Arch Intern Med* 143:753-755, 1983.
80. Sapirstein W, Alpert S, Callahan TJ: The role of clinical trials in the Food and Drug Administration approval process for cardiovascular devices, *Circulation* 89:1900-1902, 1994.
81. Shaw LW, Chalmers TC: Ethics in cooperative clinical trials, *Ann NY Acad Sci* 169:487-495, 1970.
82. Sheldon TA: Please bypass the PORT, *Br Med J* 309:142-143, 1994.
83. Silverman WA: The lesson of retrolental fibroplasia, *Sci Am* 236:100-107, 1977.
84. Simon R: Composite randomization designs for clinical trials, *Biometrics* 37:723-731, 1981.
85. Snow JB Jr, Kimmelman CP: Assessment of surgical procedures for Ménière's disease, *Laryngoscope* 89:737-747, 1979.

86. Srivastava JN, ed: *A survey of statistical design and linear models,* Amsterdam, 1975, North-Holland.

87. Stamler R, Stamler J, Grimm R, et al: Nutritional therapy for high blood pressure—Final report of a four-year randomized controlled trial—The Hypertension Control Program, *JAMA* 257:1484-1491, 1987.

88. Stampfer MJ, Buring JE, Willett W et al: The 2×2 factorial design: its application to a randomized trial of aspirin and carotene in US physicians, *Stat Med* 4:111-116, 1985.

89. Starmer CF, Lee KL, Harrell FE et al: On the complexity of investigating chronic illness, *Biometrics* 36:333-335, 1980.

90. The Canadian Cooperative Study Group: A randomized trial of aspirin and sulfinpyrazone in threatened stroke, *N Engl J Med* 229:53-59, 1978.

91. The Digitalis Investigation Group: Rationale, design, implementation and baseline characteristics of patients in the DIG Trial: a large, simple trial to evaluate the effect of digitalis on mortality in heart failure, *Controlled Clin Trials* (in press).

92. The GUSTO Investigators: An international randomized trial comparing four thrombolytic strategies for acute myocardial infarction, *N Engl J Med* 329:673-682, 1993.

93. Veterans Administration Cooperative Urological Research Group: Treatment and survival of patients with cancer of the prostrate, *Surg Gynecol Obstet* 124:1011-1017, 1967.

94. Vijayaraghavan K, Radhaiah G, Prakasam BS, et al: Effect of massive dose vitamin A on morbidity and mortality in Indian children, *Lancet* 336:1342-1345, 1990.

95. Weinstein MC: Allocation of subjects in medical experiments, *N Engl J Med* 291:1278-1285, 1974.

96. Women's Health Initiative Study Protocol, National Institutes of Health, 1994.

97. Woods JR, Williams JG, Tavel M: The two-period crossover design in medical research, *Ann Intern Med* 110:560-566, 1989.

98. Zelen M: A new design for randomized clinical trials, *N Engl J Med* 300:1242-1245, 1979.

99. Zelen M: Randomized consent designs for clinical trials: an update, *Stat Med* 9:645-656, 1990.

100. Zucker DM, Lakatos E, Webber LS et al.: Statistical design of the Child and Adolescent Trial for Cardiovascular Health (CATCH): implications of cluster randomization, *Controlled Clin Trials* 16: 96-118, 1995.

CHAPTER 5

The Randomization Process

The randomized control clinical trial is the standard by which all trials are judged since other designs have certain undesirable features. In the simplest case, randomization is a process by which each participant has the same chance of being assigned to either intervention or control. An example would be the toss of a coin, in which heads indicates intervention group and tails indicates control group. Even in the more complex randomization strategies, the element of chance underlies the allocation process. Of course, neither trial participant nor investigator should know what the assignment will be before the participant's decision to enter the study. Otherwise, the benefits of randomization can be lost. The role that randomization plays in clinical trials has been discussed in Chapter 4 as well as by numerous authors.[*] While not all accept that randomization is essential,[68,91] most agree it is the best method for achieving comparability and is the basis for statistical inference.[3,20]

FUNDAMENTAL POINT

Randomization tends to produce study groups comparable with respect to known and unknown risk factors, removes investigator bias in the allocation of participants, and guarantees that statistical tests will have valid significance levels.

Several methods for randomly allocating participants are currently in use.[†] This chapter will present the most common of these methods and consider the advantages and disadvantages of each. Unless stated otherwise, it can be assumed that the randomization strategy will allocate participants into two groups, intervention and control. However, many of the methods described here can easily be generalized for use with more than two groups.

Two forms of experimental bias are of concern. The first, selection bias, occurs if the allocation process is predictable.[‡] In this case, the decision to enter a participant into a trial may be influenced by the anticipated treatment assignment. If any

---

[*]References 3, 19, 20, 38, 46, 47, 61–63, 68, 91, 95.
[†]References 10, 40, 47, 63, 95.
[‡]References 2, 46, 77, 86, 93.

bias exists as to what treatment particular types of participants should receive, then a selection bias might occur. All of the randomization procedures described avoid selection bias by not being predictable. A second bias, accidental bias, can arise if the randomization procedure does not achieve balance on risk factors or prognostic covariates. Some of the allocation procedures described are more vulnerable to accidental bias, especially for small studies. For large studies, however, the chance of accidental bias is negligible.[46]

Whatever randomization process is used, the report of the trial should contain a brief but clear description of that method. Only 20% to 30% of trials provide fair or adequate descriptions, depending on the size of the trial or whether the trial is single center or multicenter.[93] Altman and Doré[2] report a survey of four medical journals where 30% of published randomized trials gave no evidence that randomization had in fact been used. As many as 10% of these so called randomized trials in fact used nonrandom allocation procedures. Sixty percent did not report the type of randomization that was used. Descriptions need not be lengthy to inform the reader. They should clearly indicate the type of randomization method and how the randomization was implemented.

FIXED ALLOCATION RANDOMIZATION

Fixed allocation procedures assign the intervention to participants with a pre-specified probability, usually equal, and that allocation probability is not altered as the study progresses. Several methods exist by which fixed allocation is achieved,* and we will review three of these—simple, blocked, and stratified.

Our view is that allocation to intervention and control groups should be equal. Peto,[61] among others, has suggested an unequal allocation ratio, such as 2:1, of intervention to control. The rationale for a 2:1 allocation is that the study may slightly lose sensitivity but may gain more information about participant responses to the new intervention, such as toxicity and side effects. In some instances, less information may be needed about the control group and therefore fewer control participants are required. If the intervention turns out to be beneficial, more study participants would benefit than under an equal allocation scheme. However, new interventions may also turn out to be harmful, in which case more participants would receive them under the unequal allocation strategy. Although the loss of sensitivity or power may be less than 5% for allocation ratios approximately between one half and two thirds,[18,62] more often than not, studies should have the most powerful design possible. We also believe that equal allocation is more consistent with the view of indifference or equipoise toward which of the two groups a participant is assigned. Unequal allocation may indicate to the participants and their personal

---

*References 18, 40, 42, 45, 47–49, 63, 95.

physicians that one intervention is preferred over the other. In a few circumstances, the cost of one treatment may be extreme so that an unequal allocation of 2:1 or 3:1 may help to contain costs while not causing a serious loss of power. In general, equal allocation will be presumed throughout the following discussion unless otherwise indicated.

Simple Randomization

The most elementary form of randomization, referred to as simple or complete randomization, is best illustrated by a few examples.[63,95] One simple method is to toss an unbiased coin each time a participant is eligible to be randomized. For example, if the coin turns up heads, the participant is assigned to group A; if tails, to group B. Using this procedure, approximately one half of the participants will be in group A and one half in group B. In practice, for small studies, instead of tossing a coin to generate a randomization schedule, a random digit table on which the equally likely digits 0 to 9 are arranged by rows and columns is usually used to accomplish simple randomization. By randomly selecting a certain row (column) and observing the sequence of digits in that row (column) A could be assigned, for example, to those participants for whom the next digit was even and B to those for whom the next digit was odd. This process produces a sequence of assignments that is random in order, and each participant has an equal chance of being assigned to A or B.

For large studies, a more convenient method for producing a randomization schedule is to use a random number-producing algorithm, available on most digital computer systems. A simple randomization procedure might assign participants to group A with probability p and participants to group B with probability $1 - p$. One computerized process for simple randomization is to use a uniform random number algorithm to produce random numbers in the interval from 0.0 to 0.999. Using a uniform random number generator, a random number can be produced for each participant. If the random number is between 0 and p, the participant would be assigned to group A; otherwise to group B. For equal allocation, the probability cut point, p, is one half (i.e., $p = 0.50$). If equal allocation between A and B is not desired ($p \neq \frac{1}{2}$), then p can be set to the desired proportion in the algorithm and the study will have, on the average, a proportion p of the participants in group A.

This procedure can be adapted easily to more than two groups. Suppose, for example, the trial has three groups, A, B, and C, and participants are to be randomized such that a participant has a one-fourth chance of being in group A, a one-fourth chance of being in group B, and a one-half chance of being in group C. By dividing the interval 0 to 1 into three pieces of length one fourth, one fourth, and one half, random numbers generated will have probabilities of one fourth, one fourth, and one half, respectively, of falling into each subinterval. Specifically, the intervals would be 0 to 0.249, 0.25 to 0.499, and 0.50 to 0.999. Then any participant whose random number falls between 0 and 0.249 is assigned A, any participant whose random number falls between 0.25 and 0.499 is assigned *B*, and the others, *C*. For equal allocation, the interval would be divided into thirds and assignments made accordingly.

The advantage of this simple randomization procedure is that it is easy to implement. The major disadvantage is that, although in the long run the number of participants in each group will be in the proportion anticipated, at any point in the randomization, including the end, there could be a substantial imbalance.[45] This is true particularly if the sample size is small. For example, if 20 participants are randomized with equal probability to two treatment groups, the chance of a 12:8 (i.e., 60% *A*, 40% *B*) split or worse is approximately 50%. For 100 participants, the chance of the same ratio (60:40 split) or worse is only 5%. While such imbalances do not cause the statistical tests to be invalid, they do reduce ability to detect true differences between the two groups. In addition, such imbalances appear awkward and may lead to some loss of credibility for the trial, especially for the person not oriented to statistics. For this reason primarily, simple randomization is not often used, even for large studies.

Some investigators incorrectly believe that an alternating assignment of participants to the intervention and control groups (e.g., *ABABAB*...) is a form of randomization. However, no random component exists in this type of allocation except perhaps for the first participant. A major criticism of this method is that, in a single-blind or unblinded study, the investigators know the next assignment, which could lead to a bias in the selection of participants. Even in a double-blind study, if the blind is broken on one participant as sometimes happens, the entire sequence of assignments is known. Therefore this type of allocation method should be avoided.

Blocked Randomization

Blocked randomization, sometimes called permuted block randomization, was described by Hill[38] in 1951. It is used to avoid serious imbalance in the number of participants assigned to each group, an imbalance that could occur in the simple randomization procedure. Blocked randomization guarantees that at no time during randomization will the imbalance be large and that at certain points the number of participants in each group will be equal.[51,63,95]

If participants are randomly assigned with equal probability to groups *A* or *B*, then for each block of even size (e.g., 4, 6, or 8) one half of the participants will be assigned to *A* and the other half to *B*. The order in which the interventions are assigned in each block is randomized, and this process is repeated for consecutive blocks of participants until all participants are randomized. For example, the investigators may want to ensure that after every fourth randomized participant, the number of participants in each intervention group is equal. Then a block of size 4 would be used and the process would randomize the order in which two *A*'s and two *B*'s are assigned for every consecutive group of four participants entering the trial. One may write down all the ways of arranging the groups and then randomize the order in which these combinations are selected. In the case of block size 4, there are six possible combinations of group assignments: *AABB*, *ABAB*, *BAAB*, *BABA*, *BBAA*, and *ABBA*. One of these arrangements is selected at random, and the four participants are assigned accordingly. This process is repeated as many times as needed.

Another method of blocked randomization may also be used. In this method for randomizing the order of assignments within a block of size b, a random number between 0 and 1 for each of the b assignments (half of which are A and the other half B) is obtained. The example below illustrates the procedure for a block of size four (two A's and two B's). Four random numbers are drawn between 0 and 1 in the order shown.

Example:

Assignment	Random number	Rank
A	0.069	1
A	0.734	3
B	0.867	4
B	0.312	2

The assignments then are ranked according to the size of the random numbers. This leads to the assignment order of *ABAB*. This process is repeated for another set of four participants until all participants have been randomized.

The advantage of blocking is that balance between the number of participants in each group is guaranteed during the course of randomization. The number in each group will never differ by more than $b/2$ when b is the length of the block. This can be important for at least two reasons. First, if the type of participant recruited for the study changes during the entry period, blocking will produce more comparable groups. For example, an investigator may use sources of potential participants sequentially. Participants from different sources may vary in severity of illness or other crucial respect. One source, with the more seriously ill participants, may be used early during enrollment and another source, with healthier participants, late in enrollment.[20] If the randomization were not blocked, more of the seriously ill participants might be randomized to one group. Because the later participants are not as sick, this early imbalance would not be corrected. A second advantage of blocking is that if the trial should be terminated before enrollment is completed, balance will exist in terms of number of participants randomized to each group.

A potential but solvable problem with basic blocked randomization is that if the blocking factor b is known by the study staff and the study is not double-blinded, the assignment for the last person entered in each block is known before randomization of that person. For example, if the blocking factor is 4 and the first three assignments are *ABB*, then the next assignment must be *A*. This could, of course, permit a bias in the selection of every fourth participant to be entered. Clearly, there is no reason to make the blocking factor known. However, in a study that is not double-blinded, with a little ingenuity the staff can soon discover the blocking factor. For this reason, repeated blocks of size 2 should not be used. On a few occasions, perhaps as an intellectual challenge, investigators or their clinical staff have attempted to break the randomization scheme. This curiosity is natural but nevertheless can cause problems in the integrity of the randomization process. To avoid this problem in the trial that is not double-blinded, the blocking factor can be varied as the recruitment continues. In fact, after each block has been completed, the size of the next block could be determined in a random fashion from a few possibilities such as 2, 4, 6, and 8. The probabilities of selecting a block size can be set at whatever one wishes with the constraint that their sum equals one. For example, the probabilities of selecting block sizes 2, 4, 6, and 8 can be one-sixth, one-sixth, one-third, and one-third, respectively. Randomly selecting the block size makes it difficult to determine where blocks start and stop and thus determine the next assignment.

A disadvantage of blocked randomization is that, from a strictly theoretical point of view, analysis of the data is more complicated than if simple randomization were used. The data analysis performed at the end of the study should reflect the randomization process actually performed.* This requirement would complicate the analysis because many analytical methods assume a simple randomization. In their analysis of the data, most investigators ignore the fact that the randomization was blocked. Matts and McHugh[52] studied this problem and concluded that the measurement of variability used in the statistical analysis is not exactly correct if the blocking is ignored. Since blocking guarantees balance between the two groups and therefore increases the power of a study, blocked randomization with the appropriate analysis is more powerful than not blocking at all or blocking and then ignoring it in the analysis. Statisticians recognize the problem and feel that, at worst, they are being conservative by ignoring the fact that the randomization was blocked.[40] That is, the study will have probably slightly less power than it could have with the correct analysis, and the "true" significance level is more extreme than that computed.

Stratified randomization

One of the objectives in allocating participants is to achieve between-group comparability of certain characteristics known as prognostic or risk factors.† Measured at baseline, these are factors that correlate with subsequent participant response or outcome. Investigators may become concerned when prognostic factors are not evenly distributed between intervention and control groups. As indicated previously, ran-

---

*References 41, 51, 52, 74, 76, 79.
†References 24, 26, 29, 30, 34, 35, 50, 53, 54, 58, 59, 65, 70, 95, 96.

domization tends to produce groups that are, on the average, similar in their entry characteristics, both known and unknown. This is a concept likely to be true for large studies or many small studies when averaged. For any single study, especially a small study, there is no guarantee that all baseline characteristics will be similar in the two groups. In the multicenter Aspirin Myocardial Infarction Study,[5] which had 4524 participants, the top 20 cardiovascular prognostic factors for total mortality identified in the Coronary Drug Project[24] were compared in the intervention and control groups, and no major differences were found. However, individual clinics, with an average of 150 participants, showed considerable imbalance for many variables between the groups. Imbalances in prognostic factors can be dealt with either after the fact by using stratification in the analysis (Chapter 16) or before by using stratification in the randomization. Stratified randomization is a method that helps achieve comparability between the study groups for those factors considered.

Stratified randomization requires that the prognostic factors be measured either before or at the time of randomization. If a single factor is used, it is divided into two or more subgroups or strata (e.g., age 30-34 years, 35-39 years, 40-44 years). If several factors are used, a stratum is formed by selecting one subgroup from each of them. The total number of strata is the product of the number of subgroups in each factor. The stratified randomization process involves measuring the level of the selected factors for participants, determining to which stratum each belongs, and performing the randomization within that stratum.

Within each stratum, the randomization process itself could be simple randomization, but in practice most clinical trials use some blocked randomization strategy. Under a simple randomization process, imbalances in the number in each group within the stratum could easily happen and thus defeat the purpose of the stratification. Blocked randomization is, as described previously, a special kind of stratification. However, this text will restrict use of the term *blocked randomization* to mean stratifying over time, and use *stratified randomization* to refer to stratifying on factors other than time. Some confusion may arise here because early texts on design used the term *blocking* as this text uses the term *stratifying*. However, the definition herein is consistent with current usage in clinical trials.

As an example of stratified randomization with a block size of 4, suppose an investigator wants to stratify on age, sex, and smoking history. One possible classification of the factors would be three 10-year age levels and three smoking levels.

Age	Sex	Smoking history
1. 40-49 yr	1. Male	1. Current smoker
2. 50-59 yr	2. Female	2. Ex-smoker
3. 60-69 yr		3. Never smoked

Thus the design has $3 \times 2 \times 3 = 18$ strata. The randomization for this example appears in Table 5-1.

Table 5-1   Stratified randomization with block size of four

Strata	Age	Sex	Smoking	Group assignment
1	40–49	M	Current	*ABBA BABA...*
2	40–49	M	Ex	*BABA BBAA...*
3	40–49	M	Never	etc.
4	40–49	F	Current	
5	40–49	F	Ex	
6	40–49	F	Never	
7	50–59	M	Current	
8	50–59	M	Ex	
9	50–59	M	Never	
10	50–59	F	Current	
11	50–59	F	Ex	
12	50–59	F	Never	
	etc.			

Participants who were between 40 and 49 years old, male, and current smokers—that is, participants in stratum 1—would be assigned to groups *A* or *B* in the sequences *ABBA, BABA,* and so on. Similarly, random sequences would appear in the other strata.

In the example shown above, with three levels of the first factor (age), two levels of the second factor (sex), and three levels of the third factor (smoking history), 18 strata have been created. As factors are added and the levels within factors are refined, the number of strata increase rapidly. If the example with 18 strata had 100 participants to be randomized, then only five to six participants would be expected per stratum if the study population were evenly distributed among the levels. Since the population is most likely not evenly distributed over the strata, some strata would actually get fewer than five or six participants. If the number of strata were increased, the number of participants in each stratum would be even fewer. Pocock and Simon[65] showed that increased stratification in small studies can be self-defeating because of the sparseness of data within each stratum. Thus only important variables should be chosen, and the number of strata kept to a minimum.

In addition to making the two study groups appear comparable with regard to specified factors, the power of the study can be increased by taking the stratification into account in the analysis. Stratified randomization, in a sense, breaks the trial down into smaller trials. Participants in each of the smaller trials belong to the same stratum. This reduces variability in group comparisons if the stratification is used in the analysis. Reduction in variability allows a study of a given size to detect smaller group differences in response variables or a specified difference with fewer participants.[42,51]

Sometimes the variables initially thought to be most prognostic and therefore used in the stratified randomization turn out to be unimportant. Other factors may be identified later that, for the particular study, are of more importance. If randomization is done without stratification, then analysis can take into account those factors of interest and will not be complicated by factors thought to be important at the time of randomization. It has been argued[61] that a need to stratify at randomization usually does not exist because stratification at the time of analysis will achieve nearly the same expected power. This issue of stratifying prerandomization vs. postrandomization has been widely discussed.* It appears for a large study that stratification after randomization provides efficiency nearly equal to stratification before randomization.[58,59] However, for studies of 100 participants or fewer, stratifying the randomization using two or three prognostic factors may achieve greater power, although the increase may not be large.

Stratified randomization is not the complete solution to all potential problems of baseline imbalance. Another strategy for small studies with many prognostic factors is considered in the following section on adaptive randomization.

In multicenter trials, centers vary with respect to the type of participants randomized and the quality and type of care given to participants during follow-up. Thus the center may be an important factor related to participant outcome, and the randomization process should be stratified accordingly.[30] Each center then represents, in a sense, a replication of the trial, though the number of participants within a center is not adequate to answer the primary question. Nevertheless, results at individual centers can be compared to see if trends are consistent with overall results. Another reason for stratification by center is that if a center should have to leave the study, the balance in prognostic factors in other centers would not be affected.

ADAPTIVE RANDOMIZATION PROCEDURES

The randomization procedures described in the sections on fixed allocation were nonadaptive strategies. In contrast, adaptive procedures change the allocation probabilities as the study progresses. Two types of adaptive procedures will be considered here. First, we will discuss methods that adjust or adapt the allocation probabilities according to imbalances in numbers of participants or in baseline characteristics between the two groups. Second, we will briefly review adaptive procedures that adjust allocation probabilities according to the responses of participants to the assigned intervention.

Baseline adaptive randomization procedures

The biased coin randomization procedure, originally discussed by Efron,[27] attempts to balance the number of participants in each treatment group based on

---

*References 35, 50, 53, 54, 70.

the previous assignments but does not take participant responses into consideration. Several variations to this approach have been discussed.* The purpose of the algorithm is basically to randomize the allocation of participants to groups A and B with equal probability as long as the number of participants in each group is equal or nearly equal. If an imbalance occurs and the differences in the number of participants is greater than some prespecified value, the allocation probability (p) is adjusted so that the probability is higher for the group with fewer participants. The investigator can determine the value of the allocation probability he wishes to use. The larger the value of p, the more quickly the imbalance will be corrected, while the nearer p is to 0.5, the slower the correction. Efron suggests an allocation probability of $p = \frac{2}{3}$ when a correction is indicated. Since much of the time $p > \frac{1}{2}$, the process has been named the "biased coin" method. As a simple example, suppose n_A and n_B represent the number of participants in groups A and B, respectively. If $n_A < n_B$ and the difference exceeds D, then we allocate the next participant to group A with probability $p = \frac{2}{3}$. If $n_A > n_B$ by an amount of D, we allocate to group B with probability $p = \frac{2}{3}$. Otherwise, $p = 0.50$. This procedure can be modified to include consideration of the number of consecutive assignments to the same group and the length of such a run.

This approach, from a strictly theoretical point of view, demands a cumbersome data analysis process. The correct analysis requires that the significance level for the test statistic be determined by considering all possible sequences of assignments that could have been made in repeated experiments using the same biased coin allocation rule where no group differences are assumed to exist. Although this is feasible to do with digital computers, analysis is not easy. As with the blocked randomization scheme, the analysis often ignores this requirement. Efron[27] argues that it is probably not necessary to take the biased coin randomization into account in the analysis, especially for larger studies. However, a test statistic that ignores the biased coin randomization will not provide the correct variance term. Most often, the variance will be larger than it would be with proper calculation, thus giving a conservative test in the sense that the probability of rejecting the null hypothesis is less than it would be if the proper analysis were used. One possible advantage of the biased coin approach over the blocked randomization scheme is that the investigator cannot determine the next assignment by discovering the blocking factor. However, the biased coin method does not appear to be as widely used as the blocked randomization scheme because of its complexity.

Another similar adaptive randomization method is referred to as the urn design, following the work of Wei et al.[84,88,89,90] This method also attempts to keep the number of participants randomized to each group reasonably balanced as the trial progresses. The name *urn design* refers to the conceptual process of randomization.

---

*References 6, 11, 12, 28, 31, 32, 36, 37, 43, 66, 73, 75, 78, 82, 83, 87, 92.

Imagine an urn filled with m red balls and m black balls. If a red ball is drawn at random, assign the participant to group A, return the red ball, and add a black ball to the urn. If a black ball is drawn, assign the participant to group B, return the ball, and add a red ball to the urn. This process will keep the number of participants in each group reasonably close because it adjusts the allocation probability. From a theoretical point of view, this method, like the biased coin design, would require the analyses to account for the randomization.[88] While this is possible, these analyses are not straightforward. It seems likely, as for the biased coin design, that if this randomization method is used, but ignored in the analyses, the p value will be slightly conservative, that is, slightly larger than if the strictly correct analysis were done. The urn model was used successfully in the multicenter Diabetes Control and Complications Trial.[25]

Other stratification methods are adaptive in the sense that intervention assignment probabilities for a participant are a function of the distribution of the prognostic factors for participants already randomized. This concept was suggested by Efron[27] as an extension of the biased coin method and also has been discussed in depth by Pocock and Simon,[65] among others.* In a simple example, if age is a prognostic factor and one study group has more older participants than the other, the allocation scheme is such that the next several older participants would most likely be randomized to the group that currently has fewer older participants. Various methods can be used as the measure of imbalance in prognostic factors. In general, adaptive stratification methods incorporate several prognostic factors in making an overall assessment of the group balance or lack of balance. Participants are then assigned to a group in a manner that will tend to correct an existing imbalance or cause the least imbalance in prognostic factors. This method is sometimes called *minimization* because imbalances in the distribution of prognostic factors are minimized. However, as indicated in the Appendix, the term *minimization* is also used to refer to a very specific form of adaptive stratification.[17,78] Generalization of this strategy exists for more than two groups. Development of these methods was motivated in part by the previously described problems with nonadaptive stratified randomization for small studies. Adaptive methods do not have empty or near-empty strata because randomization does not occur within a stratum although prognostic factors are used. Minimization gives unbiased estimates of treatment effect and slightly increased power relative to stratified randomization.[17] These methods are being used especially in clinical trials of cancer where several prognostic factors need to be balanced and the sample size is typically 100 to 200 participants.

The major advantage of this procedure is that it protects against a severe baseline imbalance for important prognostic factors. Overall marginal balance is maintained in

---

*References 6, 12–14, 31–33, 78, 92.

the intervention groups with respect to a large number of prognostic factors. One disadvantage is that adaptive stratification is operationally more difficult to carry out, especially if a large number of factors are considered. However, small programmable calculators can minimize most of the computational problems, although White and Freedman[92] developed a simplified version of the adaptive stratification method by using a set of specially arranged index cards. Another disadvantage is that the data analysis is complicated, from a strict viewpoint, by the randomization process. The appropriate analysis involves simulating, on a computer, the assignment of participants to groups by the actual adaptive strategy used. Replication of the simulation, assuming that no group differences exist, generates the significance level of the statistical test to be used.

Biostatisticians are not likely to go through the simulation experiments but would rather use the conventional statistical test and standard critical values to determine significance levels. As with other nonsimple randomization procedures, this strategy is probably somewhat conservative. The impact of one minimization approach on the significance level has been studied.[31] For this case, the authors concluded that if minimization adaptive stratification is used, an analysis of covariance should be employed. To obtain the proper significance level, the analysis should incorporate the same prognostic factors used in the randomization. Minimization and stratification on the same prognostic factors produce similar levels of power, but minimization may add slightly more power if stratification does not include all of the covariates.

Response adaptive randomization

Response adaptive randomization uses information on participant response to intervention during the course of the trial to determine the allocation of the next participant. Examples of response adaptive randomization models are the play-the-winner[94] and the two-armed bandit[67] models. These models assume that the investigator is randomizing participants to one of two interventions and that the primary response variable can be determined quickly relative to the total length of the study. Bailar[7] and Simon[69] review the uses of response adaptive stratification methods. Additional modifications or methods have been developed.*

The play-the-winner procedure may assign the first participant by the toss of a coin. The next participant is assigned to the same group as the first participant if the response to the intervention was a success; otherwise, the participant is assigned to the other group. That is, the process calls for staying with the winner until a failure occurs and then switching. The following illustrates a possible randomization scheme where S indicates intervention success and F indicates failure:

---

*References 4, 9, 15, 56, 71, 72, 85.

Example:

Assignment	Participant								
	1	2	3	4	5	6	7	8	...
Group A	S	F				S	F		
Group B			S	S	F			S	

Another response adaptive randomization procedure is the two-armed bandit method, which continually updates the probability of success as soon as the outcome for each participant is known. That information is used to adjust the probabilities of being assigned to either group in such a way that a higher proportion of future participants would receive the currently "better" or more successful intervention.

Both of these response adaptive randomization methods have the intended purpose of maximizing the number of participants on the superior intervention. They were developed in response to ethical concerns expressed by some clinical investigators about the randomization process. Although these methods do maximize the number of participants on the superior intervention, the possible imbalance will almost certainly result in some loss of power and require more participants to be enrolled into the study than would a fixed allocation with equal assignment probability.[72] A major limitation of these methods is that many clinical trials do not have an immediately occurring response variable. They also may have several response variables of interest with no single outcome easily identified as being the one on which randomization should be based. Furthermore, these methods assume that the population from which the participants are drawn is stable over time. If the nature of the study population should change and this is not accounted for in the analysis, the reported significance levels could be biased, perhaps severely.[71] Here, as before, the data analysis should ideally take into account the randomization process employed. For response adaptive methods, that analysis will be more complicated than it would be with simple randomization. Because of these disadvantages, response adaptive procedures are not commonly used.

One application of response adaptive allocation can be found in a trial evaluating an extracorporeal membrane oxygenator (ECMO) in a neonatal population suffering from respiratory insufficiency.* This device oxygenates the blood to compensate for the lung's inability or inefficiency in achieving this task. In this trial, the first infant was allocated randomly to control therapy. The result was a failure. The next infant received ECMO that was successful. The next 10 infants were also allocated to ECMO, and all outcomes were successful. The trial was then stopped. However, the first infant was much sicker than the ECMO-treated infants. Controversy ensued, and the benefits of ECMO remain unclear. This experience does not offer encouragement to use this adaptive randomization methodology.

---

*References 8, 57, 60, 80, 81.

MECHANICS OF RANDOMIZATION

The manner in which the chosen randomization method is actually implemented is extremely important.[64] If this aspect of randomization does not receive careful attention, the entire randomization process can easily be compromised, thus voiding any of the advantages for using it. To accomplish a valid randomization, it is recommended that an independent central unit be responsible for developing the randomization process and making the assignments of participants to the appropriate group. For a single center trial, this central unit might be a biostatistician or clinician not involved with the care of the participants. In the case of a multicenter trial, the randomization process is usually handled by the data coordinating center. Ultimately, however, the integrity of the randomization process will rest with the investigator.

Chalmers et al.[22] reviewed the randomization process in 102 clinical trials, 57 where the randomization was unknown to the investigator and 45 where it was known. The authors reported that in 14% of the 57 studies, at least one baseline variable was not balanced between the two groups. For the studies with known randomization schedules, twice as many, or 26.7%, had at least one prognostic variable maldistributed. For 43 nonrandomized studies, such imbalances occurred four times as often, or in 58%. The authors emphasized that those recruiting and entering participants into a trial should not be aware of the next intervention assignment.

In many cases when a fixed proportion randomization process is used, the randomization schedules are made before the study begins.* The investigators may call a central location, and the person at that location looks up the assignment for the next participant.[16] Another possibility, frequently used in trials involving acutely ill participants, is to have a scheme making available sequenced and sealed envelopes containing the assignments.[39] As a participant enters the trial, he receives the next envelope in the sequence, which gives him his assignment. Envelope systems, however, are more subject to errors and tampering than the former method. In one study, personnel in a clinic opened the envelopes and arranged the assignments to fit their own preferences, accommodating friends and relatives entering the trial. In another case, an envelope fell to the bottom of the box containing the envelopes, thus changing the sequence in which they were opened. Many studies prefer the telephone system to protect against this problem. In an alternative procedure that has been used in several double-blind drug studies, medication bottles are numbered with a small perforated tab.[23] The bottles are distributed to participants in sequence. The tab, which is coded to identify the contents, is torn off and sent to the central unit. This system is also subject to abuse unless an independent person is responsible for dispensing the bottles. Many clinical trials using a fixed proportion randomization schedule require that the investigator call the central location to verify that a participant is eligible to

*References 16, 21, 23, 39, 55.

be in the trial before any assignment is made. This increases the likelihood that only eligible participants will be randomized.

For many trials, logistics require a central randomization. This may be achieved by logging into a central computer or remote local computer over a computer network. In some cases, the clinic may register a participant by dialing into a central computer and entering data via touchtone, with a voice response. This concept has been used in a pediatric cancer cooperative clinical trial network.[44]

Whatever system is chosen to communicate the intervention assignment to the investigator or the clinic, the intervention assignment should be given as closely as possible to the moment when both investigator and participant are ready to begin the intervention. If the randomization occurs when the participant is first identified and the participant withdraws or dies before the intervention actually begins, several participants will be randomized without being involved in the study. An example of this occurred in a nonblinded trial of alprenolol in survivors of an acute myocardial infarction.[1] In that trial, 393 patients with a suspected myocardial infarction were randomized into the trial at the time of their admission to the coronary care unit. The alprenolol treatment was not initiated until 2 weeks later. Afterward, 231 of the randomized patients were excluded because a myocardial infarction could not be documented, death had occurred before therapy was begun, or various contraindications to therapy were noted. Of the 162 patients who remained, 69 were in the alprenolol group and 93 were in the placebo group. This imbalance raises concerns over the comparability of the two groups and possible bias in reasons for participant exclusion. By delaying the randomization until initiation of therapy, the problem of these withdrawals could have been avoided.

RECOMMENDATIONS

For large studies involving more than several hundred participants, the randomization should be blocked. If a large multicenter trial is being conducted, randomization should be stratified by center. Randomization stratified on the basis of other factors in large studies is usually not necessary because randomization tends to make the study groups quite comparable for all risk factors. The participants can still, of course, be stratified once the data have been collected and the study can be analyzed accordingly.

For small studies, the randomization should also be blocked and stratified by center if more than one center is involved. Since the sample size is small, a few strata for important risk factors may be defined to assure that balance will be achieved for at least those factors. For a larger number of prognostic factors, the adaptive stratification techniques should be considered and the appropriate analyses performed. As in large studies, stratified analysis can be performed even if stratified randomization was not done. For many situations, this will be satisfactory.

APPENDIX

Adaptive randomization algorithm

Adaptive randomization can be used for more than two intervention groups, but for the sake of simplicity only two will be used here. To describe the procedure in more detail, a minimum amount of notation needs to be defined. First, let

x_{ik} = the number of participants already assigned intervention k
(k = 1, 2) who have the same level of prognostic factor i
(i = 1, 2, ..., f) as the new participant.

and define

$$x^t_{ik} = x_{ik} \quad \text{if } t \neq k$$
$$x_{ik} + 1 \quad \text{if } t = k$$

The x^t_{ik} represents the change in balance of allocation if the new participant is assigned intervention t. Finally, let

$B(t)$ = function of the x^t_{ik}'s, which measures the lack of balance over all prognostic factors if the next participant is assigned intervention t.

Many possible definitions of $B(t)$ can be identified. As an illustrative example, let

$$B(t) = \sum_{i=1}^{f} w_i \text{Range} (x^t_{i1}, x^t_{i2})$$

where w_i = the relative importance of factor i to the other factors and the range is the absolute difference between the largest and smallest values of x^t_{i1} and x^t_{i2}.

The value of $B(t)$ is determined for each intervention (t = 1 and t = 2). The intervention with the smaller $B(t)$ is preferred, because allocation of the participant to that intervention will cause the least imbalance. The participant is assigned, with probability $p > \frac{1}{2}$, to the intervention with the smaller score, $B(1)$ or $B(2)$. The participant is assigned, with probability ($1 - p$), to the intervention with the larger score. These probabilities introduce the random component into the allocation scheme. Note that if $p = 1$ and, therefore, $1 - p = 0$, the allocation procedure is deterministic (no chance or random aspect) and has been referred to by the term "minimization."[31,78]

As a simple example of the adaptive stratification method, suppose there are two groups and two prognostic factors to control. The first factor has two levels, and the second factor has three levels. Assume that 50 participants have already been randomized and the following table summarizes the results.

TABLE A-1   Fifty randomized participants by group and level of factor (x_{ik}'s)

Factor	1		2			
Level	1	2	1	2	3	
Group						Total
1	16	10	13	9	4	26
2	14	10	12	6	6	24
	30	20	25	15	10	50

After Pocock and Simon.[65]

In addition, the function $B(t)$ as defined above will be used with the range of the x_{ik}'s as the measure of imbalance, where $w_1 = 3$ and $w_2 = 2$; that is, the first factor is 1.5 times as important as the second as a prognostic factor. Finally, suppose $p = \frac{2}{3}$ and $1 - p = 1/3$.

If the next participant to be randomized has the first level of the first factor and the third level of the second factor, then this corresponds to the first and fifth columns in the table. The task is to determine $B(1)$ and $B(2)$ for this participant as shown below.

a. Determine $B(1)$

i. Factor 1, Level 1

	k	x_{1k}	x'_{1k}	Range (x'_{11}, x'_{12})
Group	1	16	17	$\mid 17\text{-}14 \mid = 3$
	2	14	14	

ii. Factor 2, Level 3

	k	x_{2k}	x'_{2k}	Range (x'_{21}, x'_{22})
Group	1	4	5	$\mid 5\text{-}6 \mid = 1$
	2	6	6	

Using the formula given, $B(1)$ is computed as $3 \times 3 + 2 \times 1 = 11$.

b. Determine $B(2)$

i. Factor 1, Level 1

	k	x_{1k}	x^2_{1k}	Range (x^2_{11}, x^2_{12})
Group	1	16	16	$\mid 16\text{-}15 \mid = 1$
	2	14	15	

ii. Factor 2, Level 3

	k	x_{2k}	x'_{1k}	Range (x^2_{21}, x^2_{22})
Group	1	4	4	$\mid 4\text{-}7 \mid = 3$
	2	6	7	

Then $B(2)$ is computed as $3 \times 1 + 2 \times 3 = 9$.

c. Now rank $B(1)$ and $B(2)$ from smaller to larger and assign with probability p the group with the smaller $B(t)$.

t	$B(t)$	Probability of assigning t
2	$B(2) = 9$	$p = \frac{2}{3}$
1	$B(1) = 11$	$1 - p = \frac{1}{3}$

Thus this participant is randomized to group 2 with probability two-thirds and to group 1 with probability one-third. Note that if minimization were used ($p = 1$), the assignment would be group 2.

REFERENCES

1. Ahlmark G, Saetre H: Long-term treatment with ß-blockers after myocardial infarction, *Eur J Clin Pharmacol* 10:77-83, 1976.
2. Altman D, Doré CJ: Randomization and baseline comparisons in clinical trials, *Lancet* 335:149-155, 1985.
3. Armitage P: The role of randomization in clinical trials, *Stat Med* 1:345-352, 1982.
4. Armitage P: The search for optimality in clinical trials, *Int Stat Rev* 53(1):15-24, 1985.
5. Aspirin Myocardial Infarction Study Research Group: A randomized controlled trial of aspirin in persons recovered from myocardial infarction, *JAMA* 243:661-669, 1980.
6. Atkinson AC: Optimum biased coin designs for sequential clinical trials with prognostic factors, *Biometrika* 69:61-67, 1982.
7. Bailar JC: Patient assignment algorithms: an overview. In *Proceedings of the 9th international biometric conference*, vol I, Raleigh, NC, 1976, The Biometric Society.
8. Bartlett RH, Roloff DW, Cornell RG, et al: Extracorporeal circulation in neonatal respiratory failure: a prospective randomized study, *Pediatrics* 76:479-487, 1985.
9. Bather JA: Randomized allocation of treatments in sequential experiments, *J R Stat Soc Ser B* 43:265-292, 1981.
10. Bather JA: On the allocation of treatments in sequential medical trials, *Int Stat Rev* 53(1):1-13, 1985.
11. Begg CB: On inferences from Wei's biased coin design for clinical trials, *Biometrika* 77:467-484, 1990.
12. Begg CB, Iglewicz B: A treatment allocation procedure for sequential clinical trials, *Biometrics* 36:81-90, 1980.
13. Begg CB, Kalish LA: Treatment allocation in sequential clinical trials: nonlinear models, *Proc Stat Comput Sect, Am Stat Assoc*, 1982.
14. Begg CB, Kalish LA: Treatment allocation of nonlinear models in clinical trials: the logistic model, *Biometrics* 40:409-420, 1984.
15. Berry DA: Modified two-armed bandit strategies for certain clinical trials, *J Am Stat Assoc* 73:339-345, 1978.
16. Beta-Blocker Heart Attack Trial Research Group: A randomized trial of propranolol in patients with acute myocardial infarction. I. Mortality results, *JAMA* 247:1707-1714, 1982.
17. Birkett JJ: Adaptive allocation in randomized controlled trials, *Controlled Clin Trials* 6:146-155, 1985.
18. Brittain E, Schlesselman JJ: Optimal allocation for the comparison of proportions, *Biometrics* 38:1003-1009, 1982.
19. Brown BW: Statistical controversies in the design of clinical trials—some personal views, *Controlled Clin Trials* 1:13-27, 1980.
20. Byar DP, Simon RM, Friedewald WT et al: Randomized clinical trials: perspectives on some recent ideas, *N Engl J Med* 295:74-80, 1976.
21. CASS Principal Investigators and Their Associates: Coronary Artery Surgery Study (CASS): a randomized trial of coronary artery bypass surgery, survival data, *Circulation* 68:939-950, 1983.

22. Chalmers TC, Celano P, Sacks HS et al: Bias in treatment assignment in controlled clinical trials, *N Engl J Med* 309:1358-1361, 1983.
23. Collaborative Group on Antenatal Steroid Therapy: Effect of antenatal dexamethasone administration on the prevention of respiratory distress syndrome, *Am J Obstet Gynecol* 141:276-287, 1981.
24. Coronary Drug Project Research Group: Factors influencing long term prognosis after recovery from myocardial infarction—three year findings of the Coronary Drug Project, *J Chronic Dis* 27: 267-285, 1974.
25. Diabetes Control and Complications Trial Research Group: The effect of intensive treatment of diabetes on the development and progression of long-term complications in insulin-dependent diabetes mellitus, *New Engl J Med* 329:977-986, 1993.
26. Ducimetiere P: Stratification, In Boissel JP, Klimt CR, eds: *Multi-center Controlled Trials: Principles and Problems*, Paris, 1979, INSERM.
27. Efron B: Forcing a sequential experiment to be balanced, *Biometrika* 58:403-417, 1971.
28. Efron B: Randomizing and balancing a complicated sequential experiment. In Miller RG Jr, Efron B, Brown BW Jr, Moses LE, ed: *Biometrics Casebook*, Wiley, New York, 1980.
29. Feinstein AR, Landis JR: The role of prognostic stratification in preventing the bias permitted by random allocation of treatment, *J Chron Dis* 29:277-284, 1976.
30. Fleiss JL: Multicentre clinical trials: Bradford Hill's contributions and some subsequent developments, *Stat Med* 1:353-359, 1982.
31. Forsythe, AB, Stitt FW: Randomization of minimization in the treatment assignment of patient trials: validity and power of tests, Tech Rep 28, Los Angeles, 1977, Health Science Computer Facility, University of California.
32. Freedman LS, White SJ: On the use of Pocock and Simon's method for balancing treatment numbers over prognostic factors in the controlled clinical trial, *Biometrics* 32:691-694, 1976.
33. Gail MH, Wieand S, Piantadosi S: Biased estimates of treatment effect in randomized experiments with nonlinear regressions and omitted covariates, *Biometrika* 71:431-444, 1984.
34. Green SB, Byar DP: The effect of stratified randomization on size and power of statistical tests in clinical trials, *J Chronic Dis* 31:445-454, 1978.
35. Grizzle JE: A note on stratifying versus complete random assignment in clinical trials, *Controlled Clin Trials* 3:365-368, 1982.
36. Halperin J, Brown BW Jr: Sequential treatment allocation procedures in clinical trials—with particular attention to the analysis of results for the biased coin design, *Stat Med* 5:219-229, 1986.
37. Hannigan JR Jr, Brown BW Jr: Adaptive randomization based coin-design: experience in a cooperative group clinical trial, Tech Rep 74, Stanford, Calif, 1982, Div of Biostatistics, Stanford University.
38. Hill AB: The clinical trial, *Br Med Bull* 71:278-282, 1951.
39. Hypertension Detection and Follow-up Program Cooperative Group: Five-year findings of the Hypertension Detection and Follow-up Program. Reduction in mortality of persons with high blood pressure, including mild hypertension, *JAMA* 242:2562-2571, 1979.
40. Kalish LA, Begg CB: Treatment allocation methods in clinical trials: a review, *Stat Med* 4:129-144, 1985.
41. Kalish LA, Begg CB: The impact of treatment allocation procedures on nominal significance levels and bias, *Controlled Clin Trials* 8:121-135, 1987.
42. Kalish LA, Harrington DP: Efficiency of balanced treatment allocation for survival analysis, *Biometrics* 44:815-821, 1988.
43. Klotz JH: Maximum entropy constrained balance randomization for clinical trials, *Biometrics* 34:283-287, 1978.
44. Krischer J, Hurley C, Pillamarri M, et al: An automated patient registration and treatment randomization system for multicenter clinical trials, *Controlled Clin Trials* 12:367-377, 1991.
45. Lachin JM: Properties of simple randomization in clinical trials, *Controlled Clin Trials* 9:312-326, 1988.
46. Lachin JM: Statistical properties of randomization in clinical trials, *Controlled Clin Trials* 9:289-311, 1988.
47. Lachin JM, Matts JP, Wei LJ: Randomization in clinical trials: conclusions and recommendations, *Controlled Clin Trials* 9:365-374, 1988.
48. Louis TA: Optimal allocation in sequential tests comparing the means of two Gaussian populations, *Biometrika* 62:359-369, 1975.

49. Louis TA: Sequential allocation in clinical trials comparing two exponential survival curves, *Biometrics* 33:627-634, 1977.
50. Mantel N: Pre-stratification or post-stratification, *Biometrics* 40:256-258, 1984 (letter).
51. Matts JP, Lachin JM: Properties of permutated-block randomization in clinical trials, *Controlled Clin Trials* 9:327-344, 1988.
52. Matts JP, McHugh RB: Analysis of accrual randomized clinical trials with balanced groups in strata, *J Chronic Dis* 31:725-740, 1978.
53. McHugh R, Matts J: Post-stratification in the randomized clinical trial, *Biometrics* 39:217-225, 1983.
54. Meier P: Stratification in the design of a clinical trial, *Controlled Clin Trials* 1:355-361, 1981.
55. Multiple Risk Factor Intervention Trial Research Group: Multiple Risk Factor Interventional Trial, risk factor changes and mortality results, *JAMA* 248:1465-1477, 1982.
56. Nordbrock E: An improved play-the-winner sampling procedure for selecting the better of two binomial populations, *J Am Stat Assoc* 71:137-139, 1976.
57. O'Rourke PP, Crone RK, Vacanti JP et al: Extracorporeal membrane oxygenation and conventional medical therapy in neonates with persistent pulmonary hypertension of the newborn: a prospective randomized study, *Pediatrics* 84:957-963, 1989.
58. Palta M: Investigating maximum power losses in survival studies with nonstratified randomization, *Biometrics* 41:497-504, 1985.
59. Palta M, Amini SB: Magnitude and likelihood of loss resulting from nonstratified randomization, *Stat Med* 1:267-275, 1982.
60. Paneth N, Wallenstein S: Extracorporeal membrane oxygenation and the play the winner rule, *Pediatrics* 76:622-623, 1985.
61. Peto R: Clinical trial methodology, *Biomedicine* 28:24-36, 1978 (special issue).
62. Peto R, Pike MC, Armitage P et al: Design and analysis of randomized clinical trials requiring prolonged observation of each patient. 1. Introduction and design, *Br J Cancer* 34:585-612, 1976.
63. Pocock SJ: Allocation of patients to treatment in clinical trials, *Biometrics* 35:183-197, 1979.
64. Pocock SJ, Lagakos SW: Practical experience of randomization in cancer trials: an international survey, *Br J Cancer* 46:368-375, 1982.
65. Pocock SJ, Simon R: Sequential treatment assignment with balancing for prognostic factors in the controlled clinical trial, *Biometrics* 31:102-115, 1975.
66. Raghavaro D: Use of distance function in sequential treatment assignment for prognostic factors in the controlled clinical trial, *Calcutta Stat Assoc Bull* 29:99-102, 1980.
67. Robbins H: Some aspects of the sequential design of experiments, *Bull Am Math Soc* 58:527-535, 1952.
68. Royall RM: Ethics and statistics in randomized clinical trials, *Stat Sci* 6(1):52-88, 1991.
69. Simon R: Adaptive treatment assignment methods and clinical trials, *Biometrics* 33:743-749, 1977.
70. Simon R: Restricted randomization designs in clinical trials, *Biometrics* 35:503-512, 1979.
71. Simon R, Hoel DG, Weiss GH: The use of covariate information in the sequential analysis of dichotomous response experiments, *Comm Stat-Theor Meth* 8:777-788, 1977.
72. Simon R, Weiss GH, Hoel DG: Sequential analysis of binomial clinical trials, *Biometrika* 62:195-200, 1975.
73. Smith RL: Sequential treatment allocation using biased coin designs, *J R Stat Soc B* 46:519-543, 1984.
74. Smythe RT, Wei LJ: Significance tests with restricted randomization design *Biometrika* 70:496-500, 1983.
75. Soares JF, Wu CFJ: Some restricted randomization rules in sequential designs, *Comm Stat-Theor Meth A* 12:2017-2034, 1983.
76. Steele JM: Efron's conjecture on vulnerability to bias in a method for balancing sequential trials, *Biometrika* 67:503-504, 1980.
77. Stigler SM: The use of random allocation for the control of selection bias, *Biometrika* 56:553-560, 1969.
78. Taves DR: Minimization: a new method of assigning patients to treatment and control groups, *Clin Pharmacol Ther* 15:443-453, 1974.

79. Titterington DM: On constrained balance randomization for clinical trials, *Biometrics* 39:1083-1086, 1984.
80. Ware JH: Investigating therapies of potentially great benefit: ECMO, *Stat Sci* 4(4):298-340, 1989.
81. Ware JH, Epstein MF: Extracorporeal circulation in neonatal respiratory failure: a prospective randomized study, *Pediatrics* 76:849-851, 1985.
82. Wei LJ: A class of designs for sequential clinical trials, *J Am Stat Assoc* 72:382-386, 1977.
83. Wei LJ: A class of treatment assignment rules for sequential experiments, *Comm Stat-Theor Meth A* 7:285-295, 1978.
84. Wei LJ: An application of an urn model to the design of sequential controlled clinical trials, *JASA* 73:559-563, 1978.
85. Wei LJ: Exact two-sample permutation tests based on the randomized play-the-winner rule, *Biometrika* 75:603-606, 1988.
86. Wei LJ: On the random allocation design for the control of selection bias in sequential experiments, *Biometrika* 65:79-84, 1978.
87. Wei LJ: The adaptive biased coin design for sequential experiments, *Ann Stat* 6:92-100, 1978.
88. Wei LJ, Lachin JM: Properties of the urn randomization in clinical trials, *Controlled Clin Trials* 9:345-364, 1988.
89. Wei LJ, Smythe RT, Lin DY, Park TS: Statistical inferences with data–dependent treatment allocation rules, *J Am Stat Assoc* 85:156-162, 1990.
90. Wei LJ, Smythe RT, Smith RL: K-treatment comparisons with restricted randomization rules in clinical trials, *Ann Stat* 14(1):265-274, 1986.
91. Weinstein MC: Allocation of subjects in medical experiments, *N Engl J Med* 291:1278-1285, 1974.
92. White SJ, Freedman LS: Allocation of patients to treatment groups in a controlled clinical study, *Br J Cancer* 37:849-857, 1978.
93. Williams DS, Davis CE: Reporting of assignment methods in clinical trials, *Controlled Clin Trials* 15:294-298, 1994.
94. Zelen M: Play-the-winner rule and the controlled clinical trial, *J Am Stat Assoc* 64:131-146, 1969.
95. Zelen M: The randomization and stratification of patients to clinical trials, *J Chronic Dis* 27:365-375, 1974.
96. Zelen M: Aspects of the planning and analysis of clinical trials in cancer. In Srivastava JN, ed: *A Survey of Statistical Design and Linear Models*, Amsterdam, North–Holland, 1975.

CHAPTER 6

Blindness

In any clinical trial, bias is one of the main concerns. Bias may be defined as systematic error, or "difference between the true value and that actually obtained due to all causes other than sampling variability."[18] It can be caused by conscious factors, subconscious factors, or both. Bias can occur at several places in a clinical trial, from the initial design through data analysis and interpretation. The general solution to the problem of bias is to keep the participant and investigator blinded, or masked, to the identity of the assigned intervention. One can also blind several other aspects of a trial: the assessment, classification, and evaluation of the response variables.

FUNDAMENTAL POINT

A clinical trial should, ideally, have a double-blind design to avoid potential problems of bias during data collection and assessment. In studies where such a design is impossible, a single-blind approach and other measures to reduce potential bias are favored.

TYPES OF TRIALS
Unblinded trials

In an unblinded or open trial, both the participant and investigator know to which intervention the participant has been assigned. Some kinds of trials can be conducted only in this manner. Such studies include those involving most surgical procedures, comparisons of devices and medical treatment, and changes in lifestyle (e.g., eating habits, exercise, and cigarette smoking) or learning techniques.

An unblinded study is appealing for two reasons. First, all other things being equal, it is simpler to execute than other studies. The usual drug trial may be easier to design and carry out, and consequently less expensive, if blinding is not an issue. Also, it has been argued that it more accurately reflects clinical practice.[10] However, an unblinded trial need not be simple. For example, the Multiple Risk Factor Intervention Trial, which attempted to intervene on three primary risk factors for coronary heart disease simultaneously, was extraordinarily complex.[20] Second, investigators are likely to be more comfortable making decisions, such as whether or not to continue a participant on assigned medication, if they know the intervention's identity.

The main disadvantage of an unblinded trial is the possibility of bias. Participant reporting of symptoms and side effects and prescription of concomitant or compensatory treatment are all susceptible to bias. (Other problems of biased data collection and assessment by the investigator are addressed in Chapter 10.) Participants not on the new or experimental intervention may become dissatisfied and drop out of the trial in disproportionately large numbers. A trial of the possible benefits of ascorbic acid (vitamin C) in the common cold[16,17] started out as a double-blind study. However, it soon became apparent that many of the participants, most of whom were medical staff, discovered whether they were on ascorbic acid or placebo. Since evaluation of severity and duration of colds depended on the participants' reporting of their symptoms, this unblinding was important. Among those participants who claimed not to know the identity of the treatment, ascorbic acid showed no benefit over placebo. In contrast, among participants who knew or suspected what they were on, ascorbic acid did better than placebo. Therefore preconceived notions about the benefit of a treatment, coupled with a subjective response variable, may have yielded biased reporting. Only the alertness of the investigators prevented them from arriving at probably false conclusions. In addition, as more participants became aware of their medication's identity, the dropout rate increased. This was especially so in the placebo group.

In a trial of coronary artery bypass surgery vs. medical treatment,[6] the number of participants who smoked was equal in the two study groups at baseline. During follow-up there were significantly fewer smokers in the surgical group than in the medical group. The effect of this group difference on the outcome of the trial is difficult, if not impossible, to assess.

Single-blind trials

In a single-blind study, only the investigators are aware of which intervention each participant is receiving. The advantages of this design are similar to those of an unblinded study: it is usually simpler to carry out than a double-blind design, and knowledge of the intervention may help the investigators exercise their best judgment when caring for the participants. Indeed, certain investigators are reluctant to participate in studies in which they do not know the study group assignment. They recognize that bias is partially reduced by keeping the participants blinded but feel that the participants' health and safety are best served if they themselves are not blinded.

The disadvantages of a single-blind design are similar to, though not as pronounced as, those of an unblinded design. The investigators avoid the problems of biased participant reporting, but they themselves can affect the administration of nonstudy therapy, data collection, and data assessment. For example, a single-blind study reported benefits from zinc administration in a group of people with taste disorders.[23] Because of the possibility of bias in a study using a response variable as subjective and hard to measure as taste, the study was repeated, using a type of crossover, double-blind design.[11] This second study showed that zinc, when compared with placebo, did not relieve the taste disorders of the study group. The extent of the blinding of the participants did not change; therefore, presumably, knowledge of drug identity by the investigator was important. The results of treatment crossover were equally revealing. In the single-blind study, participants who did not improve on placebo were placed on zinc. Improvement was then noted. However, in all four double-blind, cross-over procedures (placebo to zinc, placebo to placebo, zinc to zinc, and zinc to placebo), the participants who had previously shown no improvement did show benefit when given the second medication. Thus the expectation that the participants who failed to respond to the first drug were now being given an active drug may have been sufficient to produce a positive response.

Both unblinded and single-blind trials are vulnerable to another source of potential bias introduced by the investigators. This relates to group differences in concomitant and compensatory treatment. Concomitant treatment means any nonstudy therapy administered to participants during a trial. If such treatment is likely to influence the response variable, this needs to be considered when determining sample size. Of more concern is the bias that can be introduced if concomitant treatment is applied unequally in the two groups. Investigators may feel that the control group is not being given the same opportunity as the intervention group and, as a result, may prescribe additional treatment as compensation. This may be in the form of advice or therapy. For example, several studies have attempted blood pressure lowering as either the sole intervention or as part of a broader effort. In each, the investigators made an intensive effort to persuade participants in the intervention group to take their medication and to reduce their weight. To persuade successfully the investigators themselves had to believe that blood pressure reduction was beneficial. In other words, they had not suspended judgment regarding the possible efficacy of the intervention. When they were seeing participants who had been assigned to the control group, this conviction was difficult to suppress. Therefore participants in the control group were likely to have been instructed about ways by which to lower their blood pressures. The result of compensatory treatment is a diminution of the difference between the intervention group and the "untreated" or control group. Working against this is the fact that investigators prefer to be associated with a study that gives positive findings. They may, therefore, subconsciously favor those in the intervention group when they deal with participants, collect data, and assess results.

To bias the outcome of a trial, concomitant treatment must be effective, and it must be used in a high proportion of the participants. When this is the case, bias is a possibility and may occur in either direction, depending on whether the concomitant treatment is preferentially used in the control, or in the intervention group. It is usually impossible to determine the direction and magnitude of such bias in advance or its impact after it has occurred.

Double-blind trials

In a double-blind study, neither the participants nor the investigators responsible for following the participants know the identity of the intervention assignment. Such designs are usually restricted to trials of drug efficacy. It is theoretically possible to design a study comparing two surgical procedures in which the surgeon performing the operation knows the type of surgery, but neither the participant nor the study investigators knows. Similarly, one might be able to design a study comparing two diets in which the food looks identical. However, such trials are uncommon.

The main advantage of a truly double-blind study is that the risk of bias is reduced. Preconceived ideas of the investigators will be less important, because they will not know which intervention a particular participant is receiving. Any effects of their actions, therefore, would theoretically occur equally in the intervention and control groups. As discussed later, the possibility of bias may never be completely eliminated. However, a well-designed and properly run double-blind study can minimize bias. As in the example of the trial of zinc and taste impairment, double-blind studies have at times led to results that differ from unblinded or single-blind studies. Such cases underline the importance of bias as a factor in clinical trials.

In a double-blind trial certain functions, which in open or single-blind studies could be accomplished by the investigators, must be taken over by others to maintain the blindness. Thus an outside body needs to monitor the data for toxicity and benefit, especially in long-term trials. (Chapter 15 discusses data monitoring in greater detail.) A person other than the investigator who sees the participants needs to be responsible for assigning the interventions to the participants.

In many single-blind and double-blind drug trials the control group is placed on a placebo. Much debate in the past has centered on the ethics of using a placebo.[2] Conducting a placebo-control trial is justified if two situations pertain. First, if the investigator seeks to evaluate a new intervention without the participant receiving any other therapy for the condition being studied, there should be no standard intervention clearly superior to placebo. If a standard therapy is known to be beneficial, the placebo and the intervention being assessed would be used in conjunction with the standard therapy. Second, the participants should fully understand that a placebo is being used and be aware of what their chances are of receiving either it or the alternative. Rothman and Michels[22] argue that in many cases a placebo has been inappropriately used because a proven standard therapy exists. Whether that is the case and whether short-term discontinuation of standard therapy is harmful is not always clear. However, as noted, in many studies, the new intervention or placebo are added to the standard therapy and do not replace it. Also, Spodick[24] has succinctly pointed out that, despite persistent views to the contrary,[27] placebo therapy has at times been as effective as standard therapy. For example, an overview of placebo-controlled trials of antianginal agents with stable angina showed no difference in clinical events between active intervention and placebo.[9] In another instance, even investigators who had initially considered use of a placebo as unethical have been persuaded of its value as a result of their clinical trial experience.[21]

Triple-blind trials

A triple-blind study is an extension of the double-blind design; the committee monitoring response variables is not told the identity of the groups. The committee is simply given data for groups A and B. A triple-blind study has the theoretical advantage of allowing the monitoring committee to evaluate the response variable results more objectively. This assumes that appraisal of efficacy and harm, as well as requests for special analyses, may be biased if group identity is known. However, in a trial where the data monitoring committee has an ethical responsibility to ensure participant safety, such a design may be counterproductive. When hampered in the safety-monitoring role, the committee cannot carry out its responsibility to minimize harm to the participants. In addition, even if the committee could discharge its duties adequately while being kept blinded, many investigators would be uneasy participating in such a study. Although in most cases the data monitoring committee looks only at group data and can rarely make informed judgments about individuals, the investigators still rely on the committee to safeguard their study participants. This may not be a completely rational approach because, by the time a monitoring committee receives data, often any emergency situation has long passed. Nevertheless, the discomfort many investigators feel about participating in double-blind studies would be magnified should the data monitoring committee also be kept blinded.

Finally, people tend not to accept beneficial outcomes unless a statistically significant difference has been achieved. Rarely, though, will investigators continue a study to achieve a clearly significant difference in an adverse direction; that is, until the intervention is statistically significantly worse than the control. Therefore many monitoring committees demand to know which study groups are on which intervention.

A triple-blind study can be conducted ethically if the data monitoring committee asks itself at each meeting whether the direction of observed trends matters. If not, then the triple-blind can be maintained, at least for the time being. This implies that the monitoring committee can ask to be unblinded at any time it chooses.[25] This has been done successfully in many studies in different fields and has been reported in the Cardiac Arrhythmia Suppression Trial.[8]

SPECIAL PROBLEMS IN DOUBLE-BLIND STUDIES

Double-blind studies are usually more complex and therefore more difficult to carry out than other trials. One must ensure that investigators remain blinded and that any data that conceivably might endanger blindness be kept from them during the study. An effective data-monitoring scheme must be set up, and emergency unblinding procedures must be established. These requirements pose their own problems and can increase the cost of a study. In the Aspirin-Myocardial Infarction Study,[1] a double-blind trial of aspirin in people with coronary heart disease, the investigators wished to monitor the action of aspirin on platelets. A postulated beneficial effect of aspirin relates to its ability to reduce the aggregation of platelets. Therefore measuring platelet aggregation provided both an estimate of whether the aspirin-treated group was getting a sufficient dose and a basis for measurement of participant compliance. However, tests of platelet aggregation needed to be performed shortly after the blood sample was drawn. The usual method was to have a laboratory technician insert the specimen in an aggregometer, add a material such as epinephrine, which, in the absence of aspirin, causes platelets to aggregate, and analyze a curve that is printed on a paper strip. To maintain the blind, the study needed to find a way to keep the technician from seeing the curve. Therefore a cassette tape recorder was substituted for the usual paper strip recorder, and the indicator needle was covered. These changes required a modification of the aggregometer. All of the 30 clinics required this equipment, so the adjustment was expensive. However, it helped ensure the maintenance of the blind.

Drug studies, in particular, lend themselves to double-blind designs. One of the surest ways to unblind a drug study is to have dissimilar appearing medications. When the treatment identity of one participant becomes known to the investigator, the whole trial is unblinded.

Naturally, participants want to be on the better intervention. In a drug trial, the better intervention usually is presumed to be the new one; in the case of a placebo-control trial, it is presumed to be the active medication. Investigators may also be curious about a drug's identity. For these reasons, consciously or unconsciously, both participants and investigators may try to unblind the medication. Unblinding can be done deliberately by going so far as to have the drug analyzed, or in a less purposeful manner by accidently breaking open capsules, holding pills up to the light, carefully testing them, or making any of numerous other tests. In the first case, which may have occurred in the vitamin C study discussed earlier, little can be done to ensure blinding absolutely. Curious participants and investigators can discover numerous ways to unblind the trial, whatever precautions are taken. Probably, however, the less purposeful unblinding is more common.

Matching of drugs

Proper matching has received little attention in the literature. Most reports of drug studies do not indicate how closely tablets or capsules resembled one another, or how great a problem was caused by imperfect matching. However, one report[12] is disturbing. The authors noted that of 22 studies surveyed, only five had excellent matching between the drugs being tested. Several features of matching must be considered.[15] Cross-over studies, where each subject sees both medications, require the most care in matching. Visual discrepancies can occur in size, shape, color, sheen, and texture. Ensuring that these characteristics are identical may not be simple. In the case of tablets, dyes or coatings may adhere differently to the active ingredient than to the placebo, causing slight differences in color or sheen. Agents can also differ in odor. The taste and the local action on the tongue of the active medication are likely to be different from those of the placebo. For example, propranolol is a topical anesthetic that causes lingular numbness if held in the mouth. Farr and Gwaltney[7] reported on problems in matching zinc lozenges against placebo. Because zinc lozenges are difficult to blind, the authors questioned whether studies using zinc for common cold prevention were truly valid. They conducted trials illustrating that if a placebo is inadequately matched, the "unpleasant side effects of zinc" may reduce the perception of cold symptoms.

Differences may become evident only after some time because of degradation of the active ingredient. Freshly prepared aspirin is relatively odor free, but after a while, tell-tale acetic acid accumulates. Less obviously, the weight or specific gravity of the tablets may differ. Matching the agents on all of these characteristics may be impossible. However, if a great deal of effort and money are being spent on the trial, a real attempt to ensure matching makes sense. The investigators also need to make sure that the containers are identical. Bottles and vials need to be free of any marks other than codes that are indecipherable except with the key.

Drug preparations should be pretested if it is possible. One method is to have a panel of observers unconnected with the study compare samples of the medications. Perfect matches are almost impossible to obtain, and some differences are to be expected. However, beyond detecting differences, it is important to assess whether the observers can actually identify the agents. If not, slightly imperfect matches may be tolerated. The investigator must remember that, except in cross-over studies, each participant has only one drug and is therefore not able to make a comparison. On the other hand, participants may meet and talk in waiting rooms, or in some other way compare notes or pills. Of course, staff always have the opportunity to compare different preparations and undermine the integrity of a study.

Use of substances to mask characteristic taste, color, or odor is often advocated. Adding vanilla to the outside of tablets may mask an odor; adding dyes will mask dissimilar colors. A substance such as quassin will impart a bitter taste to the preparations. Not only will quassin mask differences in taste, but it will also effectively discourage participants from biting into a preparation more than once. However, the possibility that chemical substances may have toxic effects after long-term use or even cause allergic reactions in a small percentage of the participants[5] must be considered. It is usually prudent to avoid using extra substances unless absolutely essential to prevent unblinding of the study.

Rarely do publications of trial results discuss possible inadequate matching. An exception is the vitamin C study[16,17] that suffered from a breakdown of the double-blind design. One possible reason given by the investigators was that, in the rush to begin the study, the contents of the capsules were not carefully produced. The lactose placebo could easily be distinguished from ascorbic acid by taste, as the study participants quickly discovered.

Sometimes, two or more active drugs are being compared. The ideal method of blinding is to have the active agents look alike, either by formulating them appropriately or by enclosing them in identical capsules. The former may not be possible, and the latter may be expensive or require capsules too large to be practical. One option is to implement a double-dummy. Each active agent has a placebo identical to it. Each study participant would then take one active and one placebo pill. This may be feasible for two medications. It becomes more unreasonable if multiple dosing regimens are used or if several active drugs are being compared.

If two or more active agents are being compared against placebo, and it is not feasible to make all drugs appear identical, nor is it reasonable to have each participant take more than one pill, another option is to create a placebo for each active drug. In this case, however, the number of participants in the placebo group assigned to each form of the placebo is a fraction of the total placebo group. For example, assume the study consists of placebo groups and active drugs A, B, and C. If each group is the same size, one third of placebo groups will take a placebo designed to look like active drug A, one third will take a placebo designed to look like active drug B, and one third will take a placebo designed to look like active drug C. The major disadvantage of this design is that participants and investigators can correctly assume that there is a 75% chance of any particular kind of pill being active. This design, however, was successfully implemented in at least one reported study.[26]

Coding of drugs

Drug coding means the labeling of individual drug bottles or vials so that the identity of the drug is not disclosed. Coding is usually done by means of assigning a random set of numbers to the active drug and a different set to the control. As many different drug codes as are logistically feasible should be used. At least in smaller studies, each participant should have a unique drug code that remains with him for the duration of the trial. If only one code were used for each study group, unblinding a single participant would result in unblinding everybody. Furthermore, many drugs have specific side effects. One side effect in one participant may not be attributable to the drug, but a constellation of several side effects in several participants with the same drug code may easily unblind the study.

Unfortunately, in large studies it becomes cumbersome to make up and stock drugs under many different codes. This is true for the investigators dispensing the medication as well as for the person labeling and coding. When several participants have the same code, there is less chance that a particular participant will run out of medication, because in emergencies, drugs can be borrowed from another participant's supply. One compromise is to have each participant assigned an individual code, but have several replacement supplies of medication, with different codes, available in emergency. Investigators need to balance the various logistic concerns against the risks of unblinding when determining the number of drug codes.

Unblinding trials

The phrase *truly double-blind study* was used earlier in the text. While many studies are designed as double- or single-blind, it is unclear how many, in fact, are truly blind. The intended physiologic effect of a drug may be readily observable. Certainly, drugs have side effects, some of which are fairly characteristic. Existence or absence of side effects does not necessarily unblind drug assignment, since all people on drugs do not develop reactions and some people on placebo develop events that can be mistaken for drug side effects. It is well known that aspirin is associated with gastrointestinal problems. In the Coronary Drug Project Aspirin Study,[4] 5.4% of the participants in the aspirin group developed gastritis. On the other hand, 3.9% of the placebo participants had the same complaints. To have made definite claims regarding study group identity based on presence or absence of gastritis would have led to many errors.

Occasionally, accidental unblinding occurs. In some studies, a special center labels and distributes drugs to the clinic where participants are seen. Obviously, each carton of drugs sent from the pharmaceutical company to this distribution center must contain a packing slip identifying the drug. The distribution center puts coded labels on each bottle and removes the packing slip before sending the drugs to the investigator. In one instance, one carton contained two packing slips by mistake. The distribution center, not realizing this, shipped the carton to the investigator with the second packing slip enclosed. Thus it is advisable to empty cartons completely before re-using them.

Laboratory errors have also occurred. These are particularly likely when, to prevent unblinding, only some laboratory results are given to the investigators. Occasionally investigators have received the complete set of laboratory results. This usually happens at the beginning of a study before "bugs" have been worked out or when the laboratory hires new personnel who are unfamiliar with the procedures. If a commercial laboratory performs the study determinations, the tests should be done in a special area of the laboratory, with safeguards to prevent study results from getting intermingled with routine work.

In addition, monitoring the use of study medication prescribed outside the study is essential. Any group differences might be evidence of a deficiency in the blind. Another way of estimating the success of a double-blind design is to monitor specific intermediate effects of the study medication. The use of platelet aggregation in the Aspirin Myocardial Infarction Study is an example. An unusually large number of subjects with nonaggregating platelets in the placebo group would raise the suspicion that the blind had been broken.

Official breaking of the blind may be necessary. There are bound to be situations that require disclosures, especially in long-term studies. Perhaps the study drug requires tapering the dosage. In an emergency, knowledge that a participant is or is not on the active drug would indicate whether tapering is necessary. Usually, most emergencies can be handled by withdrawing the medication without breaking the blind. When the treating physician is different from the study investigator, a third party can obtain the blinded information from the pharmacy or central data repository and relate the information to the treating physician. In this way, the participant and investigator need not be unblinded. When unblinding does occur, the investigator should review and report the circumstances that led to it. Knowledge of the kind of intervention seldom influences emergency care of the participant, and such reviews have helped reduce the frequency of further unblinding.

A procedure should be developed to break the blind quickly for any individual participant at any time should it be in his best interest. Such systems include having labels on file in the hospital pharmacy or other accessible locations, or having "on call" 24 hours a day someone who can decode the assignment. To avoid needless breaking of the code, someone other than the investigator could hold a list that reveals the identity of each drug code. Alternatively, each study medication bottle label might have a sealed tear-off portion that would be filed in the pharmacy or with the participant's records. In an emergency, the seal could be torn and the drug identity revealed. Care should be taken to ensure that the sealed portion is of appropriate color and thickness to prevent reading through it. In one study, the sealed labels attached to the medication bottles were transparent when held up to strong light.

In summary, double-blind trials require careful planning and constant monitoring to ensure that the blind is maintained and that participant safety is not jeopardized.

Assessment of blindness

After a study is completed, estimating the degree to which the blind was maintained may be worthwhile. One way of estimating before officially disclosing drug identity is to ask the participant and the clinic staff to guess to which group the participant was assigned. Ideally, in a trial with one half of the participants on active medication and one half on control, the guesses would be correct 50% of the time in each group. To the degree that 50% is exceeded, the amount of unblinding can be estimated. If substantially fewer than half of the guesses in each group are correct, one might suspect that people did know but were trying not to admit it.

Shortly before the end of the Aspirin Myocardial Infarction Study, 380 of the 4524 participants were asked whether they knew if they were taking aspirin or placebo.[13] Slightly over half correctly identified what they were taking, a little over one fourth chose the wrong agent, and the remainder either refused to guess or selected a drug not being tested. Most of those who guessed correctly were not certain of their selection. Those who made special efforts to break the blind did better. Adherence to the study medication did not seem to be related to guessing correctly. Even though blinding was found to be imperfect, it clearly contributed to the integrity of the trial. Other examples of assessment of adequacy of blindness have also been reported.[3,14,19]

REFERENCES

1. Aspirin Myocardial Infarction Study Research Group: A randomized controlled trial of aspirin in persons recovered from myocardial infarction, *JAMA* 243:661-669, 1980.
2. Bok S: The ethics of giving placebos, *Sci Am* 231:17-23, (Nov) 1974.
3. Byington RP, Curb JD, Mattson ME: Assessment of double-blindness at the conclusion of the Beta-Blocker Heart Attack Trial, *JAMA* 253:1733-1736, 1985.
4. Coronary Drug Project Research Group: Aspirin in coronary heart disease, *J Chronic Dis* 29:625-642, 1976.
5. Tartrazine: a yellow hazard, *Drug and Therapeutics Bulletin*: 18:53-55, 1980.
6. European Coronary Surgery Study Group: Coronary-artery bypass surgery in stable angina pectoris: survival at two years, *Lancet* i:889-893, 1979.
7. Farr BM, Gwaltney JM Jr: The problems of taste in placebo matching: an evaluation of zinc gluconate for the common cold, *J Chronic Dis* 40:875-879, 1987.
8. Friedman LM, Bristow JD, Hallstrom A, et al: Data monitoring in the Cardiac Arrhythmia Suppression Trial, *Online J Curr Clin Trials Doc* 79, 1993.
9. Glasser SP, Clark PI, Lipicky RJ et al: Exposing patients with chronic, stable, exertional angina to placebo periods in drug trials, *JAMA* 265:1550-1554, 1991.
10. Hansson L, Hedner T, Dahlöf B: Prospective randomized open blinded end-point (PROBE) study. A novel design for intervention trials, *Blood Pressure* 1:113-119, 1992.
11. Henkin RI, Schechter PJ, Friedewald WT et al: A double-blind study of the effects of zinc sulfate on taste and smell dysfunction, *Am J Med Sci* 272:285-299, 1976.
12. Hill LE, Nunn AJ, Fox W: Matching quality of agents employed in "double-blind" controlled clinical trials, *Lancet* i:352-356, 1976.
13. Howard J, Whittemore AS, Hoover JJ et al: How blind was the patient blind in AMIS? *Clin Pharmacol Ther* 32:543-553, 1982.
14. Jespersen CM and the Danish Study Group on Verapamil in Myocardial Infarction: Assessment of blindness in the Danish Verapamil Infarction Trial II (DAVIT II), *Eur J Clin Pharmacol* 39:75-76, 1990.
15. Joyce CRB: Psychological factors in the controlled evaluation of therapy. In Balint E, ed: *Psychopharmacology: dimensions and perspectives,* London, 1968, Tavistock.
16. Karlowski TR, Chalmers TC, Frenkel LD et al: Ascorbic acid for the common cold: a prophylactic and therapeutic trial, *JAMA* 231:1038-1042, 1975.
17. Lewis TL, Karlowski TR, Kapikian AZ et al: A controlled clinical trial of ascorbic acid for the common cold, *Ann NY Acad Sci* 258:505-512, 1975.
18. Mausner JS, Bahn AK: *Epidemiology: an introductory text,* Philadelphia, 1974, WB Saunders.
19. Moscucci M, Byrne L, Weintraub M, Cox C: Blinding, unblinding, and the placebo effect: an analysis of patients' guesses of treatment assignment in a double-blind clinical trial, *Clin Pharmacol Ther* 41:256-265, 1987.
20. Multiple Risk Factor Intervention Trial Research Group: Multiple Risk Factor Intervention Trial: risk factor changes and mortality results, *JAMA* 248:1465-1477, 1982.
21. Prout GR Jr, Bross IDJ, Slack NH, Ausman RK: Carcinoma of the bladder. 5-fluorouracil and the critical role of a placebo, *Cancer* 22:926-931, 1968.
22. Rothman KJ, Michels KB: The continuing unethical use of placebo controls. (Sounding Board), *N Engl J Med* 331:394-398, 1994.
23. Schechter PJ, Friedewald WT, Bronzert DA et al: Idiopathic hypogeusia: a description of the syndrome and a single-blind study with zinc sulfate, *Int Rev Neurobiol* (suppl I):125-140, 1972.

24. Spodick DH: Letter to the editor, *N Engl J Med* 292:653, 1975.
25. Task Force of the Working Group on Arrhythmias of the European Society of Cardiology: The early termination of clinical trials: causes, consequences, and control. With special reference to trials in the field of arrhythmias and sudden death, *Circulation* 89:2892-2907, 1994.
26. The CAPS Investigators: The Cardiac Arrhythmia Pilot Study, *Am J Cardiol* 57:91-95, 1986.
27. Wilks HS: Letter to the editor, *N Engl J Med* 292:321, 1975.

CHAPTER 7

Sample Size

The size of the study should be considered early in the planning phase. Often no formal sample size is ever calculated. Instead, the number of participants available to the investigators during some period determines the size of the study. Many clinical trials that do not carefully consider the sample size requirements turn out to lack the power or ability to detect intervention effects of fairly substantial magnitude and clinical importance. Freiman et al.[40] reviewed the power of 71 published randomized controlled clinical trials that failed to find significant differences between groups. "Sixty-seven of the trials had a greater than 10% risk of missing a true 25% therapeutic improvement, and with the same risk, 50 of the trials could have missed a 50% improvement." The danger in studies with low statistical power is that interventions that could be beneficial are discarded without adequate testing and may never be considered again. Even trials with sample size calculations during the design phase may still be too small to achieve primary objectives.

This chapter presents, with some details, an overview of sample size estimation. Several general discussions of sample size can be found.* For example, Lachin[60] and Donner[29] have each written a more technical discussion of this topic. For most of the chapter, the focus is on sample size where the study is randomizing individuals. In some sections, the concept of sample size for randomizing clusters of individuals or organs within individuals is presented.

FUNDAMENTAL POINT

Clinical trials should have sufficient statistical power to detect differences between groups considered to be of clinical interest. Therefore calculation of sample size with provision for adequate levels of significance and power is an essential part of planning.

Before a discussion of sample size and power calculations, it must be emphasized that, for several reasons, a sample size calculation provides only an estimate of the needed size of a study.[13] First, parameters used in the calculation are estimates, and as such, have an element of uncertainty. Often parameter estimates are based

---

*References 2, 13, 26, 29, 47, 60, 87, 96, 104, 111.

on very small prior studies. Second, the estimate of the relative effectiveness of the intervention over the control may be based on a population different from that intended to be studied. Third, the estimated effectiveness is often overly optimistic since published pilot studies may be highly selected and researchers are vulnerable to wishful thinking. Fourth, during the final planning stage of a trial, revisions of inclusion and exclusion criteria may influence the type of participant entering the study and thus alter earlier assumptions used in the sample size calculation. Assessing the impact of such changes in criteria and the screening effect is usually impossible. Experience indicates that participants enrolled into control groups do better than the population from which the participants were drawn. The reasons are not entirely clear. One factor could be that participants with the highest risk of developing the outcome of interest are excluded in the screening process. In trials involving chronic diseases, because of the research protocol, participants might receive more care and attention than they would normally be given, thus improving their prognosis. Participants assigned to the control group, may, therefore, be better off than if they had not been in the trial at all. Finally, sample size calculations are based on mathematical models that may only approximate the true, but unknown, distribution of the response variables.

Because of the approximate nature of sample size calculations, the investigator should be as conservative as can be justified while still being realistic in estimating the parameters used in the calculation. If a sample size is drastically overestimated, the trial may be judged as unfeasible. If the sample size is underestimated, there is a good chance the trial will fall short of demonstrating any effectiveness of the intervention. In general, as long as the calculated sample size is realistically obtainable, it is better to overestimate the size and possibly terminate the trial early (Chapter 15) than to underestimate and need to justify an increase or extension in follow-up, or worse, to arrive at incorrect conclusions.

STATISTICAL CONCEPTS

An understanding of the basic statistical concepts of hypothesis testing, significance level, and power is essential for a discussion of sample size estimation. A brief review of these concepts follows. Further discussion can be found in many basic medical statistics textbooks* and selected review papers.[29,40,60]

Except where indicated, studies of one intervention group and one control group will be discussed. With some adjustments, sample size calculations can be made for studies with more than two groups. Before computing sample size, the primary response variable used to judge the effectiveness of intervention must be identified. This chapter will consider three basic kinds: (1) dichotomous response

---

*References 4, 14, 28, 36, 37, 89, 102, 113.

variables, such as success and failure; (2) continuous response variables, such as blood pressure level or a change in blood pressure; and (3) time to failure (or occurrence of a clinical event).

For the dichotomous response variables, the event rates in the intervention group (p_I) and the control group (p_C) are compared. For continuous response variables, the true but unknown mean level in the intervention group (μ_I) is compared with the mean level in the control group (μ_C). For survival data, a hazard rate, λ, is often compared for the two study groups or at least is used for sample size estimation. Sample size estimates for response variables that do not exactly fall into any of the three categories can usually be approximated by one of them.

In terms of the primary response variable, p_I will be compared with p_C or μ_I will be compared with μ_C. This discussion will use only the event rates, p_I and p_C, although the same concepts will hold if response levels μ_I and μ_C are substituted appropriately. Of course, the investigator does not know the true values of the event rates. The clinical trial will yield only estimates of the event rates, denoted by $\hat{p}_I$ and $\hat{p}_C$. Typically, an investigator tests whether or not a true difference exists between the event rates of participants in the two groups. The traditional way of stating this is in terms of a null hypothesis, denoted H_0, which states that no difference between the true event rates exists (H_0: $p_C - p_I = 0$). The goal is to test H_0 and decide whether or not to reject it. That is, the null hypothesis is assumed to be true until proven otherwise.

Since only estimates of the true event rates are obtained, it is possible that, even if the null hypothesis is true ($p_C - p_I = 0$), the observed event rates might by chance be different. If the observed differences in event rates are large enough by chance alone, the investigator might reject the null hypothesis incorrectly. This false positive occurrence or type I error should be made as few times as possible. The probability of this type I error is called the significance level and is denoted by α. The probability of observing differences as large as or larger than the difference actually observed given that H_0 is true is called the "p value," denoted as p. The decision will be to reject H_0 if $p \leq \alpha$. While the level of α chosen is somewhat arbitrary, the ones used and accepted traditionally are 0.01 or 0.05. As will be shown later, as α is set smaller, the required sample size increases.

If the null hypothesis is not true, then another hypothesis, called the *alternative hypothesis*, denoted by H_A, must be true. That is, the true difference between the event rates p_I and p_C is some value δ where $\delta \neq 0$. The observed difference, $\hat{p}_C - \hat{p}_I$, can be quite small by chance alone even if the alternative hypothesis is true. Therefore, the investigator could, on the basis of small observed differences, fail to reject H_0 when he should. This is called a type II error or a false-negative result. The probability of a type II error is denoted by β. The value of β depends on the specific value of δ, the true but unknown difference in event rates between the two groups, as well as on the sample size and α. The probability of correctly rejecting H_0 is denoted $1 - \beta$

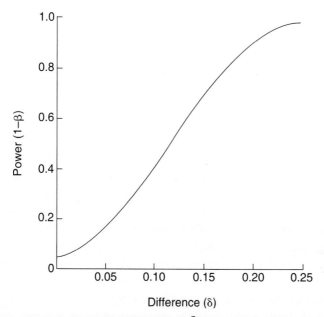

Fig. 7-1 A power curve for increasing differences (δ) between the control group rate of 0.5 and the intervention group rate with a one-sided significance level of 0.05 and a total sample size ($2N$) of 200.

and is called the power of the study. Power quantifies the ability of the study to find true differences of various values of δ. Since β is a function of α, the sample size, and δ, $1 - \beta$ is also a function of these parameters. The plot of $1 - \beta$ vs. δ for a given sample size is called the power curve and is depicted in Fig. 7-1. On the horizontal axis, values of δ are plotted from 0 to an upper value, δ_A (0.25 in this figure). On the vertical axis, the probability or power of detecting a true difference δ is shown for a given significance level and sample size. In constructing this specific power curve, a sample size of 100 in each group, a one-sided significance level of 0.05, and a control group event rate of 0.5 (50%) were assumed. Note that as δ increases, the power to detect δ also increases. For example, if $\delta = 0.10$ the power is approximately 0.40. When $\delta = 0.20$ the power increases to about 0.90. Typically, investigators like to have a power ($1 - \beta$) of at least 0.80, but often around 0.90 or 0.95 when planning a study; that is to have an 80%, 90%, or 95% chance of finding a statistically significant difference between the event rates, given that a difference, δ, actually exists.

Since the significance level α should be small, say 0.05 or 0.01, and the power ($1 - \beta$) should be large, say 0.90 or 0.95, the only quantities that are left to vary are δ and the total sample size. In planning a clinical trial, the investigator hopes to detect a difference of specified magnitude δ or larger. One factor that enters into the selection of δ is the minimum difference between groups that is judged to be clinically important. In addition, previous research may provide estimates of δ. The exact nature of the calculation of the sample size, given α, $1 - \beta$, and δ, is considered here. It can be assumed that the randomization strategy will allocate an equal number (N) of participants to each group. If the variability in the responses for the two groups is approximately the same, equal allocation provides a more powerful design than does unequal allocation. If the variable is substantially different in the groups,[12] unequal allocation may yield an appreciable increase in power. Since equal allocation is usually easier to implement and variability is usually assumed to be similar, it is the more frequently used strategy.

Before a sample size can be calculated, classical statistical theory says that the investigator must decide whether he is interested in differences in one direction only (one-sided test), say improvements in intervention over control, or in differences in either direction (two-sided test). This latter case would represent testing the hypothesis that the new intervention is either better or worse than the control. In general, two-sided tests should be used unless there is strong justification for expecting a difference in only one direction. An investigator should always keep in mind that any new intervention could be harmful and helpful. However, as discussed in Chapter 15, some investigators may not be willing to prove the intervention harmful and would terminate a study if the results are only suggestive of harm. A classic example of this issue is provided by the Cardiac Arrhythmia Suppression Trial or CAST.[16] This trial was initially designed as a one-sided, 0.025 significance level hypothesis test that antiarrhythmic drug therapy would improve survival. Since the drugs were already marketed, harmful effects were not expected. Despite the one-sided hypothesis in the design, the monitoring process used a two-sided, 0.05 significance level approach. As it turned out, the trial was terminated early because of harm. (See Chapter 15.)

If a one-sided test of hypothesis is chosen, in most circumstances the significance level ought to be half what the investigator would use for a two-sided test. For example, if 0.05 is the two-sided significance level typically used, 0.025 would be used for the one-sided test. This requires the same degree of evidence or scientific documentation to declare a treatment effective, regardless of the one-sided vs. two-sided question. In this circumstance, a test for negative or harmful effects might also be done at the 0.025 level. This in effect provides two one-sided 0.025 hypothesis tests for an overall 0.05 significance level.

As mentioned above, the total sample size $2N$ (so denoted because two study groups of equal size are assumed) is a function of the significance level (α), the power ($1 - \beta$), and the size of the difference in response (δ) that is to be detected. Changing α, $1 - \beta$, or δ will result in a change in $2N$. As the magnitude of the difference δ decreases, the larger the sample size must be to guarantee a high probability of finding that difference. If the calculated sample size is larger than can be realistically obtained, then one or more of the parameters in the design must be modified. Since the significance level is usually fixed at 0.05 or 0.01, the investigator should generally reconsider the value selected for δ and increase it, or keep δ the same and settle for a less powerful study. If neither of these alternatives is satisfactory, serious consideration should be given to abandoning the trial.

Rothman[94] among others has argued that journals should encourage using confidence intervals to report clinical trial results instead of significance levels. Several researchers[14,70,94] discuss sample size formulas from this confidence interval approach. Confidence intervals are constructed by computing the observed difference in event rates and then adding and subtracting a constant times the standard error of the difference. This provides an interval surrounding the observed estimated difference obtained from the trial. The constant is determined so as to give the confidence interval the correct probability of including the true, but unknown, difference. This constant is related directly to the critical value used to evaluate test statistics. Trials often use a two-sided α level test (e.g., $\alpha = 0.05$) and a corresponding $(1-\alpha)$ confidence interval (e.g., 95%). If the $1-\alpha$ confidence interval excludes zero, or no difference, we would conclude that the intervention has an effect. If the interval contains zero difference, no treatment effect would be claimed. However, differences of importance might exist but not be detected or statistically significant because the sample size was too small. For testing the null hypothesis of no treatment effect, hypothesis testing and confidence intervals give the same conclusions. However, confidence intervals provide more information on the range of the likely difference that might actually exist. For sample size calculations, a desired confidence interval width must be selected. This typically would be determined by the smallest difference, for example, between two event rates that would be clinically meaningful and important. Under the null hypothesis of no treatment effect, half the desired interval width is equal to the minimal difference specified in the alternative hypothesis. The sample size calculation methods presented here do not preclude the presentation of results as confidence intervals and, in fact, investigators ought to do so. However, unless there is an awareness of the relationship between two approaches, as McHugh and Le[70] have pointed out, the confidence interval method might yield a power of only 50% to detect a specified difference. This can be seen later, when the sample size calculation for comparing proportions is presented. Thus some care needs to be taken in using the confidence interval method.

So far, it has been assumed that the data will be analyzed only once at the end of the trial. However, as discussed in Chapter 15, the response variable data may be reviewed periodically during the course of a study. Thus the probability of finding significant differences by chance alone is increased.[5] This means that the significance level α may need to be adjusted to compensate for the increase in the probability of a type I error.

The sample size calculation should also employ the statistic that will be used in data analysis. Thus there are many sample size formulations. Methods that have proven useful will be discussed.

DICHOTOMOUS RESPONSE VARIABLES

We shall consider two cases for response variables that are dichotomous, that is, yes or no, success or failure, presence or absence. The first case assumes two independent groups or samples.[*] The second case is for dichotomous responses within an individual, or paired responses.[†]

Two independent samples

Suppose the primary response variable is the occurrence of an event over some fixed period. The sample size calculation should be based on the specific test statistic that will be employed to compare the outcomes. The null hypothesis H_0 ($p_C - p_I = 0$) is compared to an alternative hypothesis H_A ($p_C - p_I \neq 0$). The estimates of p_I and p_C are $\hat{p}_I$ and $\hat{p}_C$ where $\hat{p}_I = r_I/N_I$ and $\hat{p}_C = r_C/N_C$ with r_I and r_C being the number of events in the intervention and control groups and N_I and N_C being the number of participants in each group. The usual test statistic for comparing such dichotomous or binomial responses is:

$$Z = (\hat{p}_C - \hat{p}_I) / \sqrt{\bar{p}(1 - \bar{p})(1/N_C + 1/N_I)}$$

where $\bar{p} = (r_I + r_C)/(N_I + N_C)$. The square of the Z statistic is algebraically equivalent to the chi-square statistic that is often employed as well. For large values of N_I and N_C, the statistic Z has approximately a normal distribution with mean 0 and variance 1. If the test statistic Z is larger in absolute value than a constant Z_α, the investigator will reject H_0 in the two-sided test.

The constant Z_α is often referred to as the critical value. The probability of a standard normal random variable being larger in absolute value than Z_α is α. For a one-sided hypothesis, the constant Z_α is chosen such that the probability that Z is greater (or less) than Z_α is α. For a given α, Z_α is larger for a two-sided test than for a one-sided test (Table 7-1). Z_α for a two-sided test with $\alpha = 0.10$ has the same value as Z_α for a one-sided test with $\alpha = 0.05$.

Table 7-1 Z_α for sample size formulas for various values of α

	Z_α	
α	One-sided test	Two-sided test
0.10	1.282	1.645
0.05	1.645	1.960
0.025	1.960	2.240
0.01	2.326	2.576

[*]References 11, 17, 25, 35, 38, 41–43, 51, 59, 71, 107, 108.
[†]References 20, 30, 45, 92, 93.

The sample size required for the design to have a significance level α and a power of $1 - \beta$ to detect true differences of at least δ between the event rates p_I and p_C can be expressed by the formula[60]:

$$2N = 2\left\{Z_\alpha\sqrt{2\bar{p}(1 - \bar{p})} + Z_\beta\sqrt{p_C(1 - p_C) + p_I(1 - p_I)}\right\}^2 \Big/ (p_C - p_I)^2$$

where $2N$ = total sample size (N participants/group) with $\bar{p} = (p_C + p_I)/2$; Z_α is the critical value that corresponds to the significance level α; and Z_β is the value of the standard normal value not exceeded with probability β. Z_β corresponds to the power $1 - \beta$ (e.g., if $1 - \beta = 0.90$, $Z_\beta = 1.282$). Values of Z_α and Z_β are given in Tables 7-1 and 7-2 for several values of α and $1 - \beta$ and may be found in most introductory texts.* Note that the definition of $\bar{p}$ given earlier is equivalent to the definition of $\bar{p}$ given here when $N_I = N_C$; that is, when the two study groups are of equal size. An alternative to the above formula is given by:

$$2N = 4(Z_\alpha + Z_\beta)^2\,\bar{p}(1 - \bar{p}) / (p_C - p_I)^2$$

These two formula give approximately the same answer, and either may be used for the typical clinical trial.

Example

As an example, suppose the annual event rate in the control group is anticipated to be 20%. The investigator hopes that the intervention will reduce the annual rate to 15%. The study is planned so that each participant will be followed for 2 years. Therefore, if the assumptions are accurate, approximately 40% of the participants in the control group and 30% of the participants in the intervention group will develop an event. Thus the investigator sets $p_C = 0.40$, $p_I = 0.30$, and, therefore, $\bar{p} = (0.4 + 0.3)/2 = 0.35$. The study is designed as two-sided with a 5% significance level and 90% power. From Tables 7-1 and 7-2, the two-sided 0.05 critical value is 1.96 for Z_α and 1.282 for Z_β. Substituting these values into the right-hand side of the first sample size formula yields $2N$ to be:

$$2\left\{1.96\sqrt{2(0.35)(0.65)} + 1.282\sqrt{0.4(0.6) + 0.3(0.7)}\right\}^2 \Big/ (0.4 - 0.3)^2$$

Evaluating this expression, $2N = 952.3$. Therefore the calculated total sample size is 960, rounding up to the nearest 10, or 480 in each group. Using the second formula, $2N$ is $4(1.96 + 1.282)^2 (0.35)(0.65)/(0.4 - 0.3)^2$, or $2N = 956$, or 960 after rounding up.

---

*References 4, 14, 28, 36, 37, 89, 102, 113.

Table 7-2 Z_β for sample size formulas for various values of power $(1 - \beta)$

$1 - \beta$	Z_β
0.50	0.00
0.60	0.25
0.70	0.53
0.80	0.84
0.85	1.036
0.90	1.282
0.95	1.645
0.975	1.960
0.99	2.326

Table 7-3 Approximate* total sample size for comparing various proportions in two groups with significance level (α) of 0.05 and power $(1 - \beta)$ of 0.80 and 0.90

True proportions		α = 0.05 (one-sided)		α = 0.05 (two-sided)	
p_C Control group	p_I Intervention group	$1 - \beta$ 0.90	$1 - \beta$ 0.80	$1 - \beta$ 0.90	$1 - \beta$ 0.80
0.60	0.50	850	610	1040	780
	0.40	210	160	260	200
	0.30	90	70	120	90
	0.20	50	40	60	50
0.50	0.40	850	610	1040	780
	0.30	210	150	250	190
	0.25	130	90	160	120
	0.20	90	60	110	80
0.40	0.30	780	560	960	720
	0.25	330	240	410	310
	0.20	180	130	220	170
0.30	0.20	640	470	790	590
	0.15	270	190	330	250
	0.10	140	100	170	130
0.20	0.15	1980	1430	2430	1810
	0.10	440	320	540	400
	0.05	170	120	200	150
0.10	0.05	950	690	1170	870

*Sample sizes are rounded up to the nearest 10.

Sample size tables for independent samples

Sample size estimates using the first formula are given in Table 7-3 for a variety of values of p_I and p_C, for both one-sided and two-sided tests, and for α = 0.05 and $1 - \beta$ = 0.80 or 0.90. For the example just considered with α = 0.05 (two-sided), $1 - \beta$ = 0.90, p_C = 0.4, and p_I = 0.3, the total sample size using Table 7-3 is 960. This table shows that, as the difference in rates between groups increases, the sample size decreases. As the power $(1 - \beta)$ increases, the sample size also increases.

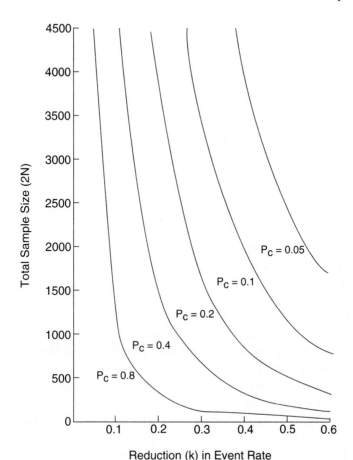

Fig. 7-2 Relationship between total sample size (2N) and reduction (k) in event rate for several control group event rates (p_C), with a two-sided significance level of 0.05 and power of 0.90.

Finally, although not shown in the table, as the significance level α decreases, the sample size increases.

The event rate in the intervention group can be written as $p_I = (1 - k)p_C$ where k represents the proportion that the control group event rate is expected to be reduced by the intervention. Figure 7-2 shows the total sample size 2N vs. k for several values of p_C using a two-sided test with α = 0.05 and 1 − β = 0.90. In the example where $p_C = 0.4$ and $p_I = 0.3$, the intervention is expected to reduce the control rate by 25% or k = 0.25. In Fig. 7-2 locate k = 0.25 on the horizontal axis and move up vertically until the curve labeled p_C = 0.4 is located. The point on this curve corresponds to a 2N of approximately 960. Notice that as the control group event rate p_C decreases, the sample size required to detect the same proportional reduction increases. Studies with small event rates (e.g., p_C = 0.1) require large sample sizes unless the interventions are dramatically effective.

To make use of the sample size formula or table, it is necessary to know something about p_C and k. The estimate for p_C is usually obtained from a previous study of similar people. In addition, the investigator must choose k based on preliminary evidence of the potential effectiveness of the intervention or be willing to specify some minimum difference or reduction that he wants to detect. Obtaining this information is difficult in many cases. Frequently, estimates may be based on a small amount of data. In such cases, several sample size calculations based on a range of estimates help to assess how sensitive the sample size is to the uncertain estimates of p_C, k, or both. The investigator may want to be conservative and take the largest, or nearly largest, estimate of sample size to be sure the study has sufficient power. The power $(1 - \beta)$ for various values of δ can be compared for a given sample size $2N$, significance level α, and control rate p_C. By examining a power curve such as in Fig. 7-1, one can see what power the trial has for detecting various differences in rates, δ. If the power is high, say 0.80 or larger, for the range of values of δ that are of interest, the sample size is probably adequate. The power curve can be especially helpful if the number of available participants is relatively fixed and the investigator wants to assess the probability that the trial can detect any of a variety of reductions in event rates.

Investigators often overestimate the number of eligible participants who can be enrolled in a trial. The actual number enrolled may fall short of the goal. To examine the effects of smaller sample sizes on the power of the trial, the investigator may find it useful to graph power as a function of various sample sizes. If the power falls far below 0.8 for a sample size that is very likely to be obtained, he can expand the recruitment effort, hope for a larger intervention effect than was originally assumed, accept the reduced power and the consequences, or abandon the trial.

Power for independent samples

To determine the power, the first sample size equation is solved for Z_β:

$$Z_\beta = \frac{-Z_\alpha \sqrt{2p(1-p)} + \sqrt{N}(p_C - p_I)}{\sqrt{p_C(1-p_C) + p_I(1-p_I)}}$$

where $\bar{p}$ as before is $(p_C + p_I)/2$. The term Z_β can be translated into a power of $1 - \beta$ by use of Table 7-2. For example, let $p_C = 0.4$ and $p_I = 0.3$. For a significance level of 0.05 in a two-sided test of hypothesis, $Z_\alpha = 1.96$. In a previous example, it is shown that a total sample of approximately 960 participants or 480 per group is necessary to achieve a power of 0.90. Substituting $Z_\alpha = 1.96$, $N = 480$, $p_C = 0.4$, and $p_I = 0.3$, 1.295 is obtained. The closest value of Z_β in Table 7-2 is 1.282, which corresponds to a power of 0.90. (If the exact value of $N = 476$ were used, the value of Z would be 1.282.) Suppose an investigator thought he could get only 350 participants per group instead of the estimated 480. Then $Z_\beta = 0.818$, which means that the power is somewhat less than 0.80. If the value of Z_β is negative, the power is less than

0.50. For more details of power calculations, a standard text in biostatistics* should be consulted.

For a given $2N$, α, $1 - \beta$, and p_C the reduction in event rate that can be detected can also be calculated. This function is nonlinear and therefore the details will not be presented here. Approximate results can be obtained by scanning Table 7-3, by using the formula for several p_I until the sample size approaches the planned number, or by using a figure where sample sizes have been plotted. In Fig. 7-2, $\alpha = 0.05$ and $1 - \beta = 0.90$. If sample size is selected as 1000, with $p_C = 0.4$, k is determined to be about 0.25. This means that the expected p_I would be 0.3. As can be seen in Table 7-3, the actual sample size for these assumptions is 960.

The above approach yields an estimate that is more accurate as the sample size increases. Modifications† have been developed that give some improvement in accuracy to the approximate formula presented for small studies. However, given that sample size estimation is somewhat imprecise because of assumptions of intervention effects and event rates, the formulation presented is probably adequate for most clinical trials.

Confidence interval approach for independent samples

If we were to design a trial comparing proportions using the confidence interval approach, we would need to make a series of assumptions as well.[11,13,70] A $100(1 - \alpha)\%$ confidence interval for a treatment comparison θ would be of the general form $\hat{\theta} \pm Z_\alpha SE(\hat{\theta})$, where $\hat{\theta}$ is the estimate for θ and $SE(\hat{\theta})$ is the standard error. In this case, the specific form would be:

$$\left(\hat{p}_I - \hat{p}_C\right) \pm Z_\alpha \sqrt{\bar{p}(1-\bar{p})(1/N_I + 1/N_C)}.$$

If we want the width of the confidence interval (CI) not to exceed W_{CI}, where W_{CI} is the difference between the upper confidence limit and the lower confidence limit, then if $N = N_I = N_C$, the width W_{CI} can be expressed simply as:

$$W_{CI} = 2Z_\alpha \sqrt{\bar{p}(1-\bar{p})(2/N)}$$

or

$$N = \frac{8 Z_\alpha^2 \bar{p}(1-\bar{p})}{(W_{CI})^2}.$$

Thus, if $\alpha = 0.05$ for a 95% confidence interval, $p_C = 0.4$, and $p_I = 0.3$ or $\bar{p} = 0.35$, $N = 8(1.96)^2(0.35)(0.65)/W_{CI}^2$. If we desire the upper limit of the confidence interval to not be more than 0.10 from the estimate or the width to be twice that, then

---

*References 4, 14, 28, 36, 37, 89, 102, 113.
†References 17, 35, 38, 41–43, 51, 107, 108.

W_{CI} = 0.20 and N = 175 or $2N$ = 375. Notice that even though we are essentially looking for differences in $p_C - p_I$ to be the same as our previous calculation, the sample size is smaller. If we let $p_C - p_I = W_{CI}/2$ and substitute this into the previous sample size formula, we obtain:

$$2N = 2\left\{Z_\alpha + Z_\beta\right\}^2 \bar{p}(1-\bar{p})/\left(W_{CI}/2\right)^2$$

$$= 8\left\{Z_\alpha + Z_\beta\right\}^2 \bar{p}(1-\bar{p})/\left(W_{CI}\right)^2.$$

This formula is very close to the confidence interval formula for two proportions. If we select 50% power, β = 0.50 and Z_β = 0, which would yield the confidence interval formula. Thus a confidence interval approach gives 50% power to detect differences of $W_{CI}/2$. This may not be adequate, depending on the situation. In general, we prefer to specify greater power (e.g., 80% to 90%) and use the previous approach.

Analogous sample size estimation using the confidence interval approach may be used for comparing means, hazard rates, or regression slopes. We do not present details of these since we prefer to use designs that yield power greater than that obtained from a confidence interval approach.

Paired dichotomous response

For designing a trial where the paired outcomes are binary, the sample size estimate is based on McNemar's test.* We want to compare the frequency of success on intervention with the frequency of success on control (i.e., $p_I - p_C$). McNemar's test compares difference in discordant responses within an individual $p_I - p_C$, between intervention and control.

In this case, the number of paired observations, N_p, may be estimated by:

$$N_p = \left|Z_\alpha\sqrt{f} + Z_\beta\sqrt{f-d^2}\right|^2/d^2$$

where d = difference in the proportion of successes ($d = p_I - p_C$) and f is the proportion of participants whose response is discordant; that is, the pair of outcomes are not the same. An alternative approximate formula for N_p is:

$$N_p = \frac{\left[Z_\alpha + Z_\beta\right]^2 f}{d^2}.$$

Example

Consider an eye study where one eye is treated for loss in visual acuity by a new laser procedure and the other eye is treated by standard therapy. The failure rate on

---

*References 20, 30, 45, 92, 93.

the control, p_C, is estimated to be 0.40, and the new procedure is projected to reduce the failure rate to 0.20. The discordant rate f is assumed to be 0.50. Using the latter sample size formula for a two-sided 5% significance level and 90% power, the number of pairs N_p is estimated as 132 since:

$$N_p = \frac{(1.96 + 1.282)^2 (0.5)}{(0.4 - 0.2)^2} = 262 \times 0.5 = 132.$$

If the discordant rate is 0.8, then 210 pairs of eyes will be needed.

Adjusting sample size to compensate for nonadherence

During the course of a clinical trial, participants will not always adhere to their prescribed intervention schedule. The reason is often that the participant cannot tolerate the dosage of the drug or the degree of intervention prescribed in the protocol. The investigator or the participant may then decide to follow the protocol with less intensity. At all times during the conduct of a trial, the participant's welfare must come first, and meeting those needs may not allow some aspects of the protocol to be followed. This is true for primary or secondary prevention trials and for acute or chronic disease trials regardless of the disease. Planners of clinical trials must recognize this phenomenon and attempt to account for it in their design. Examples of adjusting for nonadherence with dichotomous outcomes can be found in several clinical trials.*

In the intervention group a participant who does not adhere to the intervention schedule is often referred to as a "drop-out." Participants who stop the intervention regimen lose whatever potential benefit the intervention might offer. Similarly, a participant on the control regimen may at some time begin to use the intervention that is being evaluated. This participant is referred to as a "drop-in." In the case of a drop-in, a physician may decide, for example, that surgery is required for a participant assigned to medical treatment in a clinical trial of surgery vs. medical care.[18] Drop-in participants from the control group who start the intervention regimen will receive whatever potential benefit or harm that intervention might offer. Therefore both the drop-out and drop-in participants must be acknowledged because they tend to dilute any difference between the two groups that might be produced by the intervention. This simple model does not take into account the situation in which one level of an intervention is compared with another level of the intervention. More complicated models can be developed. Regardless of the model, it must be emphasized that the assumed event rates in the control and intervention groups are modified by participants who do not adhere to the study protocol.

---

*References 6, 8, 18, 22, 55, 57, 74, 81.

People who do not adhere should remain in the assigned groups and be included in the analysis. The rationale for this is discussed in Chapter 16. The basic point to be made here is that eliminating participants from analysis or transferring participants to the other group could easily bias the results of the study. However, the observed δ is likely to be less than projected because of nonadherence, and thus have an impact on the power of the clinical trial. A reduced δ, of course, means that either the sample size must be increased or the study will have smaller power than intended. Lachin[60] has proposed a simple formula to adjust crudely the sample size for a drop-out rate of proportion R_O. This can be generalized to adjust for drop-in rates, R_I, as well. The unadjusted sample size N should be multiplied by the factor $\{1/(1 - R_O - R_I)^2\}$. Thus if $R_O = 0.20$ and $R_I = 0.05$, the originally calculated sample should be multiplied by 16/9 or increased by 78%. This formula gives some quantitative idea of the effect of drop-out on the sample size.

However, more refined models to adjust sample sizes for drop-outs from the intervention to the control[†] and for drop-ins from the control to the intervention regimen[115] have been developed. These models adjust for the resulting changes in p_I and p_C, the adjusted rates being denoted p_I^* and p_C^*. These models also allow for another important factor, which is the time required for the intervention to achieve maximum effectiveness. For example, an antiplatelet drug may have an immediate effect; conversely, even though a cholesterol-lowering drug reduces serum cholesterol levels quickly, it may require years to produce a maximum effect on coronary heart disease.

Example

A drug trial[8] in postmyocardial infarction patients illustrates the effect of drop-outs and drop-ins on sample size. In this trial, total mortality over a 3-year follow-up period was the primary response variable. The mortality rate in the control group was estimated to be 18% ($p_C = 0.18$), and the intervention was believed to have the potential for reducing p_C by 28% ($k = 0.28$), yielding $p_I = 0.1296$. These estimates of p_C and k were derived from previous studies. Those studies also indicated that the drop-out rate might be as high as 26% over the 3 years; 12% in the first year, an additional 8% in the second year, and an additional 6% in the third year. For the control group, the drop-in rate was estimated to be 7% each year for a total drop-in rate of 21%.

Using these models for adjustment, $p_C^* = 0.1746$ and $p_I^* = 0.1375$. Therefore, instead of $\delta = 0.0504$ (0.18 − 0.1296), $\delta^* = 0.0371$ (0.1746 − 0.1375). For a two-sided test with $\alpha = 0.05$ and $1 - \beta = 0.90$, the adjusted sample size was 4020 participants compared with an unadjusted sample size of 2160 participants. The adjusted sample size almost doubled in this example because of the expected drop-out and drop-in experience and the recommended policy of analyzing participants in the originally

---

[†]References 7, 50, 63, 65, 77, 100, 115.

assigned study groups. The remarkable increases in sample size because of drop-outs and drop-ins strongly argue for major efforts to keep nonadherence to a minimum during trials.

SAMPLE SIZE CALCULATIONS FOR CONTINUOUS RESPONSE VARIABLES

Similar to dichotomous outcomes, we consider two sample size cases for response variables that are continuous.[29,60,86] The first case is for two independent samples. The other case is for paired data.

Two independent samples

For a clinical trial with continuous response variables, the previous discussion is conceptually relevant, but not directly applicable, to actual calculations. "Continuous" variables such as length of hospitalization, blood pressure, spirometric measures, neuropsychologic scores, and level of a serum component may be evaluated. Distributions of such measurements frequently can be approximated by a normal distribution. When this is not the case, a transformation of values, such as taking their logarithm, can still make the normality assumption approximately correct.

Suppose the primary response variable, denoted as x, is continuous with N_I and N_C participants randomized to the intervention and control groups, respectively. Assume that the variable x has a normal distribution with mean μ and variance σ^2. The true levels of μ_I and μ_C for the intervention and control groups are not known, but it is assumed that σ^2 is known. (In actual practice, σ^2 is not known and must be estimated from some data. If the data set used is reasonably large, the estimate of σ^2 can be used in place of the true σ^2. If the estimate for σ^2 is based on a small set of data, it is necessary to be cautious in the interpretation of the sample size calculations.)

The null hypothesis is H_0: $\delta = \mu_C - \mu_I = 0$, and the two-sided alternative hypothesis is H_A: $\delta = \mu_C - \mu_I \neq 0$. If the variance is known, the test statistic is:

$$Z = \left(\bar{x}_C - \bar{x}_I\right) / \sigma\sqrt{1/N_C + 1/N_I}.$$

This statistic has approximately a standard normal distribution where $\bar{x}_I$ and $\bar{x}_C$ represent mean levels observed in the intervention and control groups, respectively. The hypothesis-testing concepts previously discussed apply to the above statistic. If $|Z| > Z_\alpha$, then an investigator would reject H_0 at the α level of significance. By use of the above test statistic it can be determined how large a total sample $2N$ would be needed to detect a true difference δ between μ_I and μ_C with power $(1 - \beta)$ and significance level α by the formula:

$$2N = \frac{4\left(Z_\alpha + Z_\beta\right)^2 \sigma^2}{\delta^2}.$$

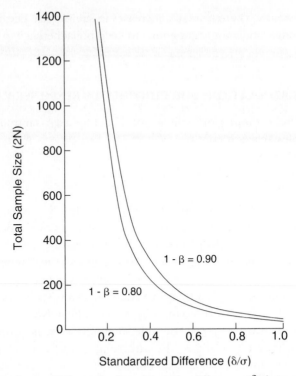

Fig. 7-3 Total sample size (2*N*) required to detect the difference (δ) between control group mean and intervention group mean as a function of the standardized difference (δ/σ) where σ is the common standard deviation, with two-sided significance level of 0.05 and power (1 - β) of 0.80 and 0.90.

For example, suppose an investigator wishes to estimate the sample size necessary to detect a 10 mg/dl difference in cholesterol level in a diet intervention group compared to the control group. The variance from other data is estimated to be (50 mg/dl)². For a two-sided 5% significance level, Z_α = 1.96, and for 90% power, Z_β = 1.282. Substituting these values into the above formula, $2N = 4(1.96 + 1.282)^2(50)^2/10^2$ or approximately 1050 participants. As δ decreases the value of 2*N* increases, and as σ² increases the value of 2*N* increases. This means that the smaller the difference in intervention effect an investigator is interested in detecting and the larger the variance, the larger the study must be. As with the dichotomous case, setting a smaller α and larger 1 - β also increases the sample size. Figure 7–3 shows total sample size 2*N* as a function of δ/σ. As in the example, if δ = 10 and σ = 50, then δ/σ = 0.2 and the sample size 2*N* for 1 - β = 0.9 is approximately 1050.

Paired data

In some clinical trials, paired outcome data may add power to detecting differences because individual variation is reduced. Trial participants may be assessed at baseline and the end of follow-up. Another type of pairing occurs in diseases that affect two organs such as lungs, kidneys, and eyes. In ophthalmology, for example, trials have been conducted where one eye is randomized to receive treatment and the other to receive control therapy.[30,45,92,93] Both the analysis and the sample size estimation need to take account of this special kind of stratification. For continuous outcomes, a mean difference in outcome between a treated and untreated eye would measure the treatment effect and could be compared using a paired t-test,[29,60] $Z = \bar{d}/S_d\sqrt{1/N}$, where $\bar{d}$ is the average difference in response of N pairs and S_d is the sample standard deviation of the differences. The mean difference μ_d is equal to the mean response of the treated or intervention eye, for example, minus the mean response of the control eye; that is $\mu_d = \mu_I - \mu_C$. Under the null hypothesis, $\mu_d = \delta_d$. An estimate of δ_d, $\bar{d}$, can be obtained by taking an estimate of the average differences or by calculating $\bar{x}_I - \bar{x}_C$. The variance of the paired differences σ_d^2 is estimated by S_d^2. Thus, the formula for paired continuous outcomes within an individual is a slight modification of the formula for comparison of means in two independent samples. To compute sample size, N_d, for number of pairs, we compute:

$$N_d = \frac{(Z_\alpha + Z_\beta)^2 \sigma_d^2}{\delta_d^2}.$$

Consider another case of paired data. Instead of looking at the difference between mean levels in the groups, an investigator interested in mean levels of change might want to test whether diet intervention lowers serum cholesterol from baseline levels when compared with a control. This is essentially the same question as asked before in the two independent samples case, but each participant's initial cholesterol level is taken into account. Because of the likelihood of reduced variability, this type of design can lead to a smaller sample size if the question is correctly posed. Assume that Δ_C and Δ_I represent the true but unknown levels of change from baseline to some later point in the trial for the control and intervention groups, respectively. Estimates of Δ_C and Δ_I would be $\bar{d}_C = \bar{x}_{C_1} - \bar{x}_{C_2}$ and $\bar{d}_I = \bar{x}_{I_1} - \bar{x}_{I_2}$. These represent the differences in mean levels of the response variable at two points for each group. The investigator tests H_0: $\Delta_C - \Delta_I = 0$ vs. H_A: $\Delta_C - \Delta_I = \delta \neq 0$. The variance σ_Δ^2 in this case reflects the variability of the change, and is likely to be smaller than the variability at a single measurement. This is the case if the correlation between the first and second measurements is >0.5. Using δ and σ_Δ^2 as defined in this manner, the previous sample size formula and graph are applicable.

Example

Assume that an investigator is still interested in detecting a 10 mg/dl difference in cholesterol between the two groups, but that the variance of the change is now (20 mg/dl)². The question being asked in terms of δ is approximately the same, because randomization should produce baseline mean levels in each group that are almost equal. The comparison of differences in change essentially is a comparison of the difference in mean levels of cholesterol at the second measurement. Using Fig. 7-3, where $\delta/\sigma_\Delta = 10/20 = 0.5$, the sample size is 170. This impressive reduction in sample size from 1050 is due to a reduction in the variance from $(50 \text{ mg/dl})^2$ to $(20 \text{ mg/dl})^2$.

Adjustment for nonadherence

As discussed previously, participants in clinical trials do not always fully adhere to the intervention being tested. Some fraction (R_O) of participants on intervention drop out of the intervention and some other fraction (R_I) drop in and start following the intervention. If we assume that these participants who drop out respond as if they had been on control and those who drop in respond as if they had been on intervention, then the sample size adjustment is the same as for the case of proportions. That is, the adjusted sample size N^* is a function of the drop-out rate, the drop-in rate, and the sample size N for a study with fully adherent participants:

$$N^* = N / \left(1 - R_O - R_I\right)^2.$$

Therefore, if the drop-out rate were 0.20 and the drop-in 0.05, then the original sample size N must be increased by 16/9 or 1.78; that is, a 78% increase in sample size.

SAMPLE SIZE FOR REPEATED MEASURES

The previous section briefly presented the sample size calculation for trials where only two points, say a baseline and a final visit, are used to determine effect of intervention and these two points are the same for all study participants. Often, a continuous response variable is measured at each follow-up visit. Considering only the first and last values would give one estimate of change but would not take advantage of all the available data. Many models exist for the analysis of repeated measurements, and methods for sample size calculation are available for several of these methods.[†] In some cases, the response variable may be categorical. We present one of the simpler models for continuous repeated measurements. While other models are beyond the scope of this text, the basic concepts presented are still useful in thinking about the number of participants, the number of measurements per individual, and when they should be taken. In such a case, one possible approach is to assume that the change in response variable is approximately a linear function of time, so that the rate of change can be summarized by the slope. This model is fit to each participant's data by the standard least squares method, and the estimated slope is used to summarize the participant's experience. In planning such a study, the investigator must be

---

[†]References 24, 58, 62, 67, 75, 80, 91, 97.

concerned about the frequency of the measurement and the duration of the observation period. As discussed by Schlesselman,[97] the observed measurement x can be expressed as $x = a + bt + error$, where a = intercept, b = slope, t = time, and $error$ represents the deviation of the observed measurement from a regression line. This error may be due to measurement variability, biologic variability, or the nonlinearity of the true underlying relationship. On the average, this error is expected to be equally distributed around 0 and have a variability denoted as $\sigma^2_{(error)}$. Schlesselman assumes that $\sigma^2_{(error)}$ is approximately the same for each participant.

The investigator evaluates intervention effectiveness by comparing the average slope in one group with the average slope in another group. Obviously, participants in a group will not have the same slope, but the slopes will vary around some average value that reflects the effectiveness of the intervention or control. The amount of variability of slopes among participants is denoted as σ^2_b. If D represents the total time duration for each participant and P represents the number of equally spaced measurements, σ^2_b can be expressed as:

$$\sigma^2_b = \sigma^2_B + \left\{ \frac{12\,(P-1)\,\sigma^2_{(error)}}{D^2 P\,(P+1)} \right\}$$

where σ^2_B is the component of participant variance in slope not because of measurement error and lack of a linear fit. The sample size required to detect difference δ between the average rates of change in the two groups is given by:

$$2N = \frac{4\left(Z_\alpha + Z_\beta\right)^2}{\delta^2} \left| \sigma^2_B + \frac{12\,(P-1)\sigma^2_{(error)}}{D^2 P\,(P+1)} \right|.$$

As in the previous formulas, when δ decreases, $2N$ increases. The factor on the right-hand side relates D and P with the variance components σ^2_B and $\sigma^2_{(error)}$. Obviously as σ^2_B and $\sigma^2_{(error)}$ increase, the total sample size increases. By increasing P and D, however, the investigator can decrease the contribution made by $\sigma^2_{(error)}$. The exact choices of P and D will depend on how long the investigator can feasibly follow participants, how many times he can afford to have participants visit a clinic, and other features. By manipulating P and D, an investigator can design a study that will be the most cost effective for his specific situation.

Example

In planning for a trial, it may be assumed that a response variable declines at the rate of 80 units/year in the control group. Suppose a 25% reduction is anticipated in the intervention group. That is, the rate of change in the intervention group would be 60 units/year. Other studies provided an estimate for $\sigma_{(error)}$ of 150 units. Also, suppose data from a study of people followed every 3 months for 1 year ($D = 1$) and

$P = 5$ gave a value for the standard deviation of the slopes, $\sigma_b = 200$. The calculated value of σ_B is then 63 units. Thus for a 5% significance level and 90% power ($Z_\alpha = 1.96$ and $Z_\beta = 1.282$), the total sample size would be approximately 630 for a 3-year study with four visits per year ($D = 3$, $P = 13$). Increasing the follow-up time to 4 years, again with four measurements per year, would decrease the variability with a resulting sample size calculation of approximately 510. This reduction in sample size could be used to decide whether to plan a 4- or 3-year study.

SAMPLE SIZE CALCULATIONS FOR "TIME TO FAILURE"

For many clinical trials, the primary response variable is the occurrence of some event, and thus the proportion of events in each group may be compared. In these cases, the sample size methods described earlier will be appropriate. In other trials, the time to the event may be of special interest. For example, if the time to death or some other event can be increased, the intervention may be useful even though at some point the proportions of events in each group are similar. Methods for analysis of this type of outcome are generally referred to as lifetable or survival analysis methods. (See Chapter 14.) In this situation, other sample size approaches are more appropriate.* At the end of this section, we also discuss estimating the number of events required to achieve a desired power.

The basic approach is to compare the survival curves for the groups. A survival curve may be thought of as a graph of the probability of surviving, or not having an event, up to any given point in time. The methods of analysis now widely used are nonparametric; that is, no mathematical model about the shape of the survival curve is assumed. However, for the purpose of estimating sample size, some assumptions are often made. A common model assumes that the survival curve, $S(t)$, follows an exponential distribution, $S(t) = e^{-\lambda t}$, where λ is called the hazard rate or force of mortality. Using this model, survival curves are characterized by λ. Thus the survival curves from a control and an intervention group can be compared by testing H_0: $\lambda_C = \lambda_I$. An estimate of λ is obtained as the inverse of the mean survival time. If the median survival time, T_M, is known, the hazard rate may also be estimated by $-\ln(0.5)/T_M$. One simple formula is given by

$$2N = \frac{4(Z_\alpha + Z_\beta)^2}{|\ln(\lambda_C / \lambda_I)|^2}$$

where N is the size of the sample in each group and Z_α and Z_β are defined as before. As an example, suppose one assumes that the force of mortality is 0.30 in the control group and expects it to be 0.20 for the intervention being tested; that is $\lambda_C / \lambda_I = 1.5$.

---

*References 1, 15, 34, 39, 44, 46, 48, 49, 54, 61, 64, 68, 73, 82–84, 95, 98, 99, 105, 114, 116.

If $\alpha = 0.05$ (two-sided) and $1 - \beta = 0.90$, then $N = 128$ or $2N = 256$. The corresponding mortality rates for 5 years of follow-up are 0.7769 and 0.6321, respectively. Using the comparison of two proportions, the total sample size would be 412. Thus the time-to-failure method may give a more efficient design, requiring a smaller number of participants.

The method just described assumes that all participants will be followed to the event. With few exceptions, clinical trials with a survival outcome are terminated at time T before all participants have had an event. For those still event-free, the time to event is said to be censored at time T. For this situation, Lachin[60] gives the approximate formula:

$$2N = \frac{2(Z_\alpha + Z_\beta)^2 [\phi(\lambda_C) + \phi(\lambda_I)]}{(\lambda_I - \lambda_C)^2}$$

where $\phi(\lambda) = \lambda^2/(1 - e^{-\lambda T})$ and where $\phi(\lambda_C)$ or $\phi(\lambda_P)$ is defined by replacing λ in $\phi(\lambda)$ with λ_C or λ_P, respectively. This assumes instantaneous recruitment of participants or equivalently, each participant is followed for a period of time T. If a 5-year study were being planned ($T = 5$) with the same design specifications as above, then the sample size is equal to 376 ($2N = 376$). Thus the loss of information because of censoring must be compensated for by increasing the sample size.

If the participants are to be recruited continually during the 5 years of the trial, the formula given by Lachin is identical but with $\phi(\lambda) = \lambda^3 T/(\lambda T - 1 + e^{-\lambda T})$. Using the same design assumptions, we obtain $2N = 620$, showing that not having all the participants at the start requires an additional increase in sample size.

More typically participants are recruited uniformly over a period of, T_0, with the trial continuing for T years ($T > T_0$). In this situation, the sample size can be estimated as before using:

$$\phi(\lambda) = \frac{\lambda^2}{1 - [e^{-\lambda(T - T_0)} - e^{-\lambda T}]/\lambda T_0}$$

Consider a case of 3 years of recruitment ($T_0 = 3$) in a 5 year study ($T = 5$). Here, the sample size ($2N$) of 466 is between the previous two examples, suggesting that it is preferable to get participants recruited as rapidly as possible.

Further models are given by Lachin.[60] A useful series of nomograms has been published[99] for sample size considering factors such as α, $1 - \beta$, the participant recruitment time, the follow-up period, and the ratio of the hazard rates.

One of the methods used for comparing survival curves is the proportional hazards model or the Cox regression model that is discussed briefly in Chapter 14. For this method, sample size estimates have been provided.[39,98] As it turns out, the formula by Schoenfeld for the Cox model[98] is identical to that given above for the simple exponential case, although developed from a different point of view.

All of the above methods assume that the hazard rate remains constant during the course of the trial. This may not be the case. The Beta-Blocker Heart Attack Trial[8] compared 3-year survival in two groups of subjects with intervention starting 1 to 3 weeks after a myocardial infarction. The risk of death was high initially, decreased steadily, and then became relatively constant.

For cases where the event rate is relatively small and the clinical trial will have considerable censoring, most of the statistical information will be in the number of events. Thus the sample size estimates using simple proportions will be quite adequate. In the Beta-Blocker Heart Attack Trial, the 3-year control group event rate was assumed to be 0.18. For the intervention group, the event rate was assumed to be approximately 0.13. In the situation of $\phi(\lambda) = \lambda^2(1 - e^{-\lambda T})$, a sample size $2N = 2208$ is obtained. In contrast, the unadjusted sample size using simple proportions is 2160. Again, it should be emphasized that all of these methods are only approximations, and the estimates should be viewed as such.

As the previous example indicates, the power of a survival analysis still is a function of the number of events. Lachin[60,61] has shown that the expected number of events $E(D)$ is a function of sample size, hazard rate, recruitment rate, and censoring distribution. Specifically, the expected number of events in the control group can be estimated as:

$$E\left(D\right) = N\lambda_C^2 / \Phi\left(\lambda_C\right)$$

where $\Phi(\lambda_C)$ is defined as before, depending on the recruitment and follow-up strategy. If we assume a uniform recruitment over the interval $(0,T_0)$ and follow-up over the interval $(0,T)$, then $E(D)$ can be written using the most general form for $\Phi(\lambda_C)$;

$$E\left(D\right) = N\left[1 - \frac{e^{-\lambda(T - T_0)} - e^{-\lambda T}}{\lambda T_0}\right]$$

This estimate of the number of events can be used to predict the number of events at various time points during the trial, including the end of follow-up. This prediction can be compared with the observed number of events in the control group to determine if an adjustment needs to be made to the design. This is, if the number of events early in the trial is larger than expected, the trial may be more powerful than designed or may be stopped earlier than the planned T years of follow-up. (See Chapter 15.) However, more worrisome is when the observed number of events is smaller than what is expected and needed to maintain adequate power. Based on this early information, the design may be modified to attain the necessary number of events by: (1) increasing the sample size (increased T_0 or expanding recruitment effort within the same period); (2) increasing follow-up (T); or (3) a combination of both.

This method can be illustrated based on a placebo-controlled trial of congestive heart failure.[81] Severe or advanced congestive heart failure has an expected 1-year event rate of 40%, where the events are all-cause mortality and nonfatal myocardial infarction. A new drug was to be tested to reduce the event rate by 25%, using a two-sided 5% significance level and 90% power. If participants are recruited over 1.5 years ($T_0 = 1.5$) during a 2-year study ($T = 2$) and a constant hazard rate is assumed, the total sample size ($2N$) is estimated to be 820 patients with congestive heart failure. The formula $E(D)$ can be used to calculate that approximately 190 events (deaths plus nonfatal myocardial infarctions) must be observed in the control group to attain 90% power. If the first-year event rate turns out to be < 40%, fewer events will be observed by 2 years than the required 190. Table 7-4 shows the expected number of control group events at 6 months and 1 year into the study for annual event rates of 40%, 35%, 30%, and 25%. Two years is also shown to illustrate the projected number of events at the completion of the study. These numbers are obtained by calculating the number of participants enrolled by 6 months (33% of 400) and 1 year (66% of 400) and multiplying by the $\lambda_C^2/\Phi(\lambda_C)$ term in the equation for $E(D)$. If the assumed annual event rate of 40% is correct, 16 control group events should be observed at 6 months and 60 events at 1 year. However, if at 1 year only 44 events are observed, the annual event rate might be closer to 30% (i.e., $\lambda = 0.357$), and some design modification should be considered to assure achieving the desired 190 control group events. One year would be a sensible time to make this decision, based only on control group events, since recruitment efforts are still underway. For example, if recruitment efforts could be expanded to 1220 patients in 1.5 years, then by 2 years of follow-up the 190 events in the placebo group would

Table 7-4   Number of expected events (in the control group) at each interim analysis given different event rates in control group

	Number of expected events			
	Calendar time into study			
Yearly event rate in control group	6 Months (N = 138/group)	1 Year (N = 275/group)	1.5 Years (N = 412/group)	2 Years (N = 412/group)
40%	16	60	124	189
35%	14	51	108	167
30%	12	44	94	146
25%	10	36	78	123

Assumptions:
  1. Time to event is exponentially distributed.
  2. Uniform entry into the study over 1.5 years.
  3. Total duration of the study will be 2 years.

be observed and the 90% power would be maintained. If recruitment efforts were continued for another 6 months at a uniform rate ($T_0 = 2$ years), another 135 participants might be enrolled. In this case, $E(D) = 545 \times 0.285 = 155$ events, which would not be sufficient without some additional follow-up. If recruitment and follow-up continued for 27 months (i.e., $T_0 = T = 2.25$), then 605 control group participants would be recruited and $E(D) = 187$, which would provide the desired power.

SAMPLE SIZE FOR TESTING "EQUIVALENCY" OF INTERVENTIONS

In some instances, an effective intervention has already been established and is considered the standard. New interventions under consideration may be less expensive, have fewer side effects, or have less impact on an individual's general quality of life, and thus may be preferred. This issue is common in the pharmaceutical industry, where a product developed by one company may be tested against an established intervention manufactured by another company. Studies of this type are sometimes referred to as trials with positive controls.

Given that several trials have shown that certain beta-blockers are effective in reducing mortality in postmyocardial infarction patients,[8,52,79] it is likely that any new beta-blockers developed will be tested against proven agents, at least for that indication. The Nocturnal Oxygen Therapy Trial[78] tested whether the daily amount of oxygen administered to chronic obstructive lung disease patients could be reduced from 24 to 12 hours without impairing oxygenation. The Intermittent Positive Pressure Breathing Trial[57] considered whether a simple and less expensive method for delivering a bronchodilator into the lungs would be as effective as a more expensive device. A breast cancer trial compared the tumor regression rates between subjects receiving the standard, diethylstilbestrol, and the newer agent, tamoxifen.[56] As no significant difference in effectiveness was found, tamoxifen was recommended because of less toxicity.

The problem in designing positive control studies is that there can be no statistical method to demonstrate complete equivalence. That is, it is not possible to show $\delta = 0$. Failure to reject the null hypothesis is not sufficient reason to claim two interventions to be equal but merely that the evidence is inadequate to say they are different.[103] Computing a sample size assuming no difference, using the previously described formulas, results in an infinite sample size.

While demonstrating complete equivalence is an impossible task, one possible approach has been discussed.[9,10,69] The strategy is to specify some value, δ, such that interventions with differences that are less than this might be considered equally effective or equivalent. Specification of δ may be difficult, but without it, no study can be designed. The null hypothesis states that differences are greater than δ, while the alternative specifies differences less than δ. The methods developed require that if the two interventions really are equally effective, the upper $100(1 - \alpha)$% confidence interval for the intervention difference will not exceed δ with the probability of 1 - β. One can alternatively approach this from a hypothesis-testing point of view, stating the null hypothesis that the two interventions differ by less than δ.

For studies with a dichotomous response, one might assume the event rate for the two interventions to be equal to p (i.e., $p = p_C = p_I$). This simplifies the previously shown sample size formula to the following:

$$2N = 4p(1 - p)(Z_\alpha + Z_\beta)^2 / \delta^2$$

where N, Z_α, and Z_β are defined as before. (This formula differs slightly from the analogue presented earlier because of the different way the hypothesis is stated.) Makuch and Simon[69] recommend for this situation that $\alpha = 0.10$ and $\beta = 0.20$. However, for many situations, β, or type-II error needs to be 0.10 or smaller to be sure a new therapy is correctly allowed to replace an older standard. We prefer an $\alpha = 0.05$, but this is a matter of judgment and will depend on the situation. The formula for continuous variables,

$$2N = \frac{4(Z_\alpha + Z_\beta)^2}{(\sigma / \delta)^2}$$

is identical to the formula for determining sample size discussed earlier. Blackwelder and Chang[10] give graphical methods for computing sample size estimates for studies of equivalence.

Another proposed strategy for comparing a new to a standard drug is to show bioequivalence or similarity in bioavailability. Several authors have discussed this approach.[3,32,109,110] If two formulations are within specified limits for a profile of biochemical measurements and one of them has already been proven to be effective, the argument is made that further efficacy trials are not necessary. The sample size estimation for demonstrating bioequivalence poses the same problem as described above, and the approach is similar.

SAMPLE SIZE FOR CLUSTER RANDOMIZATION

So far, sample size estimates have been presented for randomizing individuals. For some prevention trials or health care studies, it may not be possible to randomize individual participants. For example, a trial of smoking prevention strategy for teenagers may be implemented most easily by randomizing schools, some schools to be exposed to the new prevention strategy while other schools remain with the standard approach. Individual students are grouped or clustered within each school. As Donner[31] et al point out, "Since one cannot regard the individuals within such groups as statistically independent, standard sample size formulas underestimate the total number of subjects required for the trial." Several authors[31,53,66] have suggested a single inflation factor to the usual sample size to account for the cluster randomization. That is, the sample size per intervention arm N computed by previous formulas will be adjusted to N^* to account for the randomization of N_m clusters, each of size m.

Continuous response

For a continuous response variable, the response is measured on each individual within a cluster. Differences of individuals within a cluster and differences of individuals between clusters contribute to the overall variability of the response. We can separate the between cluster variance σ_b^2 and within cluster variance σ_w^2. Estimates are denoted S_b^2 and S_w^2, respectively, and can be estimated by standard analysis of variance. One measure of the relationship of these components is the intraclass correlation coefficient. The intraclass correlation coefficient ρ is $\sigma_b^2/(\sigma_w^2 + \sigma_b^2)$ where $0 \le \rho \le 1$. If $\rho = 0$, all clusters respond identically, so all of the variability is within a cluster. If $\rho = 1$, all individuals in a cluster respond alike, so there is no variability within a cluster. Estimates of ρ are given by $r = S_b^2/(S_b^2 + S_w^2)$. Intraclass correlation may range from 0.1 to 0.4 in typical clinical studies. If we assume that we computed the sample size calculations assuming no clustering, the sample size per arm would be N participants per treatment arm. Now, instead of randomizing N individuals, we want to randomize N_m clusters each of size m individuals for a total of $N^* = N_m \times m$ participants per treatment arm. The inflation factor[31] is $[1 + (m - 1)r]$ so that

$$N^* = N_m \times m = N \left[1 + (m-1)\rho \right]$$

Note that the inflation factor is a function of both cluster size m and intraclass correlation. If the intraclass correlation ρ is 0, then each individual in one cluster responds like any individual in another cluster, and the inflation factor is unity ($N^* = N$). That is, no penalty is paid for the convenience of cluster randomization. At the other extreme, if all individuals in a cluster respond the same ($\rho = 1$), there is no added information within each cluster, so only one individual per cluster is needed, and the inflation factor is m. That is, our adjusted sample $N^* = N \times m$, and we pay a severe price for this type of cluster randomization. However, it is unlikely that ρ is either 0 or 1, but as indicated, ρ is more likely to be in the range of 0.1 to 0.4 in clinical studies.

Example

Donner et al.[31] provide an example for a trial randomizing households to a sodium-reducing diet to reduce blood pressure. Previous studies estimated the intraclass correlation coefficient to be 0.2; that is $\hat{\rho} = r = S_b^2/(S_b^2 + S_w^2) = 0.2$. The average household size was estimated at 3.5 ($m = 3.5$). Thus the sample size per arm N must be adjusted by $1 + (m - 1)\rho = 1 + (3.5 - 1)(0.2) = 1.5$. Thus the normal sample size must be inflated by 50% to account for this randomization indicating a small between-cluster variability. If $\rho = 0.1$, then the factor is $1 + (3.5 - 1)(0.1)$ or 1.25. If $\rho = 0.4$, indicating a larger between-cluster component of variability, the inflation factor is 2.0 or a doubling.

Binomial response

For binomial responses, a similar expression for adjusting the standard sample size can be developed. In this setting, a measure of the degree of within cluster dependency or concordancy rate in participant responses is used in place of the intraclass correlation. The commonly used measure is the kappa coefficient, denoted κ, and may be thought of as an intraclass correlation coefficient for binomial responses, analogous to ρ for continuous responses. A concordant cluster with $\kappa = 1$ is one where all responses within a cluster are identical, all successes or failures, in which a cluster contributes no more than a single individual. A simple estimate for κ is provided by Donner,[31]

$$\kappa = \frac{p^* - \left[p_C^m + \left(1 - p_C \right)^m \right]}{1 - \left[p_C^m + \left(1 - p_C \right)^m \right]}$$

where p^* is the proportion of the control group with concordant clusters, and p_C is the underlying success rate in the control group. Donner then shows that the inflation factor is $[1 + (m - 1)\kappa]$, or that the regular sample size per treatment arm N must be multiplied by this factor to attain the adjusted sample size N^*:

$$N^* = N \left[1 + \left(m - 1 \right) \kappa \right].$$

Example

Donner[31] continues the sodium diet example where couples ($m = 2$) are randomized to either a low-sodium or a normal diet. The outcome is the hypertension rate. Other data suggest the concordancy of hypertension status among married couples is 0.85 ($p^* = 0.85$). The control group hypertension rate is 0.15 ($p_C = 0.15$). In this case, $\hat{\kappa} = 0.41$, so that the inflation factor is $1 + (2 - 1)(0.41) = 1.41$; that is, the regular sample size must be inflated by 41% to adjust for the couples being the randomization unit. If there is perfect control group concordance, $p^* = 1$ and $\kappa = 1$, in which case $N^* = 2N$.

Cornfield[21] proposed another adjustment procedure. Consider a trial where m clusters will be randomized, each cluster of size c_i (i = 1, 2, ..., m) and each having a different success rate of p_i (i = 1, 2, ..., m). Define the average cluster size $\bar{c} = \Sigma\, c_i/m$ and $\bar{p} = \Sigma\, c_i\, p_i / \Sigma\, c_i$ as the overall success rate weighted by cluster size. The variance of the overall success rate $\sigma_p^2 = \Sigma\, c_i(p_i - \bar{p})^2/m\bar{c}^2$. In this setting, the efficiency of simple randomization to cluster randomization is $E = \bar{p}\,(1 - \bar{p})\bar{c}\ \sigma_p^2$. The inflation factor for this design is IF $= 1/E = \bar{c}\, \sigma_p^2/(1 - \bar{p})$. Note that if the response rate varies across clusters, the normal sample size must be increased.

While cluster randomization may be logistically required, the process of making the cluster the randomization has serious sample size implications. It would be unwise to ignore this consequence in the design phase. As shown, the sample size adjustments can easily be factors of 1.5 or higher. For clusters that are schools or cities, the intraclass correlation is likely to be quite small. However, the cluster size is multiplied by the intraclass correlation, so the impact might still be nontrivial. Not making this adjustment would substantially reduce the study power if the analyses were done properly, taking into account the cluster effect. Ignoring the cluster effect would be critically viewed in most cases and is not recommended.

ESTIMATING SAMPLE SIZE PARAMETERS

As shown in the methods presented, sample size estimation depends on assumptions made about variability of the response, level of response in the control group, and difference anticipated or judged to be clinically relevant.* Obtaining reliable estimates of variability or levels of response can be challenging since the information is often based on very small studies or studies not exactly relevant to the trial being designed. Sometimes, pilot or feasibility studies may be conducted to obtain these data. In such cases, the term *external pilot* has been used.[112]

In some cases, the information may not exist before starting the trial, as was the case for early trials in AIDS; that is, no baseline incidence rates were available in an evolving epidemic. Even in cases where data are available, other factors affect the variability or level of response observed in a trial. Typically, the variability observed in the planned trial is larger than expected or the level of response is smaller or lower than planned. Numerous examples of these phenomena exist.[19] One example is provided by the Physicians' Health Study.[88] In this trial, 22,000 U.S. male physicians were randomized into a 2×2 factorial design. One factor was aspirin vs. placebo in reducing cardiovascular mortality. The other factor was beta-carotene vs. placebo for reducing cancer incidence. The aspirin portion of the trial was terminated early, in part because of a substantially lower mortality rate than assumed for in the design. In the design, the cardiovascular mortality rate was assumed to be approximately 50% of the U.S. age-adjusted rate in men. However, after 5 years of follow-up, the cardiovascular mortality rate was approximately 10% of the U.S. rate in men. This substantial difference reduced the power of the trial dramatically. To compensate for the extremely low event rate, the trial would have had to be extended another 10 years to get the necessary number of events.[88] The trial was terminated early in part because of very low power for the primary comparison. One can only speculate about reasons for low event rates, but screening of participants before entry almost certainly played a part. That is, participants had to complete a run-in period and be able to tolerate aspirin. Participants at risk for other

---

*References 19, 33, 76, 85, 101, 111, 112.

competing events were also excluded. This type of effect is referred to as a screening effect. Also, physicians who begin to develop cardiovascular symptoms may obtain care earlier than the typical U.S. man. Finally, in general, volunteers tend to be healthier than the general age-specific population, a phenomenon often referred to as the healthy volunteer effect.

Another approach to obtaining estimates for ultimate sample size determination is to design so-called internal pilot studies.[112] In this approach, a small study is initiated based on the best available information. A general sample target for the full study may be proposed, but the goal of the pilot is to refine the sample size estimate based on screening and healthy volunteer effects. The pilot study uses a protocol very close or identical to the protocol for the full study, and thus parameter estimates will reflect screening and volunteer effects. If the protocol for the pilot and the main study are essentially identical, then the small pilot can become an internal pilot. That is, the data from the internal pilot become part of the data for the overall study. This approach, in fact, was used successfully in the Diabetes Control and Complications Trial.[27] If data from the internal pilot are used only to refine estimates of variability or control group response rates, and the study design incorporates no changes in intervention effect, then the impact of this two-step approach on the significance level is negligible. The benefit is that the design will more likely have the desired power than if data from external pilots and other sources are relied on exclusively.[101] It must be emphasized that pilot studies, either external or internal, should not be viewed as instructive about intervention effect.[112] Small or no differences in intervention effect may erroneously be viewed as reason not to continue because power is too small in pilots to be sure that no effect exists. A positive trend may also be viewed as evidence that a large study is not necessary, or that clinical equipoise no longer exists.

Our experience indicates that both external and internal pilot studies are quite helpful. Internal pilot studies should be used if at all possible in prevention trials, where screening and healthy volunteer effects seem to cause major design problems. Design modifications based on an internal pilot are more prudent than allowing an inadequate sample size to create problems several years later.

Another approach is to specify the number of outcome events needed for a desired power level. Obtaining the specified number of events requires some number of individuals followed for some period. The number of participants and the duration of the follow-up period can be adjusted during the early part of the trial or during an internal pilot study, but the target number of outcome events does not change. This is discussed in more detail in Chapter 15.

MULTIPLE RESPONSE VARIABLES

We have stressed the advantages of having a single primary question and a single primary response variable, but clinical trials occasionally have more than one of each. More than one question may be asked because investigators cannot agree about which factor is most important. As an example, one clinical trial involving two schedules of oxygen administration to patients with chronic obstructive lung disease had three major questions in addition to comparing the mortality rate.[78] Measures of pulmonary function, neuropsychologic status, and quality of life were evaluated. For the participants, all three are important.

Sometimes more than one primary response variable is used to assess a single primary question. A clinical trial involving patients with pulmonary embolism[106] employed three methods of assessing a drug's ability to resolve emboli. They were: lung scanning, arteriography, and hemodynamic studies. Another trial involved the use of drugs to limit myocardial infarct size.[90] Precordial electrocardiogram mapping, radionuclide studies, and enzyme levels all were used to evaluate the effectiveness of the drugs.

Computing a sample size for such clinical trials is not easy. One could attempt to define a single model for the multidimensional response and use one of the previously discussed formulas. Such a method would require several assumptions about the model and its parameters and might require information about correlations between different measurements. Such information is rarely available. A more reasonable procedure would be to compute sample sizes for each individual response variable. If the results give about the same sample size for all variables, then the issue is resolved. However, more commonly, a range of sample sizes will be obtained. The most conservative strategy would be to use the largest sample size computed. The other response variables would then have even greater power to detect the hoped-for reductions or differences (since they required smaller sample sizes). Unfortunately, this approach is the most expensive and difficult to undertake. Of course, one could also choose the smallest sample size of those computed. That would probably not be desirable, because the other response variables would have less power than usually required, or only larger differences than expected would be detectable. It is possible to select a middle-range sample size, but there is no assurance that this will be appropriate. An alternative approach is to look at the difference between the largest and smallest sample sizes. If this difference is very large, the assumptions that went into the calculations should be reexamined, and an effort should be made to resolve the difference.

As will be discussed in Chapter 16, when multiple comparisons are made, the chance of finding a significant difference in one of the comparisons (when, in fact, no real differences exist between the groups) is greater than the stated significance level. To maintain an appropriate significance level α for the entire study, the significance level required for each test to reject H_0 should be adjusted.[5] The significance level required for rejection (α') in a single test can be approximated by α/k where k is the number of multiple response variables. For several response variables this can make α' fairly small (e.g., $k = 5$ implies $\alpha' = 0.01$ for each of k response variables with an overall $\alpha = 0.05$). If the correlation between response variables is known, then the adjustment can be made more precisely.[72] In all cases, the sample size would be much larger than if the use of multiple response variables were ignored, so that most studies have not strictly adhered to this solution of modifying the significance level. Some investigators, however, have attempted to be conservative in the analysis of results.[23] There is a reasonable limit as to how much α' can be decreased to give protection against false rejection of the null hypothesis. Some investigators have chosen $\alpha' = 0.01$ regardless of the number of tests. In the end, there are no easy solutions. A somewhat conservative value of α' needs to be set, and the investigator needs to be aware of the multiple testing problem during the analysis.

REFERENCES

1. Akazawa K, Nakamura T, Moriguchi S, et al: Simulation program for estimating statistical power of Cox's proportional hazards model assuming no specific distribution for the survival time, *Comput Methods Programs Biomed* 35:203-212, 1991.
2. Altman DG: Statistics and ethics in medical research: 111. How large a sample? *Br Med J* 281:1336-1338, 1980.
3. Anderson S, Hauck WW: A new procedure for testing equivalence in comparative bioavailability and other clinical trials, *Commun Statist-Theory Meth* A12(23):2663-2692, 1983.
4. Armitage P: *Statistical Methods in Medical Research,* New York, 1971, John Wiley & Sons.
5. Armitage P, McPherson CK, Rowe BC: Repeated significance tests on accumulating data, *J R Stat Soc Ser A* 132:235-244, 1969.
6. Aspirin Myocardial Infarction Study Research Group: A randomized controlled trial of aspirin in persons recovered from myocardial infarction, *JAMA* 243:661-669, 1980.
7. Barlow W, Azen S, The Silicone Study Group: The effect of therapeutic treatment crossovers on the power of clinical trials, *Controlled Clin Trials* 11:314-326, 1990.
8. Beta-Blocker Heart Attack Trial Research Group: A randomized trial of propranolol in patients with acute myocardial infarction. 1. Mortality results, *JAMA* 247:1701-1714, 1982.
9. Blackwelder WC: "Proving the null hypothesis" in clinical trials, *Controlled Clin Trials* 3:345-353, 1982.
10. Blackwelder WC, Chang MA: Sample size graphs for "proving the null hypothesis," *Controlled Clin Trials* 5:97-105, 1984.
11. Bristol DR: Sample sizes for constructing confidence intervals and testing hypotheses, *Stat Med* 8:803-811, 1989.
12. Brittain E, Schlesselman JJ: Optimal allocation for the comparison of proportions, *Biometrics* 38:1003-1009, 1982.
13. Brown BW Jr: Statistical controversies in the design of clinical trials—some personal views, *Controlled Clin Trials* 1:13-27, 1980.
14. Brown BW, Hollander M: *Statistics-A Biomedical Introduction,* New York, 1977, John Wiley & Sons.
15. Cantor AB: Power estimation for rank tests using censored data: conditional and unconditional, *Controlled Clin Trials* 12:462-473, 1991.
16. Cardiac Arrhythmia Suppression Trial (CAST) Investigators: Preliminary report: effect of encainide and flecainide on mortality in a randomized trial of arrhythmia suppression after myocardial infarction, *N Engl J Med* 321:406-412, 1989.
17. Casagrande JT, Pike MC, Smith PG: An improved approximate formula for calculating sample sizes for comparing two binomial distributions, *Biometrics* 34:483-486, 1978.
18. CASS Principal Investigators and Their Associates: Coronary Artery Surgery Study (CASS): A randomized trial of coronary artery bypass surgery: survival data, *Circulation* 68:939-950, 1983.
19. Church TR, Ederer F, Mandel JS, et al: Estimating the duration of ongoing prevention trials, *Am J Epidemiol* 137:797-810, 1993.
20. Connor RJ: Sample size for testing differences in proportions for the paired-sample design, *Biometrics* 43:207-211, 1987.
21. Cornfield J: Randomization by group: a formal analysis, *Am J Epidemiol* 108:100-102, 1978.
22. Coronary Drug Project Research Group: The Coronary Drug Project. Design, methods, and baseline results, *Circulation* 47(suppl I):I1-I79, 1973.
23. Coronary Drug Project Research Group: Clofibrate and niacin in coronary heart disease, *JAMA* 231:360-381, 1975.

24. Dawson JD, Lagakos SW: Size and power of two-sample tests of repeated measures data, *Biometrics* 49:1022-1032, 1993.

25. Day SJ: Optimal placebo response rates for comparing two binomial proportions, *Stat Med* 7:1187-1194, 1988.

26. Day SJ, Graham DF: Sample size estimation for comparing two or more treatment groups in clinical trials, *Stat Med* 10:33-43, 1991.

27. Diabetes Complications and Control Trial Research Group: The effect of intensive treatment of diabetes on the development and progression of long-term complications in insulin-dependent diabetes mellitus, *N Engl J Med* 329:977-986, 1993.

28. Dixon WJ, Massey FJ Jr: *Introduction to Statistical Analysis*, ed 3, New York, 1969, McGraw-Hill.

29. Donner A: Approaches to sample size estimation in the design of clinical trials—a review, *Stat Med* 3:199-214, 1984.

30. Donner A: Statistical methods in ophthalmology: an adjusted chi-square approach, *Biometrics* 45:605-611, 1989.

31. Donner A, Birkett N, Buck C: Randomization by cluster, sample size requirements and analysis, *Am J Epidemiol* 114:906-914, 1981.

32. Dunnett CW, Gent M: Significance testing to establish equivalence between treatments, with special reference to data in the form of 2 × 2 tables, *Biometrics* 33:593-602, 1977.

33. Ederer F, Church TR, Mandel JS: Sample sizes for prevention trials have been too small, *Am J Epidemiol* 137:787-796, 1993.

34. Emerich LJ: Required duration and power determinations for historically controlled studies of survival times, *Stat Med* 8:153-160, 1989.

35. Feigl P: A graphical aid for determining sample size when comparing two independent proportions, *Biometrics* 34:111-122, 1978.

36. Fisher L, Van Belle G: *Biostatistics—a Methodology for the Health Sciences,* New York, 1993, John Wiley & Sons.

37. Fleiss JL: *Statistical Methods for Rates and Proportions*, ed 2, New York, 1981, John Wiley & Sons.

38. Fleiss JL, Tytun A, Ury HK: A simple approximation for calculating sample sizes for comparing independent proportions, *Biometrics* 36:343-346, 1980.

39. Freedman LS: Tables of the number of patients required in clinical trials using the logrank test, *Stat Med* 1:121-129, 1982.

40. Frieman JA, Chalmers TC, Smith H Jr, Kuebler RR: The importance of beta, the type II error and sample size in the design and interpretation of the randomized control trial: survey of 71 "negative" trials, *N Engl J Med* 299:690-694, 1978.

41. Fu YX, Arnol J: A table of exact sample sizes for use with Fisher's exact test for 2 × 2 tables, *Biometrics* 48:1103-1112, 1992.

42. Gail M: The determination of sample sizes for trials involving several independent 2 × 2 tables, *J Chronic Dis* 26:669-673, 1973.

43. Gail M, Gart JJ: The determination of sample sizes for use with the exact conditional test in 2 × 2 comparative trials, *Biometrics* 29:441-448, 1973.

44. Gail MH: Applicability of sample size calculations based on a comparison of proportions for use with the logrank test, *Controlled Clin Trials* 6:112-119, 1985.

45. Gauderman WJ, Barlow WE: Sample size calculations for ophthalmologic studies, *Arch Ophthalmol* 110:690-692, 1992.

46. George SL, Desu MM: Planning the size and duration of a clinical trial studying the time to some critical event, *J Chronic Dis* 27:15-24, 1974.

47. Gore SM: Assessing clinical trials—trial size, *Br Med J* 282:1687-1689, 1981.

48. Gross AJ, Hunt HH, Cantor AB, Clark BC: Sample size determination in clinical trials with an emphasis on exponentially distributed responses, *Biometrics* 43:875-883, 1987.

49. Halperin M, Johnson NJ: Design and sensitivity evaluation of follow-up studies for risk factor assessment, *Biometrics* 37:805-810, 1981.

50. Halperin M, Rogot E, Gurian J, Ederer F: Sample sizes for medical trials with special reference to long-term therapy, *J Chronic Dis* 21:13-24, 1968.

51. Haseman JK: Exact sample sizes for use with the Fisher-Irwin Test for 2 × 2 tables, *Biometrics* 34:106-109, 1978.

52. Hjalmarson A, Herlitz J, Malex I, et al: Effect on mortality of metoprolol in acute myocardial infarction: a double-blind randomized trial, *Lancet* II:823-827, 1981.

53. Hsieh FY: Sample size formulae for intervention studies with the cluster as unit of randomization, *Stat Med* 8:1195-1201, 1988.

54. Hsieh FY: Sample size tables for logistic regression, *Stat Med* 8:795-802, 1989.

55. Hypertension Detection and Follow-up Program Cooperative Group: Five-year findings of the Hypertension Detection and Follow-up Program. Reduction in mortality of persons with high blood pressure, including mild hypertension, *JAMA* 242:2562-2571, 1979.

56. Ingle JN, Ahmann DL, Green SJ, et al: Randomized clinical trial of diethylstilbestrol versus tamoxifen in postmenopausal women with advanced breast cancer, *N Engl J Med* 304:16-21, 1981.

57. The Intermittent Positive Pressure Breathing Trial Group: Intermittent positive pressure breathing therapy of chronic obstructive pulmonary disease—a clinical trial, *Ann Intern Med* 99:612-620, 1983.

58. Kirby AJ, Galai N, Muñoz A: Sample size estimation using repeated measurements on biomarkers as outcomes, *Controlled Clin Trials* 15:165-172, 1994.

59. Lachenbruch PA: A note on sample size computation for testing interactions, *Stat Med* 7:467-469, 1988.

60. Lachin JM: Introduction to sample size determination and power analysis for clinical trials, *Controlled Clin Trials* 2:93-113, 1981.

61. Lachin JM, Foulkes MA: Evaluation of sample size and power for analyses of survival with allowance for nonuniform patient entry, losses to follow-up, noncompliance, and stratification, *Biometrics* 42:507-519, 1986. (Correction: 42:1009, 1986.)

62. Laird NM, Wang F: Estimating rates of change in randomized clinical trials, *Controlled Clin Trials* 11:405-419, 1990.

63. Lakatos E: Sample size determination in clinical trials with time-dependent rates of losses and noncompliance, *Controlled Clin Trials* 7:189-199, 1986.

64. Lakatos E: Sample sizes based on the log-rank statistic in complex clinical trials, *Biometrics* 44:229-241, 1988.

65. Lavori P: Statistical issues: sample size and drop out. In Benkert O, Maier W, Rickels K, eds: *Methodology of the Evaluation of Psychotropic Drugs*, Berlin, 1990, Springer-Verlag.

66. Lee EW, Dubin N: Estimation and sample size considerations for clustered binary responses, *Stat Med* 13:1241-1252, 1994.

67. Lipsitz SR, Fitzmaurice GM: Sample size for repeated measures studies with binary responses, *Stat Med* 13:1233-1239, 1994.

68. Lui KJ: Sample size determination under an exponential model in the presence of a confounder and type I censoring, *Controlled Clin Trials* 13:446-458, 1992.

69. Makuch R, Simon R: Sample size requirements for evaluating a conservative therapy, *Cancer Treat Rep* 62:1037-1040, 1978.

70. McHugh RB, Le CT: Confidence estimation and the size of a clinical trial, *Controlled Clin Trials* 5:157-163, 1984.

71. McMahon RP, Proschan M, Geller NL, et al: Sample size calculation for clinical trials in which entry criteria and outcomes are counts of events, *Stat Med* 13:859-870, 1994.

72. Miller RG: *Simultaneous Statistical Inference,* New York, 1966, McGraw-Hill.

73. Morgan TM: Nonparametric estimation of duration of accrual and total study length for clinical trials, *Biometrics* 43:903-912, 1987.

74. Multiple Risk Factor Invention Trial Research Group. Multiple Risk Factor Intervention Trial: Risk factor changes and mortality results, *JAMA* 248:1465-1477, 1982.

75. Nam J: A simple approximation for calculating sample sizes for detecting linear trend in proportions, *Biometrics* 43:701-705, 1987.

76. Neaton JD, Bartsch GE: Impact of measurement error and temporal variability on the estimation of event probabilities for risk factor intervention trials, *Stat Med* 11:1719-1729, 1992.

77. Newcombe RG: Explanatory and pragmatic estimates of the treatment effect when deviations from allocated treatment occur, *Stat Med* 7:1179-1186, 1988.

78. Nocturnal Oxygen Therapy Trial Group: Continuous or nocturnal oxygen therapy in hypoxemic chronic obstructive lung disease: a clinical trial, *Ann Intern Med* 93:391-398, 1980.

79. The Norwegian Multicenter Study Group: Timolol-induced reduction in mortality and reinfarction in patients surviving acute myocardial infarction, *N Engl J Med* 304:801-807, 1981.

80. Overall JE, Doyle SR: Estimating sample sizes for repeated measurement designs, *Controlled Clin Trials* 15:100-123, 1994.
81. Packer M, Carver JR, Rodeheffer RJ, et al for the PROMISE Study Research Group: Effect of oral milrinone on mortality in severe chronic heart failure, *N Engl J Med* 325:1468-1475, 1991.
82. Palta M, Amini SB: Consideration of covariates and stratification in sample size determination for survival time studies, *J Chronic Dis* 38:801-809, 1985.
83. Pasternack BS: Sample sizes for clinical trials designed for patient accrual by cohorts, *J Chronic Dis* 25:673-681, 1972.
84. Pasternack BS, Gilbert HS: Planning the duration of long-term survival time studies designed for accrual by cohorts, *J Chronic Dis* 24:681-700, 1971.
85. Patterson BH: The impact of screening and eliminating preexisting cases on sample size requirements for cancer prevention trials, *Controlled Clin Trials* 8:87-95, 1987.
86. Pentico DW: On the determination and use of optimal sample sizes for estimating the difference in means, *Am Statistician* 35(1):40-42, 1981.
87. Phillips AN, Pocock SJ: Sample size requirements for prospective studies, with examples for coronary heart disease, *J Clin Epidemiol* 42:639-648, 1989.
88. Physicians' Health Study Research Group: Final report on the aspirin component of the ongoing Physicians' Health Study, *N Engl J Med* 321:129-135, 1989.
89. Remington RD, Schork MA: *Statistics with Applications to the Biological and Health Sciences,* Englewood Cliffs, NJ, 1970, Prentice-Hall.
90. Roberts R, Croft C, Gold HK et al: Effect of propranolol on myocardial infarct size in a randomized blinded multicenter trial, *N Engl J Med* 311:218-225, 1984.
91. Rochon J: Sample size calculations for two-group repeated-measures experiments, *Biometrics* 47:1383-1398, 1991.
92. Rosner B: Statistical methods in ophthalmology: an adjustment for the intraclass correlation between eyes, *Biometrics* 38:105-114, 1982.
93. Rosner B, Milton RC: Significance testing for binary correlated outcome data, *Biometrics* 44:505-512, 1988.
94. Rothman KJ: A show of confidence, *N Engl J Med* 299:1362-1363, 1978.
95. Rubenstein LV, Gail MH, Santner TJ: Planning the duration of a comparative clinical trial with loss to follow-up and a period of continued observation, *J Chronic Dis* 34:469-479, 1981.
96. Schlesselman JJ: Planning a longitudinal study: I. Sample size determination, *J Chronic Dis* 26:553-560, 1973.
97. Schlesselman JJ: Planning a longitudinal study: II. Frequency of measurement and study duration, *J Chronic Dis* 26:561-570, 1973.
98. Schoenfeld DA: Sample-size formula for the proportional-hazards regression model, *Biometrics* 39:499-503, 1983.
99. Schoenfeld DA, Richter JR: Nomograms for calculating the number of patients needed for a clinical trial with survival as an endpoint, *Biometrics* 38:163-170, 1982.
100. Schork MA, Remington RD: The determination of sample size in treatment-control comparisons for chronic disease studies in which drop-out or non-adherence is a problem, *J Chronic Dis* 20:233-239, 1967.
101. Shih WJ: Sample size reestimation in clinical trials. In Peace KE, ed: *Biopharmaceutical Sequential Statistical Applications,* New York, 1992, Marcel Dekker.
102. Snedecor GW, Cochran WG: *Statistical Methods,* ed 6, Ames, Iowa, 1967, Iowa State University Press.
103. Spriet A, Beiler D: When can "nonsignificantly different" treatments be considered as equivalent? (letter to the editors), *Br J Clin Pharmacol Ther* 7:623-624, 1979.
104. Steiner DL: Sample size and power in psychiatric research, *Can J Psychiatry* 35:616-620, 1990.
105. Taulbee JD, Symons MJ: Sample size and duration for cohort studies of survival time with covariables, *Biometrics* 39:351-360, 1983.
106. Urokinase Pulmonary Embolism Trial Study Group: Urokinase-streptokinase embolism trial: phase II results, *JAMA* 229:1606-1613, 1974.

107. Ury HK, Fleiss JL: On approximate sample sizes for comparing two independent proportions with the use of Yates' Correction, *Biometrics* 36:347-351, 1980.

108. Wacholder S, Weinberg CR: Paired versus two-sample design for a clinical trial of treatments with dichotomous outcome: power considerations, *Biometrics* 38:801-812, 1982.

109. Westlake WJ: Statistical aspects of comparative bioavailability trials, *Biometrics* 35:273-280, 1979.

110. Westlake WJ: Response to "Bioequivalence testing—a need to rethink," *Biometrics* 37:591-593, 1981.

111. Whitehead J: Sample sizes for phase II and phase III clinical trials: an integrated approach, *Stat Med* 5:459-464, 1986.

112. Wittes J, Brittain E: The role of internal pilot studies in increasing the efficiency of clinical trials, *Stat Med* 9:65-72, 1990.

113. Woolson RF: *Statistical Methods for the Analysis of Biomedical Data,* New York, 1987, John Wiley & Sons.

114. Wu M: Sample size for comparison of changes in the presence of right censoring caused by death, withdrawal, and staggered entry, *Controlled Clin Trials* 9:32-46, 1988.

115. Wu M, Fisher M, DeMets D: Sample sizes for long-term medical trials with time-dependent dropout and event rates, *Controlled Clin Trials* 1:111-121, 1980.

116. Zhen B, Murphy JR: Sample size determination for an exponential survival model with an unrestricted covariate, *Stat Med* 13:391-397, 1994.

CHAPTER 8

Baseline Assessment

In clinical trials, baseline refers to the status of a participant before the start of intervention. Baseline data may be measured by interview, questionnaire, physical examination, and laboratory tests. Measurement need not be only numerical in nature. It can also mean classification of study participants into categories based on factors such as absence or presence of some trait or condition.

As discussed in Chapter 3, baseline data describe the people studied, enabling the scientific community to compare the trial results with those of other studies. Different results from different studies may be attributed to seemingly minor differences in the study participants. These differences, in turn, can lead to the creation of new hypotheses, which may be tested.

Valid inferences about benefits of therapy depend on the kinds of people enrolled, as well as on study design. Complete reporting of baseline data allows clinicians to evaluate a new therapy's chance of success in their patients. On the other hand, judgment should be used in determining the factors to be measured at baseline. Evaluating factors that are unlikely to be pertinent to the trial is not only wasteful of money and time but may reduce participant cooperation. This chapter is concerned with the uses of baseline data, what constitutes a baseline measure, and assessment of baseline comparability.

FUNDAMENTAL POINT

Relevant baseline data should be measured in all study participants before the start of intervention.

USES OF BASELINE DATA

Although baseline data may be used to determine the eligibility of participants, it is assumed that any participants who are found unable to meet entrance criteria have been excluded from the study before assignment to either intervention or control. The characteristics of people not enrolled are of interest when attempting to generalize the trial results (Chapter 3). For the discussion in this chapter, however, only data from enrolled participants are considered.

The amount of data collected at baseline depends on the nature of the trial and purpose for which the data will be used. As mentioned elsewhere, some trials have simple protocols and collect limited amounts of data. If such trials are large, it is reasonable to expect that good balance between groups will be achieved. Because the goals of the trial are restricted to answering the primary question and one or two secondary questions, the other uses for baseline data are unnecessary. The investigators do not intend to perform stratification and subgroup analyses or conduct natural history studies. The simple design of the study means that detailed documentation of baseline variables is omitted and only a few key demographic and medical variables are ascertained.

Analysis of baseline comparability

Baseline data allow people to evaluate whether the study groups were comparable before intervention was started. The assessment of comparability should include risk or prognostic factors, pertinent demographic and socioeconomic characteristics, and medical history. This assessment is necessary in both randomized and nonrandomized trials. Altman and Doré,[2] in a review of 80 published randomized trials, noted considerable variation in the quality of the reporting of baseline characteristics. Half of those reporting continuous covariates did not use appropriate measures of variability. While randomization on the average produces balance between comparison groups, it does not guarantee balance in any specific trial. This may even be true in large studies. In the Aspirin Myocardial Infarction Study,[5] which had more than 4500 participants, the aspirin group was at slightly higher risk than the placebo group when baseline characteristics were examined. In assessing comparability in any trial, the investigators can look at only factors about which they are aware. Obviously, those which are unknown cannot be compared.

Stratification and subgrouping

If there is concern that one or two key prognostic factors may not "balance out" during randomization, thus yielding imbalanced groups at baseline, the investigators may stratify on the basis of these factors. Stratification can be done at the time of randomization or during analysis. Chapters 5 and 16 review the advantages and disadvantages of stratified randomization and stratified analysis. The point here is that to stratify at either time, the relevant characteristics of the participants at baseline must be known. For nonrandomized trials, these factors must also be measured to select properly the control group and analyze results by strata.

Often, investigators are interested not only in the response to intervention in the total study group, but also in the response in one or more subgroups. Particularly, in studies in which an overall intervention effect is present, analysis of results by appropriate subgroup may help to identify the specific population most likely to benefit from, or be harmed by, the intervention. Subgrouping may also help to elucidate the mechanisms of action of the intervention. Definition of such subgroups should rely only on baseline data, not data measured after initiation of intervention (except for factors such as age or sex that cannot be altered by the intervention). An example of establishing subgroups is the Canadian Cooperative Study Group trial[17] of aspirin and sulfinpyrazone in people with cerebral or retinal ischemic attacks. After noting an overall benefit from aspirin in reducing continued ischemic attacks or stroke, the authors observed that the benefit was restricted to men. Any conclusions drawn from subgroup hypotheses not explicitly stated in the protocol, however, should be given much less credibility than those from hypotheses stated a priori. Retrospective subgroup analysis should serve primarily to generate new hypotheses for subsequent testing (Chapter 16). In approving aspirin for the indication of transient ischemic attacks in men, the FDA relied on the Canadian Cooperative Study Group. A later meta-analysis of platelet active drug trials in cardiovascular disease, however, concluded that the effect is similar in men and women.[4]

Evaluation of change

Making use of baseline data will usually add sensitivity to a study. For example, an investigator may want to evaluate a new antihypertensive agent. She can either compare the mean change in blood pressure from baseline to some subsequent time in the intervention group against the mean change in the control group, or simply compare the mean blood pressures of the two groups at the end of the study. The former method usually is a more powerful statistical technique because it can reduce the variability of the response variables. As a consequence, it may permit either fewer participants to be studied or a smaller difference between groups to be detected.

Evaluation of possible unwanted reactions requires knowledge, or at least tentative ideas, about what effects might occur. The investigators should record at baseline those clinical or laboratory features that are likely to be adversely affected by the intervention. Unexpected adverse reactions might be missed, but the hope is that animal studies or earlier clinical work will have identified the important factors to be measured.

Natural history analyses

Baseline measurements enable investigators to perform natural history analyses in a control group that is on either placebo or no uniformly administered intervention. The prognostic importance of suspected risk factors for a variety of fatal and nonfatal events can be evaluated, particularly in large, long-term trials. This evaluation can include verifying previously ascertained risk factors and identifying others not considered earlier. Such analyses, although peripheral to the main objectives of a clinical trial, may be important for future research efforts. Their potential importance is especially true if variables that are subject to intervention can be identified.[8] Even if they are not variables that can be studied in future trials, they can be used in future stratification or subgroup analyses.

WHAT IS A TRUE BASELINE MEASUREMENT?

To describe accurately the study participants, baseline data should ideally reflect the true condition of the participants. Certain information can be obtained accurately by means of one measurement or evaluation at a baseline interview and examination. However, for many variables, accurately determining the participant's true state is difficult, since the mere fact of impending enrollment in a trial or the baseline examination itself may alter a measurement. For example, is true blood pressure reflected by a single measurement taken at baseline? If more than one measurement is made, which one should be used as the baseline value? Is the average of repeated measurements recorded over some extended period more appropriate? Does the participant need to be taken off all medications or be free of other factors that might affect the determination of a true baseline level? When resolving these questions, the screening required to identify eligible potential participants, the time and cost entailed in this identification, and the specific uses for the baseline information must be considered.

In almost every clinical trial, some sort of screening of potential participants is necessary. Screening eliminates participants who, based on the entrance criteria, are ineligible for the study. Occasionally, entrance criteria require repeated measurements over a period. A prerequisite for inclusion is the participant's willingness to comply with a possibly long and arduous study protocol. The participant's commitment, coupled with the need for repeated measurements of eligibility criteria, means that intervention allocation usually occurs later than the time of the investigator's first contact with the participant. An added problem may result from the fact that discussing a study with people or inviting them to participate in a clinical trial may alter their state of health. For instance, people asked to join a study of lipid-lowering agents because they had an elevated serum cholesterol at a screening examination might change their diet on their own initiative just because they were invited to join the study. Therefore, their serum cholesterol as determined at baseline, perhaps 1 month after the initial screen, may be somewhat lower than usual. Improvement could happen in many potential candidates for the trial and could affect the validity of the assumptions used to calculate sample size. If the study calls for a special dietary regimen, this might not be as effective at the new, lowered cholesterol level. As a result of the modification in participant behavior, there may be less room for change because of the intervention.

Although it may be impossible to avoid altering the behavior of potential participants, in study design it is often possible to adjust for such changes. Special care can be taken when discussing studies with people to avoid sensitizing them. Time between invitation to join a study and baseline evaluation can be kept to a minimum. People who have greatly changed their eating habits between the initial screen and baseline, as determined by a questionnaire at baseline, can be declared ineligible to join. Alternatively, they can be enrolled and the required sample size increased. Whatever is done, these are expensive ways to compensate for the reduced expected effectiveness of the intervention.

Sometimes a person's eligibility for a study is determined by measuring continuous variables, such as blood pressure or cholesterol level. If the entrance criterion is a high or low value, a phenomenon referred to as regression toward the mean is encountered.[14] Regression toward the mean occurs because measurable characteristics of an individual do not have constant values but vary above and below the average value for that individual. Because of this variability, although the population mean for a characteristic may be relatively constant over time, the locations of individuals within the population change. If two sets of measurements are made on individuals within the population, therefore, the correlation between the first and second series of measurements will not be perfect. That is, depending on the variability, the correlation will be something less than 1. In addition, it is often the case that the more distant a measured characteristic is from the population mean of that characteristic, the more variable the measurement tends to be.

Therefore, whenever participants are selected from a population on the basis of some measured characteristic, the mean of a subsequent measurement will be closer to the population mean than is the first measurement mean. Furthermore, the more extreme the initial selection criterion (that is, the further from the population mean), the greater will be the regression toward the mean at the time of the next measurement. The floor-and-ceiling effect used as an illustration by Schor[16] is helpful in understanding this concept. If all the flies in a closed room are near the ceiling in the morning, then at any subsequent time during the day more flies will be below where they started than above. Similarly, if the flies start close to the floor, the more probable it is for them to be higher, rather than lower, at any subsequent time.

Cutter[9] gives some nonbiologic examples of regression toward the mean. He presents the case of a series of three successive tosses of two dice. The average of the first two tosses is compared with the average of the second and third tosses. If no selection or cut-off criterion is used, the average of the first two tosses would, in the long run, be close to the average of the second and third tosses. However, if a cut-off point is selected which restricts the third toss to only those instances where the average of the first and second tosses is nine or greater, regression toward the mean will occur. The average of the second and third tosses for this selected group will be less than the average of the first two tosses for this group.

As with the example of the participants changing their diets between screening and baseline, this phenomenon of regression toward the mean can complicate assessment of intervention. In another case, an investigator may wish to evaluate the effects of an antihypertensive agent. She measures blood pressure once at the baseline examination and enters into her study only those people with diastolic pressures over 95 mm Hg. She then gives a drug and finds when she rechecks that most people have responded with lowered blood pressures. However, when she re-examines the control group, she finds that most of those people also have lower pressures. The value of a control group is obvious in such situations. An investigator cannot simply compare preintervention and postintervention values in the intervention group. She must compare postintervention values in the intervention group with values obtained at similar times in the control group. This regression toward the mean phenomenon can also lead to a problem discussed previously. People are screened initially for high or low values. Because of regression, the values at baseline are less extreme than the investigator had planned on, and there is less room for improvement from the intervention. In the blood pressure example, after randomization, many of the patients may have diastolic blood pressures in the low 90s or even 80s rather than above 95 mm Hg. There may be a reluctance to use antihypertensive agents in people with these lower pressures and, certainly, the opportunity to demonstrate full effectiveness of the agent may be lost.

Two approaches to reducing the impact of regression toward the mean were used by the trial of antihypertensive agents in the Hypertension Detection and Follow-up Program.[12] One approach was to use a more extreme value than the entrance criterion when the investigators screened people before baseline. Second, to enroll participants with diastolic blood pressure greater than 90 mm Hg, each potential participant had his or her pressure recorded three times. Only those whose second and third measure averaged 95 mm Hg or greater were invited to the clinic for further evaluation. The average of two recordings at the second evaluation was the baseline value, which was used for comparison with subsequent determinations. The Systolic Hypertension in the Elderly Program[19] used similar techniques in measuring isolated systolic hypertension.

When baseline data are measured too far in advance of intervention assignment, an event may occur in the interim. Investigators might not be able to determine whether this response occurred before or after the beginning of intervention. An effective treatment may reduce the frequency of complications of a disease from 15% to 10% in 3 months. The investigators should be able to detect this improvement. If, however, responses occur in the 1-month interval between baseline examination and start of intervention at a rate of 5% per month in each group, they would see a reduction from nearly 20% to nearly 15%. This relative reduction of about 25%, instead of 33%, might not be statistically significant, and the investigators could arrive at a different conclusion. The participants having events in the interval between allocation and the actual initiation of intervention would dilute the results and decrease the chances of finding a significant difference. In the European Coronary Surgery Study,[10] coronary artery bypass surgery should have occurred within 3 months of intervention allocation. However, the mean time until surgery was 3.9 months. Consequently, of the 21 deaths in the surgical group in the first 2 years, 6 occurred before surgery could be performed. If the response, such as death, is nonrecurring and this occurs between baseline and the start of intervention, the number of participants at risk of having the event later is reduced. Therefore, investigators need to be alert to any event occurring after baseline but before intervention is instituted. When such an event occurs before allocation to intervention or control, they can exclude the participant from the study. When the event occurs after allocation, but before start of intervention, participants should nevertheless be kept in the study and the event counted in the analysis. Removal of such participants from the study may bias the outcome. For this reason, the European Coronary Surgery Study Group[10] kept these participants in the trial for analysis purposes. In an unblinded trial of alprenolol in survivors of an acute myocardial infarction[1], a large number of participants were excluded between randomization and start of therapy. Since the study was not blinded, bias could have entered into the decision to exclude participants. Bias seems more likely since the investigators excluded many more patients from the alprenolol group than from the control group. The appropriateness of withdrawing participants from data analysis is discussed more fully in Chapter 16.

Particularly troublesome are those studies where baseline factors cannot be completely ascertained until after intervention has begun. The Multi-Institutional Study to Limit Infarct Size[15] investigated whether the size of a myocardial infarct could be reduced by propranolol or hyaluronidase administered within hours of onset of the infarction. Unfortunately, because of the requirement to start intervention early, the investigators could not fully characterize the infarct in the time available. Determination of the initial extent of the infarct became extraordinarily difficult, if not impossible, afterward, especially since the interventions were postulated to alter its course. In this instance, the investigators needed to be satisfied with more limited baseline information than they would have liked. Another solution is for the study to include patients who are suspected, but not proven, to have the condition, recognizing that as reflecting what is done in clinical practice.[13,18]

Even an investigator who can get baseline information just before initiating intervention, may need to compromise. For instance, serum cholesterol level, an important prognostic factor, is obtained in most heart disease studies. These levels, however, are temporarily lowered during the acute phase of a myocardial infarction. Therefore, in any trial using people who have just had a myocardial infarction, baseline serum cholesterol data relate poorly to their usual levels. Usual cholesterol levels would be known only if the investigator has data on participants from a time before the myocardial infarction. Cholesterol levels obtained at the time of the infarction might not allow her to evaluate natural history or make reasonable observations about changes in cholesterol that occurred because of the intervention. On the other hand, because the investigator has no reason to expect that one group would have greater lowering of cholesterol at baseline than the other group, such levels can certainly indicate whether the study groups are initially comparable.

Medications that participants are taking may also complicate the interpretation of the baseline data and restrict the uses to which an investigator can put baseline data. Hospitalized patients with severe cardiac arrhythmias may be given short-acting antiarrhythmic drugs. The investigator may want to evaluate the efficacy of a new drug in the long-term suppression of cardiac arrhythmias. However, for the purpose of obtaining a baseline estimate of the arrhythmias, to discontinue the present medication may be difficult. This issue came up in the Beta-Blocker Heart Attack Trial.[6] Although the primary response variable was mortality, the effect of propranolol on cardiac arrhythmias was obviously of interest. However, at baseline, several patients were being prescribed antiarrhythmic agents such as lidocaine. These could not be withdrawn simply to obtain an uncontaminated estimate of baseline arrhythmia. Some baseline data, therefore, became the number of participants on lidocaine and other antiarrhythmic drugs, rather than the frequency of severe arrhythmias.

Appreciating that, for many measurements, baseline data may not reflect the participant's true condition at the time of baseline, investigators perform the examination as close to the time of intervention allocation as possible. Baseline assessment may, in fact, occur shortly after allocation but prior to the actual start of intervention. The advantage of such timing is that the investigator does not spend extra time and money performing baseline tests on participants who may turn out to be ineligible. The baseline examination then occurs immediately after randomization and is performed not to exclude participants, but solely as a baseline reference point. Since allocation has already occurred, all participants remain in the trial regardless of the findings at baseline. This reversal of the usual order is not recommended in single-blind or unblinded studies, because it raises the possibility of bias during the examination. An investigator who knows to which group the participant belongs may subconsciously measure characteristics differently, depending on the group assignment. Furthermore, the order reversal may unnecessarily prolong the interval between intervention allocation and its actual start.

BALANCE AND IMBALANCE

As mentioned earlier, assessment of baseline comparability is one of the reasons for measuring baseline variables. Imbalance in important characteristics can yield misleading results. Assessment of baseline comparability is important in all trials, and particularly so in nonrandomized studies. The investigator needs to look at baseline variables in several ways. The simplest way is to compare each variable to make sure that it has reasonably similar distribution in each study group. Means, medians, and ranges are all convenient measures. The investigator can also combine the variables, giving each one an appropriate weight or coefficient, but doing this presupposes a knowledge of the relative prognostic importance of the variables. This kind of knowledge can come only from another study with a very similar population or by looking at the control group after the present study is completed. The weighting technique has the advantage that it can take into account numerous small differences between groups. If imbalances between most of the variables are in the same direction, the overall imbalance can turn out to be large, even though differences in individual variables are small.

In small studies especially, randomization may not yield entirely comparable groups. Treatment and control groups may differ in one or more baseline variables. In the 30-center Aspirin Myocardial Infarction Study that involved more than 4500 participants,[5] each center can be thought of as a small study with about 150 participants. When the baseline comparability within each center was reviewed, substantial differences in almost half the centers were found, some favoring intervention and some, control.* The difference between intervention and control groups in predicted 3-year mortality, using the Coronary Drug Project model,[7] exceeded 20% in 5 of the 30 clinics. Therefore, all factors that are known or suspected to be important in the subsequent course of the condition under study should be looked at when interpreting results. Identified imbalances do not invalidate a randomized trial, but they may make interpretation of results more complicated. In nonrandomized trials, the credibility of the findings may be compromised because selection bias may have occurred.

When comparing baseline factors, groups can never be shown to be identical. Only absence of significant differences can be demonstrated. In fact, 5% of the comparisons would be expected to show differences at the 0.05 significance level. In studies with small sample sizes, clinically important differences might be missed because there is insufficient power to demonstrate statistically significant differences. Yet, in numerous reports, authors state that the groups are similar because no statistically significant differences have been detected. Such a statement is an unwarranted interpretation of the data.

Of course, all important prognostic factors have probably not been identified, nor can all of them be measured. For example, ability to predict coronary heart disease occurrence has increased impressively in recent years.[3,11] Nevertheless, there are still large gaps in knowledge. This is one of the reasons for randomization, and why the process of identifying imbalances in known risk factors may not give a complete, or even true, picture of baseline comparability.

---

*Furberg, unpublished data 1981.

REFERENCES

1. Ahlmark G, Saetre H: Long-term treatment with β-blockers after myocardial infarction, *Eur J Clin Pharmacol* 10:77-83, 1976.
2. Altman DG, Doré CJ: Randomisation and baseline comparisons in clinical trials, *Lancet* 335:149-153, 1990.
3. Anderson KM, Wilson PWF, Odell PM, Kannel WB: An updated coronary risk profile. A statement for health professionals, *Circulation* 83:356-362, 1991.
4. Antiplatelet Trialists Collaboration: Collaborative overview of randomised trials of antiplatelet therapy—I: Prevention of death, myocardial infarction, and stroke by prolonged antiplatelet therapy in various categories of patients, *BMJ* 308:81-106, 1994.
5. Aspirin Myocardial Infarction Study Research Group: A randomized, controlled trial of aspirin in persons recovered from myocardial infarction, *JAMA* 243:661-669, 1980.
6. Beta-Blocker Heart Attack Trial: Protocol. National Heart, Lung, and Blood Institute, Division of Heart and Vascular Diseases, Clinical Trials Branch, Bethesda, MD, 1978.
7. Coronary Drug Project Research Group: Factors influencing long-term prognosis after recovery from myocardial infarction—three year findings of the Coronary Drug Project, *J Chronic Dis* 27:267-285, 1974.
8. Coronary Drug Project Research Group: Treatable risk factors—hypercholesterolemia, smoking, and hypertension—after myocardial infarction: implications of the Coronary Drug Project data for clinical management, *Primary Care* 7:175-179, 1980.
9. Cutter GR: Some examples for teaching regression toward the mean from a sampling viewpoint, *Am Stat* 30:194-197, 1976.
10. European Coronary Surgery Study Group: Coronary-artery bypass surgery in stable angina pectoris: survival at two years, *Lancet* i:889-893, 1979.
11. Gordon T, Kannel WB, Halperin M: Predictability of coronary heart disease, *J Chronic Dis* 32:427-440, 1979.
12. Hypertension Detection and Follow-up Program Cooperative Group: Five-year findings of the Hypertension Detection and Follow-up Program. I. Reduction in mortality of persons with high blood pressure, including mild hypertension, *JAMA* 242:2562-2571, 1979.
13. ISIS-2 (Second International Study of Infarct Survival) Collaborative Group: Randomised trial of intravenous streptokinase, oral aspirin, both, or neither among 17 187 cases of suspected acute myocardial infarction:ISIS-2, *Lancet* ii:349-360, 1988.
14. James KE: Regression toward the mean in uncontrolled clinical studies, *Biometrics* 29:121-130, 1973.
15. Roberts R, Croft C, Gold HK et al: Effect of propranolol on myocardial-infarct size in a randomized blinded multicenter trial, *N Engl J Med* 311:218-225, 1984.
16. Schor SS: The floor-and-ceiling effect, *JAMA* 207:120, 1969.
17. The Canadian Cooperative Study Group: A randomized trial of aspirin and sulfinpyrazone in threatened stroke, *N Engl J Med* 299:53-59, 1978.
18. The GUSTO Investigators: An international randomized trial comparing four thrombolytic strategies for acute myocardial infarction, *N Engl J Med* 329:673-682, 1993.
19. The Systolic Hypertension in the Elderly Program (SHEP) Cooperative Research Group: Rationale and design of a randomized clinical trial on prevention of stroke in isolated systolic hypertension, *J Clin Epidemiol* 41:1197-1208, 1988.

CHAPTER 9

Recruitment of
Study Participants

Often the most difficult task in a clinical trial involves obtaining sufficient study participants within a reasonable time. Time is a factor for both scientific and logistic reasons. From a scientific viewpoint, there is an optimal window of time within which a clinical trial should be completed. Changing medical practice and advances in understanding the condition under study may make the trial outdated. Other investigators may answer the questions sooner. In terms of logistics, the longer recruitment extends beyond the initially allotted recruitment period, the greater the pressure becomes to meet the goal. Costs increase, and frustrations and discouragement often follow. The primary reasons for recruitment failure include failure to start on time, inadequate planning, insufficient effort, and over-optimistic expectations. Invariably, participant recruitment is more difficult than originally planned. As Pocock[26] reported, among 39 international trials in oncology, only 2 achieved the projected number of patients within 2 years.

Although Hunninghake et al.[19] reviewed approximately 900 citations during a careful literature search in 1986, the amount of published information on recruitment is limited. Most information comes from large multicenter studies.[1,18,22]

In response to a relative paucity of clinical trial data on women and minorities, the U.S. Congress recently directed the NIH to establish guidelines for inclusion of these groups in clinical research.[15] The charge to the Director of NIH to "ensure that the trial is designed and carried out in a manner sufficient to provide valid analysis of whether the variables being studied in the trial affect women and members of minority groups, as the case may be, differently than other subjects in the trial" may have major implications depending on the interpretation of the term "valid analysis." A requirement to document a similar effect, beneficial or harmful, separately for both men and women, and separately for various racial/ethnic groups could increase the sample size by a factor ranging from 4 to 16.[15] We support adequate representation of women and minorities in clinical trials but suggest that the scientific question being posed be the primary determinant of the composition of the study population.

Approaches to recruitment of participants vary depending on the type and size of the trial, the length of time available, the setting (hospital, physician's office, and community), whether the trial is single or multicenter, and numerous other factors. Because of the broad spectrum of possibilities, this chapter summarizes concepts and general methods rather than elaborating on specific techniques. Emphasis is placed on anticipating and preventing problems. Sections of the text address plans for the recruitment effort, major recruitment problems, and participants' motives for volunteering for research projects. Obtaining institutional review board approval for the trial from all participating institutions is part of the planning process. Such approval must be granted prior to initiating any recruitment efforts.

FUNDAMENTAL POINT

Successful recruitment depends on developing a careful plan with multiple strategies, maintaining flexibility, establishing interim goals, and preparing to devote the necessary effort.

PLANNING

In the planning stage of a trial, an investigator needs to evaluate the likelihood of obtaining sufficient study participants within the allotted time. This planning effort entails obtaining realistic estimates of the number of available potential participants meeting the study entry criteria. Available data may be inadequate. Census tract data or hospital and physician records may be out of date, incomplete, or incorrect. People may have moved or died since the records were last updated. Information about current use of drugs or frequency of surgical procedures may not reflect what will occur in the future, when the trial is actually conducted. Records may not give sufficient, or even accurate, details about potential participants. Available data certainly do not reflect the willingness of people to enroll in the trial or comply with the intervention.

After initial record review, an investigator may find it necessary to expand the population base by increasing the geographical catchment area, canvassing additional hospitals, relaxing one or more of the study entrance criteria, increasing the planned recruitment time, or combining some of these factors. The preliminary survey of participant sources should be as thorough as possible, since these determinations are better made before, rather than after, a study begins.

The sample size calculation typically assumes a constant rate of enrollment. A slow start can reduce the statistical power of the trial.[27]

Planning also involves setting up a clinic structure for recruitment with interested and involved co-investigators, an experienced and organized coordinator in charge of recruitment, and other staff required for the operations. A close working relationship between the clinic staff and the investigators with regular clinic meetings is crucial from the very beginning to enrollment of the last participant. Careful planning and clear delineation of staff responsibilities are essential features of a well-performing recruitment unit.

The investigator also needs support from his institution and colleagues. Other investigators in the same institution or at nearby institutions may compete for similar participants. Since participants should not be in more than one trial at a time, competing studies may decrease the likelihood that the investigator will meet his recruitment goal. Competition for participants in turn may necessitate reappraising the entry criteria, study time line, or perhaps even the feasibility of conducting the study.

Announcements of the trial should precede initiation of recruitment. The courtesy of informing area health professionals about the trial in advance can facilitate cooperation, reduce misconceptions and opposition, and avoid local physicians' surprise at first hearing about the study from their patients rather than from the investigator. Professional talks or notices should indicate whether the investigator is simply notifying physicians about the study or whether he is actively seeking their support in recruiting participants.

Recruitment should begin no later than the first day of the designated recruitment period. Commitment and willingness to spend a considerable amount of time in recruiting are as important as good planning. Just as investigators usually overestimate the number of participants available, they often underestimate the time and effort needed to recruit. Investigators must accommodate themselves to the schedules of potential participants, many of whom work. Thus recruitment is sometimes done on weekends and evenings, as well as during usual working hours.

The need for multiple recruitment strategies has been well documented.[17] These strategies should be implemented on day 1 of recruitment. Because it is difficult to know which strategies will be productive, it is important to monitor effort and yield of the various strategies. In a community-based prevention trial of smokers, only 1 of 10 participating centers retained its original recruitment plan.[12] Media campaigns, mass mailings and screening are costly. It is a common experience in clinical trials that insufficient funds are allocated to these activities.

The value of multiple approaches is illustrated by one large study in which the investigator identified possible participants and wrote letters to them, inviting them to participate. He received a poor response until he publicized his study via local radio and television news and interview programs. The media coverage had apparently legitimized the study and primed the community.

If the feasibility of a recruitment approach is uncertain, a pretest may provide valuable information. Daly et al.[11] evaluated the feasibility of telephone recruitment and found that while 63% of 203 women from a health maintenance organization met the eligibility criteria for a tamoxifen trial, less than half of those eligible (45%) expressed interest in participating. Pretests of this kind are useful to estimate the yield of screening.

If data concerning recruitment of potential participants to a particular type of trial are scanty, a pilot or feasibility study may be worthwhile. Pilot studies can provide valuable information on optimal participant sources, recruitment techniques, and yield estimates. In a trial of elderly people, the question arose whether those in their 70s or 80s would volunteer and actively participate in a long-term, placebo-controlled trial. Before implementing a costly full-scale trial, a pilot study was conducted to answer these and other questions.[16] The study not only showed that the elderly were willing participants but also provided information on recruitment techniques. The success of the pilot led to a full-scale trial.

Contingency plans must be available in case recruitment lags. Experience has shown that recruitment estimates, in general, should be reduced by a factor of one third to one half. Hence, additional sources of potential study participants should be kept in reserve. Approval from hospital staff, large group practices, managed care organizations, corporation directors, or others controlling large numbers of potential participants often takes considerable time. Waiting until recruitment problems appear before initiating such approval can lead to weeks or months of inaction. Therefore it is advisable to make plans to use other sources before the study actually gets underway. If they are not needed, little is lost except for additional time used in planning. Most of the time these reserves will prove useful.

Planning for recruitment of special populations often requires special attention and strategies. For example, others have reported their experience regarding recruitment of children,[35] elderly,[30,34] minorities,[29] women from a cancer registry,[24] drug abusers,[3] and HIV-infected individuals.[29]

STRATEGIES AND SOURCES

The approach to recruitment depends on the features of the study population; sick people vs. well, hospitalized vs. not, or acute vs. chronic illness. For example, enrollment of acutely ill hospitalized patients can only be conducted in an acute care setting, while enrollment of healthy asymptomatic individuals with certain characteristics or risk factors requires a community-based screening program. This chapter will review recruitment issues in general. Many of them apply to the broad spectrum of study populations.

The first recruitment approach involves actively searching for participants. The investigator identifies target groups such as hospitalized persons, clinic patients, patients of particular physicians, census tract populations, or employees of factories or other organizations. These groups are then screened, by reviewing hospital admissions, searching records, or setting up a testing facility for rapid screening of potential participants (for instance, special laboratory tests in clinic patients or blood pressure determinations in a group of factory workers). Those passing the initial screen or chart review are invited to undergo a more detailed eligibility evaluation. This two-stage method, though time consuming and tedious, often proves more fruitful than other methods.

In one study of cholesterol reduction in men with heart disease, the investigator had an elaborate, well-organized scheme. He identified all hospitals in a specific geographic area. Letters were mailed to these hospitals asking for names and addresses of all patients who had a heart attack within the past few years. When information such as sex, age, and attending physician was available, these too were requested. A second mailing was done for hospitals failing to respond within a certain period. After receiving the names of identified patients, the investigator contacted the attending physicians to ask for permission to speak with or write to their patients. Upon approval, patients were contacted to gauge their interest in entering the study. A similar approach was employed by investigators who obtained listings from the U.S. Health Care Financing Administration. Those eligible for enrollment were invited to a screening visit. Some hospitals refused (on grounds of confidentiality) to send out names of patients. In these instances, the investigator asked the hospital to forward letters prepared by him to the attending physicians and patients. Finally, each attending physician was periodically briefed on the status of his patient. The steps, composing a long, arduous process, resulted in a low yield. However, for trials enrolling persons who are already known to have a specific diagnosis, the scheme may be the most effective or efficient way to ensure identification of potential participants.

Another strategy involves direct invitation to study participants. In contrast to the first method, no attempt is made to prescreen those who are contacted about the trial. This approach may be more appealing and require less initial work. Participant solicitation may be done through mass media, through wide dissemination of leaflets advertising the trial, or through participation by the investigator in health fairs or similar vehicles. None of these methods is foolproof. The yield is unpredictable and seems to depend predominantly on the skill with which the approach is made and the size and kind of audience it reaches. One success story featured a distinguished investigator in a large city who managed to appear on a local television station's early evening news show. Thousands of people volunteered for the screening program following this single 5-minute appeal. Experience, however, has shown that most individuals who respond to a media campaign are not eligible for the trial.

Participants may also be approached through a third party. For example, an investigator may bring the attention of physicians to his study by means of letters, telephone calls, presentations at professional society meetings, notices in professional journals, or exhibits at scientific conferences. The hope is that these physicians will identify a potential participant and either notify the investigator or ask the person to call him.

Whichever of the three methods is used, several points are worth emphasizing:

1   Success of a technique is unpredictable. What works in one city at one time may not work at the same place at another time or in another city. Therefore the investigator needs to be flexible and to leave room for modifications.
2. Investigators working especially with sick participants must maintain good relationships with participants' personal physicians. Physicians disapproving of the study or the way it is conducted are more likely to urge their patients not to participate.
3. Investigators must respect the families of potential participants. Most participants like to discuss research participation with their family and friends. Investigators should be prepared to spend time reviewing the study with them. If the study requires long-term cooperation from the participant, we encourage such discussions. Anything that increases family support is likely to lead to better recruitment and protocol adherence.
4. Recruiting should not be overly aggressive. While encouragement is necessary, excessive efforts to convince people to participate could prove harmful in the long run. Those reluctant to join may be more likely to abandon the study later or be nonadherent to study interventions after randomization. Effective work on adherence begins during the recruitment phase.
5. In most recruitment efforts for large trials, a combination of approaches is usually needed.

Several investigative groups have reported on their recruitment experiences, including the yield from various strategies.[5,7] A few studies formally compared different strategies in terms of both yield and cost.[20,33,36]

CONDUCT

Successful recruitment of participants depends not only on planning but also on the implementation of the plan. Systems must be in place to identify all potential participants from the recruitment pool and to screen these people for eligibility.

For hospital-based studies, logging all admissions to special units, wards, or clinics is invaluable. However, keeping such records complete can be difficult, especially during evenings or weekends. During such hours, those dedicated to the study are often not available to ensure accuracy and completeness. Vacation times and illness may also present difficulties in keeping the log up to date. Therefore frequent quality checks should be made.

Participant privacy is also important. At what point do the investigators obtain consent? For those who refuse to participate, what happens to the data that had been collected and used to identify them? The answer to this will vary from institution to institution and will depend on who is keeping the log and for what reason. Information recorded by code numbers can facilitate privacy.

For community-based studies, screening large numbers of people is a major undertaking, especially if the yield is low. Prescreening potential participants by telephone to identify those with major exclusion criteria (e.g., using demographics and medical history) has been employed in many projects. In the Lung Health Study,[12] investigators used prescreening to reduce the number of screening visits to approximately half of those projected.

Investigators need to identify the best times to reach the maximum number of potential participants. If they intend to make home visits or hope to contact people by telephone, they should count on working evenings or weekends. Unless potential participants are retired, or investigators plan on contacting people at their jobs (which, depending on the nature of the job, may be difficult), normal working hours may not be productive times. Vacation times and summers are additional slow periods for recruitment.

The actual mechanics of recruiting participants need to be established in advance. A smooth clinic operation is beneficial to all parties. Investigators must be certain that necessary staff, facilities, and equipment are available at appropriate times in the proper places. Keeping potential participants waiting is a poor way to earn their confidence.

The logistics of recruitment may become more difficult when follow-up of enrolled participants occurs while investigators are still recruiting. In long-term studies, the most difficult time is usually toward the end of the recruitment phase when the same staff, space, and equipment may be used simultaneously for participants seen for screening, baseline, and follow-up examinations.

Investigators and staff need to keep abreast of recruitment efforts. Conducting regular staff meetings and generating regular reports may serve as forums for discussing yields from various strategies, percentage of recruitment goal attained, and brainstorming and morale boosting. These meetings, useful for both single and multicenter trials, also provide the opportunity to remind everyone about the importance of following the study protocol, including paying careful attention to collection of valid data.

Record keeping of recruitment activities is essential to allow analyses of recruitment yields and costs from the various recruitment strategies. Recruiting large numbers of potential participants requires the creation of timetables, flow charts, and databases to ensure that screening and recruitment proceed smoothly. Such charts should include the number of people to be seen at each step in the process at a given time, the number and type of personnel and amount of time required to process each participant at each step, and the amount of equipment needed (with an allowance for "down" time). A planned pilot phase is helpful in making these assessments. One positive aspect of slow early recruitment is that the bugs in the start-up process can be worked out and necessary modifications made.

MONITORING

Successful trial recruitment often depends on establishing short-term and long-term recruitment goals. The investigator should record these goals and make every effort to achieve them. Since lagging recruitment commonly results from a slow start, timely preparation and establishment of initial goals are crucial. The investigator should be ready to recruit participants on the first official day of study opening.

The use of weekly and/or monthly interim goals in a long-term study orients the investigator and staff to the short-term and long-term recruitment needs of the study. These goals can serve as indicators for lagging recruitment and may help avoid a grossly uneven recruitment pace. Inasmuch as participant follow-up is usually done at regular intervals, uneven recruitment results in periods of peak and slack during the follow-up phase. This threatens effective use of staff time and equipment. Of course, establishing a goal in itself does not guarantee timely participant recruitment. The goals need to be realistic, and the investigator must make the commitment to meet each interim goal. Formal statistical models have been proposed to determine and assess interim recruitment goals.[21]

Centers falling behind their recruitment goals should determine the reasons for lagging recruitment. In a multicenter clinical trial, valuable insight can be obtained by comparing results from different centers. Those clinical sites with the best recruitment performance can serve as "role models" for other sites, which should be encouraged to incorporate other successful techniques into their recruitment schemes. Multicenter studies require a central office to oversee recruitment, to compare enrollment results, to facilitate communication among sites, and to lend support and encouragement. Frequent feedback to the centers by means of tables and graphs, which show the actual recruitment compared with originally projected goals, is a useful tool. Examples are shown in the following figures and table. Figure 9-1 shows the progress of an investigator who started participant recruitment on schedule and maintained a good pace during the recruitment period. The investigator and clinic staff accurately assessed participant sources and demonstrated a commitment to enrolling participants in a relatively even fashion. Figure 9-2 shows the record of an investigator who started slowly, but later improved. However, considerable effort was required to compensate for the poor start. Clinic efforts included expanding the base from which participants were recruited and increasing the time spent in enrollment. In contrast, as seen in Fig. 9-3, the investigator started slowly and never was able to improve his performance. This center was dropped from a multicenter study because it could not contribute enough participants to the study to make its continued participation efficient. Table 9-1 shows goals, actual recruitment, and projected final totals (assuming no change in enrollment pattern) for three other centers of a multicenter trial.

Such tables are useful to gauge short-term recruitment efforts and to project final numbers of participants. The tables and figures should be updated as often as necessary.

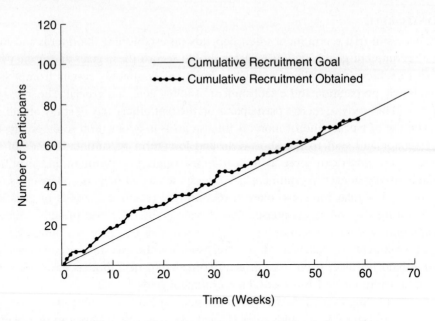

Fig. 9-1 Participant recruitment in clinic that consistently performed at goal rate.

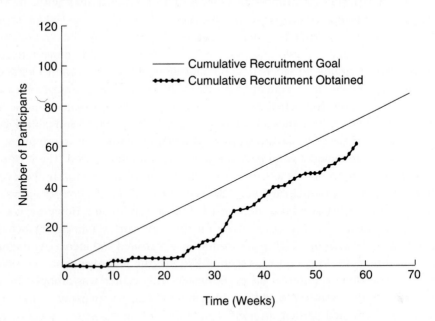

Fig. 9-2 Participant recruitment in a clinic that started slowly and then performed at greater than goal rate.

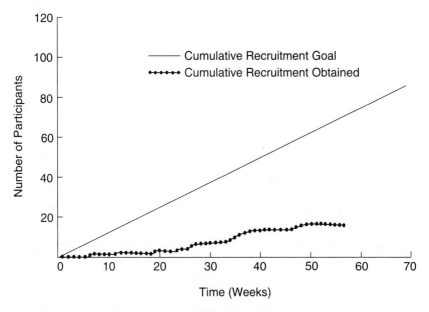

Fig. 9-3 Participant recruitment in a clinic that performed poorly

Table 9-1 Weekly recruitment status report by center

Center	(1) Contracted goal	(2) Enrollment this week	(3) Actual enrollment to date	(4) Goal enrollment to date	(5) Actual minus goal	(6) Success rate (3)/(4)	(7) Final projected intake	(8) Final Deficit or excess (7)-(1)
A	150	1	50	53.4	-3.4	0.94	140	-10
B	135	1	37	48.0	-11.0	0.77	104	-31
C	150	2	56	53.4	2.6	1.06	157	7

Table used in the Beta-Blocker Heart Attack Trial: Coordinating Center, University of Texas, Houston.

In single-center trials, investigators should monitor recruitment status at regular and frequent intervals. Review of these data with staff keeps everyone aware of recruitment progress. If recruitment lags, the delay can be noted early, the reasons identified, and appropriate action taken.

PROBLEMS

Even when carefully planned and perfectly executed, recruitment may still proceed slowly. Investigators should expect problems to occur despite their efforts. These may be completely unforeseen. In one multicenter study, there were reports of murders of inpatients at the hospital adjacent to the study clinic. It is hardly surprising that attendance at the clinic fell sharply.

The typical problems with recruitment have been summarized by Tilley et al.[32] In a trial of osteoporosis, the investigators encountered problems because of inadequate funding for the screening process, unwillingness of physicians to refer patients, overestimation of the prevalence of the condition, and overly rigorous entry criteria for the trial.

Reliance on physician referrals is common and often problematic. Usually this technique results in very few eligible participants. In one multicenter trial, an investigator invited internists and cardiologists from a large metropolitan area to a meeting. He described the study, its importance, and his need to recruit men who had had a myocardial infarction. Each of the physicians stood up and promised to contribute one or more participants. One hundred fifty participants were pledged; only five were ultimately referred. Despite this, such pleas may be worthwhile because they make the professional community aware of a study and its purpose. Investigators who stay in close contact with physicians in a community and form a referral network have more success in obtaining cooperation and support.

A similar experience was reported from the United Kingdom.[25] Of 1003 general practitioners asked if they would refer patients with heavy menstrual bleeding, 315 agreed, but only 129 of these did so. Moreover, a review of records from six practices showed that only approximately 20% of eligible patients were referred. Forgetfulness and time pressures were the reasons given for the low referral rate. Clinic visits by an investigator during the planning phase improved subsequent recruitment.

Overoptimistic recruitment projections are the rule rather than the exception. In a trial of aspirin in people with transient ischemic attacks, estimates of numbers of potential participants were made by each collaborating investigator.[14] According to the study's Manual of Instruction, approximately 300 participants would be enrolled annually. Instead, it took almost 3 years of recruitment to achieve this number. Baines[4] has reported on difficulties in recruiting participants for the Canadian National Breast Screening Study. After a comprehensive program of educating the medical profession and the public, and obtaining media support, enrollment improved markedly. The best approach involved mailing personally addressed letters to potentially eligible participants followed by telephone calls. These examples are not unusual.

When recruitment becomes difficult, one possible outcome is that an investigator will begin to interpret loosely entry criteria or deliberately change data to enroll otherwise ineligible participants. Unfortunately, this issue is not theoretical. Such practices have occurred, to a limited extent, in more than one trial. The best way to avoid the problem is to make it clear that this type of infraction harms both the study and participants, and that neither science nor the investigators are served by such practices. Random record audits by an independent person or group may serve as a deterrent.

SOLUTIONS

One possible way to deal with lagging recruitment is to accept a smaller number of participants than originally planned. Doing this is far from ideal, inasmuch as the power of the study will be reduced. In accepting a smaller number of participants than hoped for, the investigator must either alter design features such as the primary response variable, or change assumptions about intervention effectiveness and participant adherence. As indicated elsewhere, such changes midway in a trial may be liable to legitimate criticism. Only if the investigator is lucky and discovers that some of the assumptions used in calculating sample size were too pessimistic would this solution provide comparable power. The previously mentioned trial of aspirin in people with transient ischemic attacks[14] had the happy experience of finding that aspirin produced a greater effect than initially postulated. Therefore the less-than-hoped-for number of participants turned out to be adequate. Alternatively, extra effort might be made to achieve better-than-projected participant adherence to the study protocol, and thereby reduce the number of required participants.

Collins et al.[6] have reviewed ways in which investigators handled lagging recruitment in seven Veterans Administration multicenter trials. In six of the studies, the required sample size was reevaluated and lowered. The authors indicate that the recruitment problems could have been avoided had the planning of the trial been better.

A second approach is to relax the inclusion criteria. This should be done only if little expectation exists that the study design will suffer. The design can be marred when, as a result of the new type of participants, the control group event rate is altered to such an extent that the estimated sample size is no longer appropriate. Also, the expected response to intervention in the new participants may not be as great as in the original participants. Furthermore, the intervention might have a different effect or greater likelihood of being harmful in the new participants than in those originally recruited. The difference in additional participants would not matter if the proportion and type of participants randomized to each group stayed the same throughout recruitment. However, as indicated in Chapter 5, certain randomization schemes alter that proportion, depending on baseline criteria or study results. Under these circumstances, changing entry criteria may create imbalances.

In the Coronary Drug Project,[9] only people with documented transmural myocardial infarctions were originally eligible. With enrollment falling behind, the investigators decided to admit participants with nontransmural myocardial infarctions. Since there was no reason to expect that the action of lipid-lowering agents would be any different in the new group than in the original group and since the lipid-lowering agents were not contraindicated in the new participants, the modification seemed reasonable. However, there was some concern that overall mortality rate would be changed because mortality in people with nontransmural infarctions may be less than mortality in people with transmural infarctions. Nevertheless, the pressure of recruitment overrode that concern. Possible baseline imbalances did not turn out to be a problem. In this particular study, where the total number of participants was so large (8341), there was every expectation that randomization would yield comparable groups. If there had been uncertainty regarding this, stratified randomization could have been employed (Chapter 5). Including people with nontransmural infarctions may have reduced the power of the study because this group had a lower mortality rate than those with transmural infarctions in each of the treatment groups, including the placebo group. However, the treatments were equally ineffective when people with transmural infarctions were examined separately from people with nontransmural infarctions.[10]

A possible third solution to recruitment problems is to extend the time for recruitment or, in the case of multicenter studies, to add recruiting centers. Both are the preferred solutions, requiring neither modification of admission criteria nor diminution of power. However, they are also the most costly. Whether the solution of additional time or additional centers is adopted depends on cost, on the logistics of finding and training other high-quality centers, and on the need to obtain study results quickly.

A possible fourth solution involves a change in design. It has been claimed that one of the factors leading to recruitment problems is unwillingness on the part of people and their private physicians to participate in a randomized trial. Zelen[37] proposed a design where eligible patients were randomized to control or intervention before obtaining informed consent. Only those assigned to the intervention are informed of the trial and are asked to give their consent. The other group receives standard treatment and is followed by their usual source of medical care.

The technique was employed in a trial of different surgical approaches for breast cancer.[31] During the initial 44 months, only 519 participants had been enrolled, 16% of the goal. The major reasons given by the investigators were concern that randomization would impair the doctor-patient relationship, difficulty in obtaining informed consent, and difficulty separating the scientist and clinician roles. After switching to the Zelen design, recruitment increased sixfold.[13] In other trials, the experience has been encouraging but not as dramatic. However, several concerns have been raised.[2,8,13] Concerns include the ethics of not informing the participants assigned to the control group that they are in a trial and the potential dilution of results if a large number of participants decline to participate. In fact, the Cancer Research Council Working Party in Great Britain has rejected the Zelen model.[8] The long-term acceptability and use of this approach to improving recruitment remains unclear.

A fifth approach to lagging recruitment is recycling of potential participants. When a prospective participant just misses meeting the eligibility criteria, the temptation is natural to try to enroll him by repeating a measurement, perhaps under slightly different conditions. Because of variability in a screening test, many investigators argue that it is reasonable to allow one repeat test and give a person interested in the trial a second chance. In general, this recycling should be discouraged. A study is harmed by enrolling persons for whom the intervention might not be effective or appropriate.

Instances exist where, to enter a drug study, the participant needs to be off all other medication with similar actions. At baseline, he may be asked whether he has complied with this requirement. If he has not, the investigator may repeat the instructions and have the participant return in a week for repeat baseline measurements. This second chance is different from recycling. The entry criterion checks on a participant's ability to comply with a protocol and his understanding of instructions. From a design viewpoint it may be legitimate to give a candidate this second chance. However, the second-chance participant, even if he passes the repeat baseline measurement, may not be as good a candidate for the study as someone who complied on the first occasion.[28]

REASONS FOR PARTICIPATION

At the conclusion of both the Aspirin Myocardial Infarction Study and the Beta-Blocker Heart Attack Trial,[23] the participants were asked about their reaction to the project, including their perceptions of the beneficiaries of the trial. Although the scientific community and other heart patients received the highest ranking, the participants also saw a personal benefit, because their participation provided care by specialists and offered increased knowledge about their heart condition, and the trial finding would apply directly to them.

Limited information is available in the literature concerning people's reasons for participation in research projects. The finding of two surveys, one employing open-ended interviews in a random sample of participants before the end of follow-up and the other using a mail questionnaire, have been reported.[23] The participants were all survivors of a heart attack. The major conclusions were that patients valued particularly the additional monitoring, a second opinion of their condition, the emotional benefit of reassurance, the resulting peace of mind, the fact that altruistic motivations matched those considered self-directed. The perceived disadvantages (transportation problems and clinic waiting time) were infrequent, but the active trial participants obviously represent a biased sample. It was reassuring that when asked, 80% to 85% indicated they would participate again.

REFERENCES

1. Agras WS, Bradford RH, Marshall GD, eds: Recruitment for clinical trials: the Lipid Research Clinics Coronary Primary Prevention Trial experience. Its implications for future trials, *Circulation* 66 (suppl IV):IV-1–IV-78, 1982.
2. Angell M: Patients' preferences in randomized clinical trials, *N Engl J Med* 310:1385-1387, 1984 (editorial).

3. Ashery RS, McAuliffe WE: Implementation issues and techniques in randomized trials of outpatient psychosocial treatments for drug abusers: recruitment of participants, *Am J Drug Alcohol Abuse* 18:305-329, 1992.

4. Baines CJ: Impediments to recruitment in the Canadian National Breast Screening Study: response and resolution, *Controlled Clin Trials* 5:129-140, 1984.

5. Carew BD, Boichot HD, Dolan NA et al for the SOLVD Investigators: Recruitment strategies in the Studies Of Left Ventricular Dysfunction (SOLVD): strategies for screening and enrollment in two concurrent but separate trials, *Controlled Clin Trials* 13:325-338, 1992.

6. Collins JF, Bingham SF, Weiss DG, et al: Some adaptive strategies for inadequate sample acquisition in Veterans Administration cooperative clinical trials, *Controlled Clin Trials* 1:227-248, 1980.

7. Connett JE, Bjornson-Benson WM, Daniels K for the Lung Health Study Research Group: Recruitment of participants in the Lung Heart Study, II: Assessment of recruiting strategies, *Controlled Clin Trials* 14:38S-51S, 1993.

8. Consent: how informed? *Lancet* i:1445-1447, 1984 (editorial).

9. Coronary Drug Project Research Group: The Coronary Drug Project: design, methods, and baseline results, *Circulation* 47 (suppl 1):I-1-I-50, 1973.

10. Coronary Drug Project Research Group: Clofibrate and niacin in coronary heart disease, *JAMA* 231:360-381, 1975.

11. Daly M, Seay J, Balshem A et al: Feasibility of a telephone survey to recruit health maintenance organization members into a tamoxifen chemoprevention trial, *Cancer Epidemiol Biomarkers Prev* 1:413-416, 1992.

12. Durkin DA, Kjelsberg MO, Buist AS et al: Recruitment of participants in the Lung Health Study, I: description of methods, *Controlled Clin Trials* 14:20S-37S, 1993.

13. Ellenberg SS: Randomization designs in comparative clinical trials, *N Engl J Med* 310:1404-1408, 1984.

14. Fields WS, Lemak NA, Frankowski RF et al: Controlled trial of aspirin in cerebral ischemia, *Stroke* 8:301-316, 1977.

15. Freedman LS, Simon R, Foulkes MA et al: Inclusion of women and minorities in clinical trials and the NIH Revitalization Act of 1993—the perspective of NIH clinical trialists, *Controlled Clin Trials* 16:277-285, 1995.

16. Hulley SB, Furberg CD, Gurland B et al: Systolic Hypertension in the Elderly Program (SHEP): antihypertensive efficacy of chlorthalidone, *Am J Cardiol* 56:913-920, 1985.

17. Hunninghake DB: Summary conclusions, *Controlled Clin Trials* 8:1S-5S, 1987.

18. Hunninghake DB, Blaszkowski TP, eds: Proceedings of the workshop on the recruitment experience in NHLBI-sponsored clinical trials, *Controlled Clin Trials* 8 (suppl), 1987.

19. Hunninghake DB, Darby CA, Probstfield JL: Recruitment experience in clinical trials: literature summary and annotated bibliography, *Controlled Clin Trials* 8:6S-30S, 1987.

20. Kelly RB, McMahon SH, Hazey JA: Does practice location or academic connection affect recruitment of patients as research subjects? *Fam Prac Res J* 12:177-184, 1992.

21. Lee YJ: Interim recruitment goals in clinical trials, *J Chronic Dis* 36:379-389, 1983.

22. Lung Health Study Research Group: The Lung Health Study: design of the trial and recruitment of participants, *Controlled Clin Trials* 14 (suppl), 1993.

23. Mattson ME, Curb JD, McArdle R, the AMIS and BHAT Research Groups: Participation in a clinical trial: the patients' point of view, *Controlled Clin Trials* 6:156-167, 1985.

24. Newcomb PA, Love RR, Phillips JL, Buckmaster BJ: Using a population-based cancer registry for recruitment in a pilot cancer control study, *Prev Med* 19:61-65, 1990.

25. Peto V, Coulter A, Bond A: Factors affecting general practitioners' recruitment of patients into a prospective study, *Fam Prac* 10:207-211, 1993.

26. Pocock SJ: Size of cancer clinical trials and stopping rules, *Br J Cancer* 38:757-766, 1978.

27. Probstfield JL, Wittes JT, Hunninghake DB: Recruitment in NHLBI population-based studies and randomized clinical trials: data analysis and survey results, *Controlled Clin Trials* 8:141S-149S, 1987.

28. Sackett DL: A compliance practicum for the busy practitioner. In Haynes RB, Taylor DW, Sackett DL, eds: *Compliance in health care*, Baltimore, 1979, Johns Hopkins University Press.

29. El-Sadr W, Capps L: The challenge of minority recruitment in clinical trials for AIDS, *JAMA* 267:954-957, 1992.
30. Silagy CA, Campion K, McNeil JJ, et al: Comparison of recruitment strategies for a large-scale clinical trial in the elderly, *J Clin Epidemiol* 44:1105-1114, 1991.
31. Taylor KM, Margolese RG, Soskolne CL: Physicians' reasons for not entering eligible patients in a randomized clinical trial of surgery for breast cancer, *N Engl J Med* 310:1363-1367, 1984.
32. Tilley BC, Shorck MA: Designing clinical trials of treatment for osteoporosis: recruitment and follow-up, *Calcif Tissue Int* 47:327-331, 1990.
33. Turnbull D, Irwig L: Ineffective recruitment strategies for screening mammography: letterbox drops and invitations for friends, *Aust J Public Health* 16:79-81, 1992.
34. Vogt TM, Ireland CC, Black D, et al: Recruitment of elderly volunteers for a multicenter clinical trial: the SHEP pilot study, *Controlled Clin Trials* 7:118-133, 1986.
35. Vollmer WM, Hertert S, Allison MJ: Recruiting children and their families for clinical trials: a case study, *Controlled Clin Trials* 13:315-320, 1992.
36. Wadland WC, Hughes JR, Secker-Walker RH et al: Recruitment in a primary care trial on smoking cessation, *Fam Med* 22:201-204, 1990.
37. Zelen M: A new design for randomized clinical trials, *N Engl J Med* 300:1242-1245, 1979.

CHAPTER **10**

Data Collection and
Quality Control

No study is better than the quality of its data. Data in clinical trials are collected from several sources—interviews, questionnaires, participant examinations, or laboratory determinations. Also, data that have been collected and evaluated by someone outside the study may be used in a trial; for example, diagnoses obtained from death certificates or hospital records.

In the past decade there have been a disturbing number of reports of scientific misconduct, including data fabrication and plagiarism.[2,11,39,40] It is difficult to determine whether these reports reflect a true increase of the problem or a higher rate of detection. Scientific misconduct is common, according to a review of 1995 routine audits conducted by the FDA from June 1977 to April 1988.[40] Serious deficiencies were discovered in 12% of routine audits. The reduction to 8% after October 1985 was attributed to the implementation of the audit program. The most prevalent problems related to patient consent, drug accountability, protocol nonadherence, and inaccurate records. Troublesome observations were that many categories of deficiencies did not decline over time and some investigators were allowed to continue their involvement in clinical trials even after the revelation of flagrant violations of recognized research practices. The authors[40] discuss five regulatory options that could improve the quality of clinical trials: certifying clinical investigators, competitive application for research contracts (according to the model used by the NIH), limiting the investigators' level of participation in clinical trials, penalizing industry sponsors for misconduct by investigators, and permitting suspension of investigators prior to a hearing. They recognize that these options have advantages and disadvantages. Many European countries are moving toward regulations and guidelines for the clinical evaluation of new drugs.[9,10,33,36] However, implementation of so-called "Good Clinical Practice" could turn out to be a major challenge. The problems relate to establishment of properly functioning ethics committees, the practice of obtaining written informed consent, training of investigators, implementation of data verification and audits, and permission for official inspections.[36]

Quality control starts with clear definitions of response variables and procedures and with training; it ends with data collection, editing, and assessment. Any experiment based on poorly standardized procedures or ambiguous definitions, or conducted by insufficiently trained staff with limited knowledge about the study protocol, may lead to erroneous results and conclusions. This chapter will review why problems in data collection arise and provide some general solutions. The section on quality monitoring emphasizes issues that need to be considered in drug trials. The last section of the chapter deals with audits.

FUNDAMENTAL POINT

During all phases of a study, sufficient effort should be spent to ensure that all key data critical to the interpretation of the trial are of high quality.

PROBLEMS IN DATA COLLECTION

The definition of key data depends on trial type and objectives. Baseline characteristics of the enrolled participants, particularly those related to major eligibility measures, are clearly key, as are primary and secondary outcome measures. It is essential that conclusions or inferences from the trial are based on accurate and valid data. Fastidious attention to all data is not possible, nor is it necessary. Therefore the focus of any quality assurance effort should be directed to the key data. One approach is to decide in advance the degree of error one is willing to tolerate for each type of data. The key data and certain process information, such as informed consent, should be as error free as possible. The effort expended on assuring freedom from error for key data will be considerable. One may be willing to tolerate a greater error rate for other data. The confirmation, duplicate testing, and auditing that is done on data of secondary importance need not be as extensive. Perhaps only a sampling of audits is necessary.

Major types of problems

Problems in data collection can be of several sorts and can apply to the initial acquisition of data, such as physical examination, and to the recording of the data on a form or data entry into a remote computer terminal or microcomputer. There are three major types of data problems that are discussed here: (1) missing data, (2) incorrect data, and (3) excess variability.

First, incomplete and irretrievably missing data can arise, for example, from the inability of participants to provide necessary information, from inadequate physical examinations, from laboratory mishaps, or from carelessness in completing study forms or data entry. The percentage of missing data in a study is considered one indicator of the quality of the data and, therefore, the quality of the trial.

Second, erroneous data may not be recognized and, therefore, can be even more troublesome than incomplete data. For study purposes, a specified condition may be defined in a particular manner. A clinic staff member may unwittingly use a clinically acceptable definition, but one that is different from the study definition. Specimens may be mislabeled. In one clinical trial, the investigators suspected mislabeling errors when, in a glucose-tolerance test, the fasting glucose levels were higher than the 1-hour glucose levels in some participants. Badly calibrated equipment can be a source of error. In addition, the incorrect data may be entered on a form. A blood pressure of 84/142 mm Hg, rather than 142/84 mm Hg, is easy to identify as wrong. However, while 124/84 mm Hg may be incorrect, it is perfectly reasonable, and the error would not necessarily be recognized.

The third problem is variability in the observed characteristics. Variability reduces the opportunity to detect real changes. The variability between repeated assessments can be unsystematic (or random), systematic, or a combination of both. Variability can be intrinsic to the characteristic being measured, the instrument used for the measurement,or the observer responsible for obtaining the data. Patients can show substantial day-to-day variations in a variety of physiologic measures.[17] Learning effects associated with many performance tests also contribute to variability.[22] The problem of variability, recognized many decades ago, is not unique to any specific field of investigation.[24,25] Reports of studies of repeat chemical determinations, determinations of blood pressure, physical examinations, and interpretations of x-rays, electrocardiograms, and histological slides indicate the difficulty in obtaining reproducible data. People perform tasks differently, and they may vary in level of knowledge and experience. These factors can lead to interobserver variability. In addition, inconsistent behavior of the same observer between repeated measurements may also be much greater than expected, though intraobserver inconsistency is generally less than interobserver variability.

Specific examples of variability

Reports from studies of laboratory determinations illustrate that the problem of variability has not changed much during almost half a century. In 1947, Belk and Sunderman[3] reviewed the performance of 59 hospital laboratories on several common chemical determinations. Using prepared samples, they found that "unsatisfactory results outnumbered the satisfactory." In 1969, Lewis and Burgess[27] assessed interlaboratory measures of red blood cell count using two methods (visual and electronic). The ranges for both methods on identical samples were extremely broad. Results for the visual method varied from 2.2×10^6 RBC/mm^3 to 5.1×10^6 RBC/mm^3, and for the electronic method from 0.7×10^6 RBC/mm^3 to 4.7×10^6 RBC/mm^3. In 1978, others[30] looked at six selected laboratories. The overall performance was reasonably good. However, performance on simulated patient specimens was worse than on designated quality control specimens. When special attention is given to the analyses, laboratories perform better. Recently, a comparison of zidovudine levels from 23 different laboratories using four different assay methods revealed a very high rate of falsely elevated measurements at six of the laboratories.[26]

Classification of histologic specimens may also be highly variable. Feinstein et al.[12] reviewed interpretation of cellular types of lung cancer by five experienced pathologists. On second readings, pathologists disagreed with their first diagnoses up to 20% of the time. Similar experiences have been reported from studies of breast cancer[15] and "undifferentiated" lymphomas.[44] The diagnostic reproducibility was 59% in the Burkitt's and non-Burkitt's lymphoma groups.

Waters et al.[42] assessed the reproducibility of quantitative coronary angiography under four conditions: (1) same film, same frame; (2) same film, different frame; (3) same view from films obtained within 1 month; and (4) same view from films 1 to 6 months apart. The standard deviation of repeat measurements of minimum vessel diameter increased between conditions 1 and 2 and between 3 and 4. The variability between visual and quantitative measurements of the same frame was 2 to 3 times higher than the variability of paired quantitative measurements from the same frame. Large variation in mantle technique has also been reported among radiotherapists.[31]

When Davies[8] looked at the readings of electrocardiograms by nine experienced cardiologists, he found large interobserver and intraobserver disagreement. On the average, on rereading electrocardiograms, the cardiologists disagreed with one in eight of their original interpretations. A study that assessed clinical findings of the respiratory system[41] concluded that "interobserver repeatability of respiratory signs falls midway between chance and total agreement." Dermatologists differ widely in the assessment of disease progress in psoriasis.[29] Use of computer-assisted planimetry reduces variability in the calculation of the area of psoriatic skin involvement. A review of the site, stage, and compliance to the protocol for surgical treatment of patients with advanced head and neck cancer showed differences between surgeons and institutions.[18] A reliability study[4] of two toxicity scales concluded that "experienced managers, when interviewing patients, draw varying conclusions regarding toxic effects experienced by such patients." Klinkhoff et al.[20] demonstrated nicely how this problem of interobserver variability could be markedly reduced by having investigators agree on a precise method of examination and participate in discussion and patient examination aimed at producing agreement in examining techniques.

The use of technology may reduce variability. This reduction in variability has been demonstrated for a variety of procedures, for example, computerized exercise electrocardiogram digitization,[6] ambulatory blood pressure monitoring,[7] and densitometric analysis of nuclear cataracts.[28]

Regardless of the source of variability, several factors may have an impact on the magnitude of variability. Vagueness in definitions, inadequate methodology, lack of training of personnel, and carelessness all increase the variation inherent in any measurement.

MINIMIZING POOR QUALITY DATA

General approaches for minimizing potential problems in data collection are summarized in the following section. Most of these should be considered during the planning phase of the trial. Examples in the cardiovascular field are provided by Rose et al.[37] In this section, we discuss design of protocol and manual, development of forms, training, pretesting, techniques to reduce variability, and data entry.

Design of protocol and manual

Clear definitions of entry and diagnostic criteria and methodology are essential. These should be included in the protocol and written so that all investigators and staff can apply them in a consistent manner throughout the trial. The same question can be interpreted in many ways. Even the same investigator may forget how he previously interpreted a question unless he can readily refer to instructions and definitions. Accessibility of these definitions is also important. A manual of procedures should be prepared in every clinical trial. Although it may contain information about study background, design, and organization, the manual of procedures is not simply an expanded protocol. In addition to listing eligibility criteria and response variable definitions, it should indicate how the criteria and variables are determined. This document provides detailed answers to all conceivable "how to" questions. Most important, the manual needs to describe in detail the participant visits and their scheduling and content. Instructions must be accurate and complete for filling out forms; performing tasks such as laboratory determinations, drug ordering, storing, and dispensing; and adherence monitoring. Finally, recruitment techniques, informed consent, participant safety, emergency unblinding, use of concomitant therapy, and other issues need to be addressed. Updates and clarifications usually occur during the course of a study. These revisions should be made available to every staff person involved in data collection.

Descriptions of laboratory methods and the ways the results are to be reported also need to be stated in advance. In one study, plasma levels of the drug propranolol were determined by using four methods. Only after the study ended was it discovered that two laboratories routinely were measuring free propranolol and two other laboratories were measuring propranolol hydrochloride. A conversion factor allowed investigators to make simple adjustments and arrive at legitimate comparisons. Such adjustments are not always possible.

Development of forms

Ideally, the study forms should contain all necessary information. If that is not possible, the forms should outline the key information and refer the investigator to the appropriate page in a manual of procedures. Well-designed forms will minimize errors and variability. Forms should be as short and as well organized as possible, with a logical sequence to the questions. Forms should be clear, with few "write-in" answers. As little as possible should be left to the imagination of the person completing the form. This means, in general, no essay questions. The questions should elicit the necessary information and little else. Questions that are tacked on because the answers would be "nice to know" are rarely analyzed and may distract attention from pertinent questions. In several studies where death is the primary response variable, investigators have expressed interest in learning about the circumstances surrounding the death. In particular, the occurrence of symptoms before death, the time lapse from the occurrence of such symptoms until death, and the activity and location of the participant at the time of death have been considered important and helpful in classifying the cause of death. While this may be true, focusing on these details has led to the creation of extraordinarily complex forms that take considerable time to complete. Moreover, questions arise concerning the accuracy of the information, because much of it is obtained from proxy sources who may not have been with the participant when he died. Unless investigators clearly understand how these data will be used, simpler forms are preferable. General guidelines to forms design for clinical trials are also available.[21,34,45]

Training

Training sessions for investigators and staff to promote standardization of procedures are crucial to the success of any large study. Whenever more than one person is filling out forms or examining participants, training sessions help to minimize error. There may be more than one correct way of doing something in clinical practice, but for study purposes, there is only one way. Similarly, the questions on a form should always be asked in the same way. The answer to, "Have you had any chest pain in the last 3 months?" may be different from the answer to, "You haven't had any chest pain in the last 3 months, have you?" Even differences in tone or the emphasis placed on various parts of a question can alter or affect the response. Training laboratory personnel is equally important. Two technicians may use slightly different techniques. These differences can lead to confusing results. Kahn et al.[19] reviewed the impact of training procedures instituted in the Framingham Eye Study. The 2 days of formal training included duplicate examinations, discussions about differences, and the use of a reference set of fundus photographs. Neaton et al.[32] concluded that initial training is useful and should cover the areas of clinic operation, technical measurements, and delivery of intervention. Centralized interim training of new staff is less efficient and can be replaced by regional training and use of audiovisual techniques.

Mechanisms to verify that all clinic staff do things the same way should be developed. These include instituting certification procedures for specified types of data collection. If blood pressure, electrocardiograms, pulmonary function tests, or laboratory tests are important, the people performing these determinations should not only be trained, but also be tested and certified as competent. Periodic retraining and recertification are especially useful in long-term studies since people tend to forget, and personnel turnover is common. For situations where staff must conduct interviews, special training procedures to standardize the approach have been used.[38] In a study of B-mode ultrasonography[14] of the carotid arteries, marked differences in intimal-medial thickness measurements were found between the 13 readers at the reading center. Some readers changed their reading from low to high and vice versa during the 5-year study. A sharp increase in average intimal-medial thickness measurements toward the end of the study was explained by readers reading high having an increased workload, the hire of a new reader also reading high, and a reader changing from reading low to high.

Pretesting

Pretesting of forms and procedures is useful and almost always essential. Several people similar to the intended participants should participate in a simulated interview and examination to make sure procedures are properly performed and questions on the forms flow well and provide the desired information. Furthermore, by pretesting, the investigator grows familiar and comfortable with the form. Fictional case histories can be used to check form design and the care with which forms are completed. When developing forms, most investigators cannot even begin to imagine the numerous ways questions can be misinterpreted until several people have been given the same information and asked to fill out the same form. Part of the reason for different answers is undoubtedly because of carelessness by the person completing the form. The use of debriefing in the pilot test may bring to light misinterpretations that would not be detected when real participants fill out the forms. Anyone editing a form has no way of identifying errors that are not completely unreasonable. Inadequacies in form structure and logic can also be uncovered by use of pretesting. In conclusion, pretesting reveals areas where forms might be improved and where additional training might be worthwhile.

Debriefing is an essential part of the training process. This helps people completing the forms to understand how the forms are meant to be completed and what interpretations are wanted. Discussion also alerts them to carelessness. When done before the start of the study, this sort of discussion allows the investigator to modify inadequate items on forms. These case history exercises might be profitably repeated several times during the course of a long-term study to indicate when education and retraining are needed. Ideally, forms should not be changed after the study has started. Inevitably, though, modifications are made. Pretesting can help to minimize them.

Techniques to reduce variability

Both variability and bias in the assessment of response variables should be minimized through repeat assessment, blinded assessment, or (ideally) both. At the time of the examination of a participant, for example, an investigator may determine blood pressure two or more times and record the average. Performing the measurement without knowing the group assignment helps to minimize bias. In blinded or single-blinded studies, the examination might be performed by someone who is unaware of participant treatment assignment. In assessing slides, x-rays, or electrocardiograms, two individuals can make independent, blinded evaluations, and the results can be averaged or adjudicated in cases of disagreement. Independent evaluations are particularly important when the assessment requires an element of judgment. Classification of response variables such as cause of death or nonfatal events can be performed in a similar manner.

Data entry

The introduction of microcomputers into clinical trials has improved data quality. Data-entry programs identify missing, extreme, or inconsistent values and prohibit further data entry until a correction has been made. In cases where an investigator must go back to the participant to check the information, this aspect is particularly valuable, because the error is identified rapidly. Double entry of data is also used to reduce the error rate. Adequate training of staff is essential to fully realize the advantages of this technology.

An issue under debate is whether forms can be eliminated. Typically, a paper form is completed and the data transferred to the microcomputer. Thus a record trail is available for data verification and audit. If only the final entered data are available, there is no assurance that the data have not been altered inappropriately. Programs can be developed that will ensure that both original and revised data are saved. Thus a computerized audit trail can be developed. In such a case, it is conceivable that an investigator can dispense with paper forms.

In general, there has been a favorable experience with entering clinical trial data into microcomputers. Error rates have been low, and corrections have been minimal.[1,32]

QUALITY MONITORING

Even though every effort is made to obtain high-quality data, a monitoring or surveillance system is crucial. When errors are found, a monitoring system enables the investigator to take corrective action. Monitoring is most effective when it is current. Additionally, monitoring allows an assessment of data quality when interpreting study results. Numerous forms and procedures can be monitored, but monitoring all of them is usually not feasible. Rather, monitoring those areas most important to the trial is recommended. Form completion, procedures, and drug handling also need to be monitored.

Monitoring of data quality proves most valuable when there is feedback to the clinic staff and technicians. Once weaknesses and errors have been identified, performance can be improved. Chapter 19 contains several tables illustrating quality control reports. With careful planning, reports can be provided and improvement can be accomplished without unblinding the staff. All quality control measures take time and money; it is thus impossible to be compulsive about the quality of every piece of datum and every procedure. Investigators need to focus their efforts on those procedures that yield key data, those on which the conclusions of the study critically depend.

Monitoring of forms

During the study, all key forms should be checked for completeness, internal consistency, and consistency with other forms. On a follow-up visit to evaluate a participant's progress, the investigator might want to know whether the participant has had a myocardial infarction since the previous follow-up visit. If the participant has had such an event, then more information about the event can be collected on a special event form. When the forms disagree, the person or group responsible for ensuring consistent and accurate forms should question the person filling out forms. Consistency within a given form can also be evaluated. Dates and times are particularly prone to error.

It may be important to examine consistency of data over time. A participant with a missing leg on one examination was reported to have palpable pedal pulses on a subsequent examination. Cataracts that did not allow for a valid eye examination at one visit were not present at the next visit, without an interval surgery having been performed. The data forms may indicate extreme changes in body weight from one visit to the next. In such a case, changing the data after the fact is likely to be inappropriate because the correct weights may be unknown. However, the investigator can take corrective action for future visits by more carefully training his staff. Sometimes, mistakes can be corrected. In one trial, comparison of successive electrocardiographic (ECG) readings disclosed gross discrepancies in the coding of abnormalities. The investigator discovered that one of the technicians responsible for coding the ECGs was fabricating his readings. In this instance, correcting the data was possible.

Someone needs constantly to monitor completed forms to find evidence of missing participant visits or visits that are off schedule to correct any problems. Frequency of missing or late visits may be associated with the intervention. Differences between groups in missed visits may bias the study results. To improve upon results, it may be necessary to observe actual clinic procedures. Observing clinic procedures is particularly important in multicenter trials.[13]

Monitoring of procedures

Extreme laboratory values should be checked. Values incompatible with life, such as potassium of 10 mEq/L, are obviously incorrect. Other less extreme values (e.g., total cholesterol of 125 mg/dl in male adults in the United States) should be questioned. They may be correct, but it is unlikely. Finally, values should be compared with previous ones from the same participant. Certain levels of variability are expected, but when these levels are exceeded, the value should be flagged as a potential outlier. For example, unless the study involves administering a lipid-lowering therapy, any determination that shows a change in serum cholesterol of perhaps 20% or more from one visit to the next should be repeated. Repetition would require saving samples of serum until the analysis has been checked. In addition to checking results, a helpful procedure is to monitor submission of laboratory specimens to ensure that missing data are kept to a minimum.

Investigators doing special procedures (laboratory work, ECG readings) need to have an internal quality control system. Such a system should include reanalysis of duplicate specimens or materials at different times in a blinded fashion. A system of resubmitting specimens from outside the laboratory or reading center might also be instituted. As noted by McCormick et al.,[30] these specimens need to be indistinguishable from actual study specimens. An external laboratory quality control program established in the planning phase of a trial can pick up errors at many stages (specimen collection, preparation, transportation, and reporting of results), not just at the analysis stage. Thus it provides an overall estimate of quality. Unfortunately, the system most often cannot indicate at which step in the process errors may have occurred. The external quality control programs implemented in the Coronary Drug Project have been described by Canner et al.[5] Another example is provided by the National Cooperative Gallstone Study.[16]

All recording equipment should be checked periodically. Even though initially calibrated, the machines can break down or require adjustment. Scales can be checked by means of standard weights. If aneroid sphygmomanometers are used, they should be compared regularly with a mercury sphygmomanometer. Factors such as linearity, frequency response, paper speed, and time constant should be checked on electrocardiographic machines. In one long-term trial, the prevalence of specific electrocardiographic abnormalities was monitored. The sudden appearance of a threefold increase in one abnormality, without any obvious medical cause, led the investigator to suspect correctly electrocardiographic machine malfunction.

Monitoring of drug handling

In a drug study, the quality of the drug preparations should be monitored throughout the trial. Monitoring includes periodically examining containers for possible mislabeling and proper contents (both quality and quantity). It has been reported[35] that in one trial, "half of the study group received the wrong medication" because of errors at the pharmacy. Investigators should carefully look for discoloration and breaking or crumbling of capsules or tablets. When the agents are being prepared in several batches, samples from each batch should be examined and analyzed. Occasionally, monitoring the number of pills or capsules per bottle is useful. The actual bottle content of pills should not vary by more than 1% or 2%. The number of pills in a bottle is important to know because pill count may be used to measure adherence of participants.

Another aspect to consider is the storage shelf life of the preparations and whether they deteriorate over time. Even if they retain their potency, do changes in odor (as with aspirin) or color occur? If shelf life is long, preparing all agents at one time will minimize variability. Of course, in the event that the study ends prematurely, there may be a large supply of unusable drugs. Products having a short shelf life require frequent production and shipment of small batches. Complete records should be maintained for all drugs prepared, examined, and used. Ideally, a sample from each batch should be saved. After the study is over, questions about drug identity or purity may arise and samples will be useful.

The dispensing of medication should also be monitored. Checking has two aspects. First, were the proper drugs sent from the pharmacy or pharmaceutical company to the clinic? If the study is double-blind, the clinic staff will be unable to check on this. They must assume that the medication has been properly coded. However, in unblinded studies, staff should check to assure that the proper drugs and dosage strengths have been received. In one case, the wrong strength of potassium chloride was sent to the clinic. The clinic personnel failed to notice the error. An alert participant to whom the drug was issued brought the mistake to the attention of the investigator. Had the participant been less alert, serious consequences could have arisen. An investigator has an obligation to be as careful about dispensing drugs as is a licensed pharmacist. Close reading of labels and documentation of all drugs that are handed out to participants are essential.

Second, when the study is blinded, the clinic personnel need to be absolutely sure that the code number on the container is the proper one. Labels and drugs should be identical except for the code; therefore extra care is essential. If bottles of coded medication are lined up on a shelf, it is relatively easy to pick up the wrong bottle accidentally. Unless the participant noticed the different code, such errors may not be recognized. Even if he is observant, he may assume that he was meant to receive a different code number. The clinic staff should be asked to note on a study form the code number of the bottle dispensed and the code number of bottles that are returned by the participant. Theoretically, that should enable investigators to spot errors. In the end, however, investigators must rely on the care and diligence of the staff person dispensing the drugs.

It may be worthwhile periodically to send study drug samples to a laboratory for analysis. Although the center responsible for packaging and labeling drugs should have a foolproof scheme, independent laboratory analysis serves as an additional check on the labeling process.

The drug manufacturer assigns lot or batch numbers to each batch of drugs that are prepared. If contamination or problems in preparations are detected, then only those drugs from the problem batch need to be recalled. The use of batch numbers is especially important in clinical trials, since the recall of all drugs can severely delay, or even ruin, the study. When only some drugs are recalled, the study can usually manage to continue. Therefore the lot number of the drug and the name or code number should be listed in the participant's study record.

AUDITS

Some investigators have objections to random external data audits, especially in the absence of evidence of scientific misconduct. However, the magnitude of the problems detected when audits occur makes it difficult to take a position against audits. Of interest, the FDA does not perform audits of trials sponsored by the National Cancer Institute (NCI) according to a long-standing agreement.[40] An NCI-sponsored audit program has been in place for more than a decade. A recent review of four cycles of internal audits conducted over an 11-year period by the investigators of the Cancer and Leukemia Group B showed similarities with the FDA audit.[43] The deficiency rate (among main institutions) of 28% in the first cycle dropped to 13.3% in the fourth cycle. Only two cases of major scientific impropriety were uncovered during these on-site peer reviews. Compliance with Institutional Review Board requirements improved over time, as did compliance with having proper consent forms. Although compliance with eligibility improved from 90% to 94%, no changes were noted for disagreement with auditors for treatment responses (5%) and deviations from the treatment protocol (11%). The authors conclude that the audit program had been successful in "pressuring group members to improve adherence to administrative requirements, protocol compliance, and data submission. It has also served to weed out poorly performing institutions." The findings of a quality control study of institutions participating in a European radiotherapy trial in lung cancer[23] were similar and noted important clinic differences. Deviations in staging and treatment parameters occurred in one fifth of the patients. The authors strongly recommend implementation of a quality control system at the earliest possible stage in multicenter trials to improve data quality and trial conclusions. As noted earlier, however, any audit plan needs to concentrate on key information and distinguish between important and unimportant errors. For some data, informed consent, proper allocation, safety, and key outcomes, 100% verification is essential; for others, occasional sampling may be sufficient.

REFERENCES

1. Bagniewska A, Black D, Curtis C et al: Data quality control in a distributed data processing system: the SHEP Pilot Study, *Controlled Clin Trials* 7:27-37, 1986.
2. Bailey KR: Detecting fabrication of data in a multicenter collaborative animal study, *Controlled Clin Trials* 12:741-752, 1991.

3. Belk WP, Sunderman FW: A survey of the accuracy of chemical analyses in clinical laboratories, *Am J Clin Pathol* 17:853-861, 1947.

4. Brundage MD, Pater JL, Zee B: Assessing the reliability of two toxicity scales: implications for interpreting toxicity data, *J Natl Cancer Inst* 85:1138-1148, 1993.

5. Canner PL, Krol WF, Forman SA: External quality control programs, *Controlled Clin Trials* 4:441-466, 1983.

6. Caralis DG, Shaw L, Bilgere B, et al: Application of computerized exercise ECG digitization, *J Electrocardiol* 25:101-110, 1992.

7. Conway J, Coats A: Value of ambulatory blood pressure monitoring in clinical pharmacology, *J Hypertens* 7 (suppl 3):S29-S32, 1989.

8. Davies LG: Observer variation in reports on electrocardiograms, *Br Heart J* 20:153-161, 1958.

9. Dent NJ: European good laboratory and clinical practices: their relevance to clinical pathology laboratories, *Qual Assurance: Good Prac, Regul, Law* 1:82-89, 1991.

10. EEC: EEC note for guidance: good clinical practice for trials on medicinal products in the European community, *Pharmacol Toxicol* 67:361-372, 1990.

11. Engler RL, Cavell JW, Friedman PJ et al: Misrepresentation and responsibility in medical research, *N Engl J Med* 317:1383-1389, 1987.

12. Feinstein AR, Gelfman NA, Yesner R et al: Observer variability in the histopathologic diagnosis of lung cancer, *Am Rev Respir Dis* 101:671-684, 1970.

13. Ferris FL, Ederer F: External monitoring in multiclinic trials: applications from ophthalmologic studies, *Clin Pharmacol Ther* 25:720-723, 1979.

14. Furberg CD, Byington RP, Craven T: Lessons learned from clinical trials with ultrasound endpoints, *J Intern Med* 236:575-580, 1994.

15. Gilchrist KW, Kalish L, Gould VE et al: Interobserver reproducibility of histopathological features in stage II breast cancer. An ECOG study, *Breast Cancer Res Treat* 5:3-10, 1985.

16. Habig RL, Thomas P, Lippel K, et al: Central laboratory quality control in the National Cooperative Gallstone Study, *Controlled Clin Trials* 4:101-123, 1983.

17. Irvine EJ, Tougas G, Lappalainen R, Bathurst NC: Reliability and interobserver variability of ultrasound measurement of gastric emptying rate, *Dig Dis Sci* 38:803-810, 1993.

18. Jacobs JR, Pajak TF, Weymuller E et al: Development of surgical quality-control mechanisms in large-scale prospective trials: Head and Neck Intergroup report, *Head Neck* 13:28-32, 1991.

19. Kahn HA, Leibowitz H, Ganley JP et al: Standardizing diagnostic procedures, *Am J Ophthalmol* 79:768-775, 1975.

20. Klinkhoff AV, Bellamy N, Bombardier C, et al: An experiment in reducing interobserver variability of the examination of joint tenderness, *J Reumatol* 15:492-494, 1988.

21. Knatterud GL, Forman SA, Canner PL: Design of data forms, *Controlled Clin Trials* 4:429-440, 1983.

22. Knox AJ, Morrison JFJ, Muers MF: Reproducibility of walking test results in chronic airways disease, *Thorax* 43:388-392, 1988.

23. Schaake-Koning C, Kirkpatrick A, Kroger R et al: The need for immediate monitoring of treatment parameters and uniform assessment of patient data in clinical trials, *Eur J Cancer* 27:615-619, 1991.

24. Koran LM: The reliability of clinical methods, data and judgments. Part 1, *N Engl J Med* 293:642-646, 1975.

25. Koran LM: The reliability of clinical methods, data and judgments. Part 2, *N Engl J Med* 293:695-701, 1975.

26. Krogstad DJ, Eveland MR, Lim L L-Y et al: Drug level monitoring in a double-blind multicenter trial: false-positive zidovudine measurements in AIDS clinical trials group protocol 019, *Antimicrob Agents Chemother* 35:1160-1164, 1991.

27. Lewis SM, Burgess BJ: Quality control in haematology: report of interlaboratory trials in Britain, *BMJ* 4:253-256, 1969.

28. Magno BV, Freidlin V, Datiles MB: Reproducibility of the NEI Scheimpflug Cataract Imaging System, *Invest Ophthalmol Vis Sci* 35:3078-3084, 1994.

29. Marks R, Barton SP, Shuttleworth D, Finley AY: Assessment of disease progress in psoriasis, *Arch Dermatol* 125:235-240, 1989.

30. McCormick W, Ingelfinger JA, Isakson G et al: Errors in measuring drug concentrations, *N Engl J Med* 299:1118-1121, 1978.
31. Sebag-Montefiore DJ, Maher EJ, Young J et al: Variation in mantle technique: implications for establishing priorities for quality assurance in clinical trials, *Radiot Oncol* 23:144-149, 1992.
32. Neaton JD, Duchene AG, Svendsen KH, Wentworth D: An examination of the efficacy of some quality assurance methods commonly employed in clinical trials, *Stat Med* 9:115-124, 1990.
33. Nordic Council on Medicines: *Good clinical trial practice. Nordic guidelines,* Uppsala; NLN Pub 28, 1989.
34. Pocock SJ: *Clinical trials. A practical approach,* Chichester, 1983, John Wiley & Sons.
35. Quality assurance of clinical data: Discussion, *Clin Pharmacol Ther* 25:726-727, 1979.
36. Regnier B: Good clinical practice, *Eur J Clin Microbiol Infect Dis* 9:519-522, 1990.
37. Rose GA, Blackburn H, Gillum RF, Prineas RJ: *Cardiovascular survey methods,* Geneva, 1982, World Health Organization, Monograph Ser 56.
38. Russell ML, Ghee KL, Probstfield JL et al: Development of standardized simulated patients for quality control of the clinical interview, *Controlled Clin Trials* 4:197-208, 1983.
39. Shapiro MF, Charrow RP: Scientific misconduct in investigational drug trials, *N Engl J Med* 312:731-736, 1985.
40. Shapiro MF, Charrow RP: The role of data audits in detecting scientific misconduct, *JAMA* 261:2505-2511, 1989.
41. Smyllie HC, Blendis LM, Armitage P: Observer disagreement in physical signs of the respiratory system, *Lancet* 2:412-413, 1965.
42. Waters D, Lespérance J, Craven TE, et al: Advantages and limitations of serial coronary arteriography for the assessment of progression and regression of coronary atherosclerosis. Implications for clinical trials, *Circulation* 87(suppl II): II38-II47, 1993.
43. Weiss RB, Vogelzang NJ, Peterson BA et al: A successful system of scientific data audits for clinical trials. A report from the Cancer and Leukemia Group B, *JAMA* 270:459-464, 1993.
44. Wilson JF, Kjeldsberg CR, Sposto R et al: The pathology of non-Hodgkin's lymphoma of childhood: II. Reproducibility and relevance of the histologic classification of "undifferentiated" lymphomas (Burkitt's versus non-Burkitt's), *Hum Pathol* 18:1008-1014, 1987.
45. Wright P, Haybittle J: Design of forms for clinical trials, *BMJ* 2:529-530, 590-592, 650-651, 1979.

CHAPTER 11

Assessing and Reporting Adverse Effects

The assessment of adverse effects encompasses the whole spectrum of research from laboratory work during drug and device development, animal studies, and early work in small numbers of human beings, to case reports, clinical trials, and postmarketing surveillance. Carcinogenic or teratogenic adverse effects of drugs, such as noted with diethylstilbestrol[15,16] and thalidomide[21] or possible failures of devices such as cardiac pacemakers or silicone breast implants, receive considerable publicity, but other sorts of findings are undoubtedly more common.

Many have written about and developed approaches for evaluating adverse reactions, both before a drug is approved and marketed[3] and after approval, through postmarketing surveillance.* The difficulties in assessing adverse effects in the postmarketing situation have also been widely discussed.† The FDA has recently instituted "a new approach to reporting medication and device adverse effects" for marketed products.[19]

The discussion here is limited to assessment of adverse effects in clinical trials beyond the initial stages of development and testing. That is, even though the drugs may not yet be marketed, they have undergone early evaluation in human beings and are ready for larger-scale evaluation. For the purposes of this book, adverse effects are defined as any clinical event, sign, or symptom that goes in an unwanted direction. It encompasses any undesirable clinical outcome, but has the added dimensions of physical findings, complaints, and laboratory results. Adverse effects can include both objective measures and subjective responses.

FUNDAMENTAL POINT

Adequate attention needs to be given to the assessment, analysis, and reporting of adverse effects to permit valid assessment of potential risks of interventions.

Adverse effects are considered to be important, and most reports of studies present selected data. However, trials are generally not designed for the purpose of

---

*References 3, 11, 18, 25, 28, 36.

†References 11, 18, 25, 34, 36.

assessing adverse effects. The scientific standards that are used in evaluating an intervention for efficacy are rarely employed when evaluating possible adverse effects. The assessing and reporting of adverse effects have often played, and continue to play, a secondary role in clinical trials. An example is the almost complete lack of information on hematotoxicity in 314 published trials of antidepressants, despite the concern that antidepressants can cause hematotoxicity.[13]

Adverse effects can be either expected or unexpected. Expected ones are those that, based on previous knowledge about the intervention or similar drugs or devices, are known or likely to occur. Occasionally, completely unanticipated problems can occur. These may be serious enough to lead to termination of the trial, or even to withdrawal of the agent from the market.[22]

Unlike the few and generally well-defined primary or even secondary response variables, many possible adverse effects may be monitored in a trial. Because of this problem of multiple testing (Chapter 15), the intervention may appear significantly different from the control more often by chance alone than indicated by the p value. Nevertheless, investigators tend to relax their statistical requirements for declaring adverse effects to be real findings. It reflects understandable conservatism and the desire to avoid unnecessary harm to the participants.

In assessing adverse effects, it must be noted that many problems arise with some frequency in the control group. These may be due to the natural history of the disease or condition or to the nonstudy therapy the participant is receiving. In the Beta-Blocker Heart Attack Trial[4] of propranolol in participants with recent myocardial infarction, 66% of the group receiving a placebo complained of shortness of breath over the course of 2 years. At baseline, only 6% had a history of shortness of breath.[7]

As Bulpitt[6] discussed, the noting of an adverse effect by participants in an accurate way depends greatly on the setting and manner in which it is elicited and the phrasing of the question. Good questions must be clear and easily understood, have high repeatability, be valid, and be answered by the participant. These features apply to all areas in clinical trials but are perhaps most important when the investigation is dealing with subjective complaints.

This chapter will cover several determinants of adverse effects; that is, factors that can influence their observed or reported occurrence, frequency, and severity. It will also review several aspects in the reporting or presenting of adverse effects.

DETERMINANTS OF ADVERSE EFFECTS

Several factors play a role in determining adverse effects. These can affect the quality of the data, the reported frequency of the effects, and the interpretation of their meaning.

Definitions

The rationale for defining adverse effects is similar to that for defining any response variable: it enables investigators to record something in a consistent manner. Further, it allows someone reviewing a trial to better assess it and possibly to compare the results with those of other trials of similar interventions.

Because adverse effects are typically viewed as truly secondary or tertiary response variables, they are not often seriously thought about in advance. Generally, an investigator will prepare a list of potential adverse effects on a study form, using, perhaps, commonly accepted terms. These adverse effects usually are not defined, except by the way investigators apply them in their daily practice. Study protocols seldom contain written definitions of adverse effects, unlike primary or other secondary response variables. In multicenter trials, the situation may often be even worse. In those cases, an adverse effect may be simply what each investigator declares it to be. Thus intrastudy consistency may be poor.

Given the large number of possible adverse effects, it is not feasible to define clearly all of them, and many do not lend themselves to good definition. Though it is not always easy, important adverse effects that are associated with individual signs or laboratory findings, or a constellation of signs, symptoms, and laboratory results, can and should be well-defined. These include ones known to be associated with the intervention and that are clinically important. Other adverse effects that are purely based on a participant's report of symptoms may be important but are more difficult to define. These may include nausea, fatigue, or headache. Nevertheless, the fact that an adverse effect is not well-defined should be stated in the study protocol. Some adverse effects cannot be defined in that they are not listed in advance but are spontaneously mentioned by the participants. Any trial publication should indicate which events were not prespecified.

Ascertainment

The issue of whether one should elicit adverse effects by means of a checklist or rely on the participant to volunteer complaints often arises. Eliciting adverse effects has the advantage of allowing a standard way of obtaining information on a preselected list of symptoms. Thus both within and between trials, the same series of effects can be ascertained in the same way, with assurance that a "yes" or "no" answer will be present for each. This presupposes, of course, adequate training in the administration of the questions. Volunteered responses to a question such as "Have you had any health problems since your last visit?" have the possible advantage of tending to yield only the more serious episodes, while others are likely to be ignored or forgotten. In addition, only volunteered responses will give information on truly unexpected adverse effects.

Table 11-1 Percentage of patients ever reporting (volunteered and elicited) selected adverse effects, by study group, in the Aspirin Myocardial Infarction Study

	Hematemesis	Tarry stools	Bloody stools
Volunteered			
Aspirin	0.27	1.34*	1.29[†]
Placebo	0.09	0.67	0.45
Elicited			
Aspirin	0.62	2.81*	4.86*
Placebo	0.27	1.74	2.99

*Aspirin-placebo difference > 2 S.E.

[†]Aspirin-placebo difference > 3 S.E.

Aspirin group: N = 2267

Placebo group: N = 2257

In the Aspirin Myocardial Infarction Study,[1] information on several adverse effects was both volunteered by the participants and elicited. After a general question about adverse effects, the investigators asked about specific complaints. The results for three adverse effects are presented in Table 11-1. Two points might be noted. First, for each adverse effect, eliciting gave a higher percentage of participants with complaints than did asking for volunteered problems. Second, the same aspirin-placebo differences were noted, regardless of the method. Thus, the investigators could arrive at the same conclusions with each technique. In this study, little additional information was gained by the double ascertainment. Perhaps the range between the volunteered and the elicited numbers within the individual study groups provides bounds on the true incidence of the adverse effect.

Downing et al.[10] reported on a comparison of elicited vs. volunteered adverse effects in a trial of tranquilizers and antidepressants. Thirty-three participants receiving active drug volunteered complaints, as opposed to 12 receiving placebo. This contrasts with 53 elicited complaints from the active drug group and 12 elicited from the placebo group. The authors concluded that eliciting adverse effects preferentially increases the number in the active drug group, rather than the placebo group. This is contrary to the findings in the Aspirin Myocardial Infarction Study.

In the same paper, Downing et al. examined the severity of adverse effects obtained by both methods. Of 29 drug-treated participants who had complaints ascertained by both eliciting and volunteering, 26 were classified as more severe. Of 24 participants whose complaints were ascertained only by eliciting, half were called more severe. Therefore the requirement that an adverse effect be volunteered by a participant led to a preponderance of severe ones.

In a clinical trial of antirheumatic drugs, Huskisson and Wojtulewski[17] also compared elicited ("checklist") adverse effects with volunteered ("no checklist"). They created a score from the sums of the participant responses, weighted by perception of adverse effect severity. When the adverse effects were elicited, "the difference between the incidence of the significant side effect and the 'background' incidence in the control population was diminished." In addition, the volunteer approach yielded more unlisted and presumably unexpected adverse effects than did the elicited approach. Avery et al.[2] also compared checklist vs. nonchecklist ascertainment of adverse effects in a series of depressed patients. They came to the opposite conclusion concerning severity; namely, there are "significantly greater numbers and greater severity of side effects reported in the checklist group." Simpson et al.[30] also compared a checklist with event recording in a cross-over trial of an antidepressant on weight and appetite. Similar adverse effects were reported for the two methods, though additional complaints, not in the checklist, were noted with the event recording.

Because of these inconsistent findings, many researchers have continued to use both methods. Recognizing this, the National Institute of Mental Health developed a Systematic Assessment for Treatment of Emergent Events.[32] This instrument provides a standard way of asking both general and specific items for different organ systems. It allows the investigator to enter both symptoms and physical findings in a systematic way. However, perhaps because of its length or the concern that it may yield a greater number of adverse effect complaints, it has not been widely used (J. Levine, personal communication, 1994).

It has been suggested that subjective adverse effects are influenced by the amount of information provided to participants during the informed consent process. Romanowski et al.[29] compared responses of 25 people given general information about possible adverse effects in a consent form with responses from the 29 provided with a detailed listing of possible adverse effects. In this study, there was no important difference in frequency of reported subjective adverse effects (4 vs. 6). The investigators therefore concluded that "previous priming of the patient" did not affect reporting of adverse effects. Obviously, the numbers are small, and a larger study would be necessary to confirm this.

Frequency of events

Assessment of an adverse effect is also affected by the number of participants who suffer the effect. The more participants with an occurrence of an effect, the more reliable is the estimate of its true frequency. Adverse effects that occur rarely will only be detected in very large trials. Another problem with low-frequency effects (especially unexpected ones) is that investigators are unsure when to ignore them. Disregarding them may be entirely appropriate. On occasion, however, an important adverse effect may be erroneously overlooked because just one or two participants were affected.

An unavoidable difficulty in documenting drug- or device-related problems is that investigators calculate sample sizes on the basis of primary response variables, not as a result of estimates of adverse effect frequency. Even if assessment of adverse effects is a major objective of the study, a trial's size will not generally be increased in an effort to improve the likelihood of reliably detecting such effects. A possible exception is a study that aims to show no important difference in efficacy between a new intervention and a standard therapy, which serves as the control. If indeed, no clinically major difference between groups for the primary response variable is demonstrated, the ultimate choice of therapy may depend on factors such as lower cost, ease of administration, and lack of serious or annoying adverse effects. In this circumstance, an investigator should consider adverse effect assessment and primary outcome assessment in the sample-size estimate.

One major drawback of trials using surrogate response variables to limit the required sample size and duration is that the assessment of adverse effects and safety will be inadequate because of the scanty number of events.

Length of follow-up

Obviously, the duration of a trial has a substantial impact on adverse effect assessment. The longer the trial, the more opportunity one has to discover adverse effects, especially those with low frequency. Also, the cumulative number of participants in the intervention group complaining will increase, giving a better estimate of the adverse effect incidence. Of course, eventually, most participants will report some general complaint, such as headache or fatigue. However, this will occur in the control group as well. Therefore, if a trial lasts for several years, and an adverse effect is analyzed simply on the basis of cumulative number of participants suffering from it, the results may not be very informative.

Duration of follow-up is also important in that exposure time may be critical. Some drugs may not cause certain adverse effects until a person has been taking them for a minimum period. An example is the lupus syndrome with procainamide. Given enough time, a large proportion of participants will develop this syndrome, but very few will do so if followed for only several weeks.[38] Other sorts of time patterns may be important as well. Many adverse effects occur at low drug doses shortly after initiation of treatment. In such circumstance, it is useful, and indeed prudent, to carefully monitor participants for the first few hours or days. If no reactions occur, the subject may be presumed to be at a low risk of developing these effects subsequently. In the Beta-Blocker Heart Attack Trial,[4] all participants were started on a test dose of 20 mg of propranolol (or matching placebo) before being raised to the early maintenance dose of 40 mg three times a day. The purpose was to discover those participants unable to tolerate the first dose of the drug while they were still in a closely monitored hospital setting. In the Diabetes Control and Complications Trial, cotton exudates were noted in the eyes of the participants receiving tight control of glucose early after onset of the intervention. Subsequently, the progression of retinopathy in the regular control group surpassed that in the tight

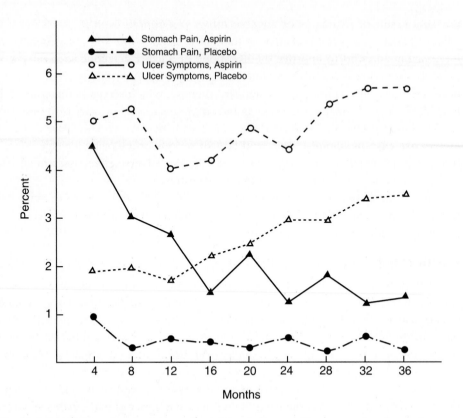

Fig. 11-1 Percentage of patients reporting selected adverse effects, over time, by study group, in the Aspirin Myocardial Infarction Study.

control group, and tight control was shown to reduce retinal complications in insulin-dependent diabetes.[35] Figure 11-1 illustrates the first occurrence of ulcer symptoms and complaints of stomach pain, over time, in the Aspirin Myocardial Infarction Study.[1] Ulcer symptoms rose fairly steadily in both the aspirin and placebo groups, peaking at 36 months. In contrast, complaints of stomach pain were maximal early in the aspirin group, then decreased. Participants on placebo had a constant, low level of stomach pain complaints. A researcher who tried to compare adverse effects in two studies of aspirin, one lasting weeks and the other months, would have different findings. To add to the complexity, the aspirin data in the study of longer duration may be confounded by changes in aspirin dosage and concomitant therapy.

An intervention may cause continued discomfort throughout a trial, and its persistence may be an important feature. Yet, unless the discomfort is considerable, such that the intervention is stopped, the participant may eventually stop complaining about it. Unless the investigator is alert to this possibility, the proportion of participants with symptoms at the final assessment in a long-term trial may be misleadingly low.

Individual susceptibility

Different kinds of people react differently to interventions, in terms of both benefit and adverse effects. Age, sex, stage of disease, and many other features of the participants or their conditions can and will affect the incidence and severity of specific effects. In addition, they may alter the perception of or actual importance of the adverse effects. Women with hypertension have been noted to report more adverse effects than men.[20] In trials of primary prevention, where the participants may be entirely asymptomatic, even relatively mild adverse effects may not be tolerated. Participants with diseases of moderate severity, who hope for recovery or remission, may accept more toxic reactions from a drug or device. While some patients with a terminal illness may accept many bothersome effects and indignities in the hope of a cure, others may refuse anything that increases their discomfort.

The dose and dosing schedule of a study medication can also have different impacts in different participants. Elderly participants often require smaller doses than younger participants. In long-term studies, participants who are employed outside the home may have difficulties complying with multiple drug-dosing regimens, especially if the drug needs to be taken mid-day. Not only is it inconvenient, but otherwise acceptable adverse effects such as flushing or drowsiness may cause embarrassment if noticed by co-workers.

Analysis of nonadherent participants

As discussed in Chapter 16, there are differing views on analyzing data from participants who fail to adhere to the study intervention regimen. For analysis of primary response variables, the "intention-to-treat" approach, which includes all participants in their originally randomized groups, is more conservative and less open to bias than the "explanatory" approach, which omits participants who stop taking their assigned intervention. When adverse effects are assessed, however, the issue is less clear. Participants are less likely to report adverse effects if they are not receiving medication (active or placebo) than if they are receiving it. Therefore the intention-to-treat principle may underestimate the true incidence of adverse effects by inflating the number of participants at risk. On the other hand, the explanatory policy makes it impossible to assess events that occur sometime after drug discontinuation but may in fact be a real adverse effect that was not recognized until later. In addition, withdrawing participants can void the benefits of randomization, resulting in invalid group comparisons. While there is no easy solution to this dilemma, it is probably safer and more reasonable to continue to assess adverse effects for the duration of the trial, even if a participant has stopped taking his study drug. The analysis and reporting might then be done both including and omitting nonadherent participants. Certainly, it is extremely important to specify what was done.

REPORTING ADVERSE EFFECTS

Adverse effects can be reported in at least four general ways. First, there may simply be an indication that participants either did or did not have a particular problem. Second, an investigator may provide an estimate of the severity of an adverse effect. Third, the frequency that the adverse effect occurs in a given participant over a given period can be presented. Fourth, time patterns may be shown.

The usual measures of adverse effects include:

a. Reasons participants are taken off study medication or device removed;
b. Reasons participants are on reduced dosage of study medication or on lower intensity of intervention;
c. Type and frequency of participant complaints;
d. Laboratory measurements, including x-rays;
e. In long-term studies, possible intervention-related reasons participants are hospitalized;
f. Combinations or variations of any of the above.

All of these can rather easily indicate the number of participants with a particular adverse effect during the course of the trial. Severity indices can be more complicated. It may be assumed that a participant who was taken off study drug because of an adverse effect had a more serious episode than one who merely had his dosage reduced. Someone who required dose reduction probably had a more serious effect than one who complained but continued to take the dose required by the study protocol. Data from the Aspirin Myocardial Infarction Study,[1] using the same adverse effects as in the previous example, are shown in Table 11-2. In the aspirin and placebo groups, the percentages of participants complaining about hematemesis, tarry stools, and bloody stools are compared with the percentages having their medication dosage reduced for those events. As expected, numbers complaining were many times the numbers with reduced dosage. Thus the implication is that most of the complaints were for relatively minor occurrences or had been transient.

The Program on the Surgical Control of the Hyperlipidemias investigators[5] reported, in different ways, various side effects of partial ileal bypass, which was used to reduce serum cholesterol. The average number of bowel movements per day and the percentage of participants with watery or frothy stools were noted. In addition, the number of participants who had their ileal bypass reversed, by reason, was indicated, the most common reason being diarrhea.

Table 11-2   Percentage of participants with drug dosage reduced or complaining of selected adverse effects, by study group, in the Aspirin Myocardial Infarction Study

	Aspirin (N = 2267)	Placebo (N = 2257)
Hematemesis		
Reasons dosage reduced	0.00	0.00
Complaints	0.27	0.09
Tarry stools		
Reasons dosage reduced	0.09	0.04
Complaints	1.34	0.67
Bloody stools		
Reasons dosage reduced	0.22	0.04
Complaints	1.29	0.45

Many clinical trials use a severity scale that requires the investigator and/or the participant to indicate on a line or series of boxes the perceived degree of severity.[17,24] It is then possible to indicate the proportion of participants with a particular adverse effect who have greater than a specified level of severity. The Eastern Cooperative Oncology Group[24] toxicity criteria have five levels of severity for each of about 20 signs or symptoms. Alternatively, a composite score, incorporating several factors, may be created. As previously mentioned, another way of reporting severity is to establish a hierarchy of consequences of adverse effects, such as permanently off study drug, which is more severe than permanently on reduced dosage, which is more severe than ever on reduced dosage, which is more severe than ever complaining about the effect. Unfortunately, few clinical trial reports present such severity data.

The frequency with which a particular adverse effect has occurred in any participant can be viewed as another measure of severity. For example, episodes of nausea occurring daily, rather than monthly, are obviously more troublesome to the participant. Presenting such data in a clear fashion is complicated. It can be done by means of frequency distributions, but these consume considerable space in tables. Another method is to select a frequency and assume that adverse effects that occur less often in a given period are less important. Thus only the number of participants with a frequency of specified adverse effects above that are reported. As an example, of 10 participants having nausea, 3 might have it at least twice a week, 3 at least once a week but less than twice, and 4 less than once a week. Only those 6 having nausea at least once a week might be included in a table. These ways of reporting assume that adequate and complete data have been collected and may require the use of a diary. Obviously, if a follow-up questionnaire asks only if nausea has occurred since the previous evaluation, frequency measures cannot be presented.

The dimension of time can complicate the reporting of adverse effects. First, participants can be listed as ever having been off medication, or on reduced doses. Second, they can also be off drug or on reduced dose at some specified time during the trial. This specified time may be the interval between two particular clinic visits. For example, the percentage of participants on reduced study medication in the first year of treatment could be presented.

A third time-related way of looking at adverse effects is to report the percentage of participants who permanently discontinued or took a reduced dose of the study drug. Depending upon the pattern of drug discontinuation and possible restarting, this measure may or may not provide results similar to the percentage of participants off drug during some specified period.

As with other response variables, adverse effects can be analyzed using survival analysis (Chapter 14). An advantage of this sort of presentation is that the time to a particular episode, in relation to when the intervention was started, is examined. Further, the frequency of a particular adverse effect will be directly related to the number of participants at risk of suffering it. This can give a higher rate of adverse effects than other measures, but this high rate may be a realistic estimate. The Hypertension Detection and Follow-Up Program[9] presented survival analyses showing decreasing discontinuation of medication because of side effects, over time, in participant subsets. Difficulties with survival analysis techniques include the problems of interpreting repeated episodes in any participant and severity of a particular adverse effect, changes in dosing pattern or adherence, and changes in sensitization or tolerance to adverse effects. Nevertheless, this technique has been underused in reporting adverse effects.

An attempt to compare adverse effects reported from several studies of similar agents, in this case beta-blockers, has been made.[12] To minimize potential difficulties, only large, placebo-controlled, long-term trials using approximately equipotent doses of beta-blockers in post–myocardial infarction patients were evaluated. Despite this, different follow-up times, severity of illness of the study participants, time from acute illness to initiation of study drug, and definitions of adverse effects made review of the published papers difficult. Even after contacting study investigators and obtaining unpublished data, only a few reasons for permanent drug discontinuation could be reasonably compared. No obvious major differences in complications of therapy were discovered, but, given the problems, the conclusions must be interpreted cautiously.

The FDA has several reporting requirements for adverse effects in submissions for New Drug Applications.[14] These require considerable detail and must be kept in mind if a New Drug Application is anticipated at the end of the trial. Other regulatory agencies have similar requirements.

OTHER ISSUES

Clinical trials are excellent mechanisms for comparing groups of participants and deciding whether a particular intervention is beneficial or harmful. For example, they can be used to show that an intervention causes 25% of the participants exposed to it to develop nausea, as compared with 10% of subjects receiving a placebo, over the follow-up period. Clinical trials, however, usually cannot say precisely which particular intervention participants are among the "expected" 10% and which are among the "excess" 15%. It is even possible that some among the expected 10% with nausea may have had their problem aggravated by the intervention. In general, only individual participant experience, such as drug rechallenge or perhaps documentation of a clear temporal relationship between drug administration or device implantation and the adverse effect or obvious device failure, can identify in which participants the intervention is the responsible agent.

Temple et al.[33] and Riegelman[27] indicated other difficulties in using clinical trials to evaluate adverse effects. They concluded that most trials are too small and of too short duration to detect uncommon adverse effects. It has been noted[33] that at most, a few thousand participants receive an intervention during a trial, with perhaps a few hundred receiving it for more than several months. Trials also include a selected type of participant. People most likely to develop adverse effects are generally excluded from clinical trials. Exclusion criteria are intentionally designed to do just that. The thalidomide tragedy[15,21] illustrates the problem that can arise when people who are likely to use a drug are not initially evaluated. Recent efforts to include the elderly and other groups, when appropriate, in clinical trials, may reduce this problem, though certainly not eliminate it.

A similar point has been made by Venning,[37] who reviewed the identification and report of 18 adverse effects in a variety of drugs. Clinical trials played a key role in identifying only 3 of the 18 adverse reactions discussed. Of course, clinical trials may not have been conducted in all of the other instances. Nevertheless, it is clear that assessment of adverse effects, historically, has not been a major contribution of clinical trials.

A clinical trial may, however, suggest that further research on adverse effects would be worthwhile. As a result of implications from the Multiple Risk Factor Intervention Trial[23] that high doses of thiazide diuretics might increase the incidence of sudden cardiac death, Siscovick et al.[31] conducted a population-based case-control study. This study confirmed that high doses of thiazide diuretics, as opposed to low doses, were associated with a higher rate of cardiac arrest.

Drugs of the same class generally are expected to have similar effects on the primary outcome of interest. For example, different angiotensin converting enzyme inhibitors will reduce blood pressure and ease symptoms of heart failure. Different calcium channel-blocking agents will treat hypertension and angina. The factors that make the drugs in the same class different, however, may mean that side effects may differ in degree if not in kind. Longer-acting preparations, or preparations that are absorbed or metabolized differently, may be administered in different doses and have greater or lesser adverse effects. It cannot be assumed in the absence of appropriate comparisons that the adverse effects from similar drugs are or are not alike. As noted, however, a clinical trial may not be the best vehicle for detecting these differences.

An important aspect in toxicity assessment is long-term follow-up monitoring of the participants after the formal trial has ended. Such follow-up is not always feasible in trials that employ continuing intervention. They have the possibility for treatment cross-over and contamination of groups. It can be useful, however, if a drug is found to have serious toxicity during the trial. It can then be assumed that few, if any, participants will remain on the drug or begin taking it. Poststudy observation can show whether adverse effects persist after cessation of the intervention. An example of the latter is the WHO clofibrate trial.[26] There, the poststudy attenuation of the observed in-study adverse mortality experience emphasized that the finding was probably real (see Chapter 17 for further discussion). Reasonable assessment of long-term effects can more easily be accomplished in studies with limited or one-time interventions. In the antenatal steroid therapy trial, the primary response was neonatal respiratory distress syndrome.[8] Even after establishing the short-term impact of therapy, for safety reasons the children were followed for a 3-year evaluation of growth and neurologic outcomes. Similarly, the Program on the Surgical Control of the Hyperlipidemias[5] will, through long-term follow-up, be able to assess continued incidence of adverse effects such as diarrhea, kidney stones, and gallstones.

CONCLUSIONS

Clinical trials have inherent methodologic limitations in the evaluation of adverse effects. These include inadequate size, duration of follow-up, and restricted participant selection. Problems in data collection and reporting, however, can be adequately addressed and solved.

The protocol should indicate how adverse effects are defined and collected. Though consistency between studies may not be achieved, what is done should at least be mentioned. Adverse effects should be presented in the main results paper, not buried in subsidiary ones. Published reports should present adverse effect results in several ways. The cumulative number of participants with a particular problem at any time during the trial and the number with that problem at a particular point are useful overall measures. Some indicator of severity, using either a scale from a questionnaire or the number of participants taken off drug or device, is also important. In long-term trials, the time course of adverse effects should be reported.

Many adverse effects may be assessed. Clearly, not all can be reported. A reasonable approach is to present adverse effects known or suspected to be caused by the intervention, any serious clinical events, and those where a significant difference between groups is observed.

REFERENCES

1. Aspirin Myocardial Infarction Study Research Group: A randomized, controlled trial of aspirin in persons recovered from myocardial infarction, *JAMA* 243:661-669, 1980.
2. Avery CW, Ibelle BP, Allison B, Mandell N: Systematic errors in the evaluation of side effects, *Am J Psychiatry* 123:875-878, 1967.
3. Bateman DN, Chaplin S: Adverse reactions. I, *BMJ* 296:761-764, 1988.
4. Beta-Blocker Heart Attack Trial Research Group: A randomized trial of propranolol in patients with acute myocardial infarction. 1. Mortality results, *JAMA* 247:1707-1714, 1982.
5. Buchwald H, Varco RL, Matts JP et al: Effect of partial ileal bypass surgery on mortality and morbidity from coronary heart disease in patients with hypercholesterolemia. Report of the Program on the Surgical Control of the Hyperlipidemias (POSCH), *N Engl J Med* 328:946-955, 1990.
6. Bulpitt CJ: *Randomised controlled clinical trials,* The Hague, 1983, Martinus Nijhoff, pp. 214-220.
7. Byington RP, for the Beta-Blocker Heart Attack Trial Research Group. Beta-Blocker Heart Attack Trial: design, methods, and baseline results, *Controlled Clin Trials* 5:382-437, 1984.
8. Collaborative Group on Antenatal Steroid Therapy: Effects of antenatal dexamethasone administration in the infant: long-term follow-up, *J Pediatr* 104:259-267, 1984.
9. Curb JD, Borhani NO, Blaszkowski TP et al: Long-term surveillance for adverse effects of antihypertensive drugs, *JAMA* 253:3263-3268, 1985.
10. Downing RW, Rickels K, Meyers F: Side reactions in neurotics: 1. A comparison of two methods of assessment, *J Clin Pharmacol* 10:289-297, 1970.
11. Edlavitch SA: Adverse drug event reporting: improving the low U.S. reporting rates, *Arch Intern Med* 148:1499-1503, 1988 (editorial).
12. Friedman LF: How do various beta blockers compare in type, frequency and severity of their adverse effects? *Circulation* 67(suppl 1):I-89-I-90, 1983.
13. Girard M, Biscos-Garreau M: Reliability of data on haematotoxicity of antidepressants. A retrospective assessment of haematological monitoring in clinical trials on tricyclics, *J Affective Disorders* 17:153-158, 1989.
14. Guideline for the Format and Content of the Clinical and Statistical Sections of New Drug Applications. Center for Drug Evaluation and Research, Food and Drug Administration, Department of Health and Human Services, July, 1988.
15. Heinonen OP, Slone D, Shapiro S: *Birth defects and drugs in pregnancy,* Littleton, MA 1977, PSG, pp 1-7.
16. Herbst AL, Ulfelder H, Poskanzer DC: Adenocarcinoma of the vagina, *N Engl J Med* 284:878-881, 1971.
17. Huskisson EC, Wojtulewski JA: Measurement of side effects of drugs, *BMJ* 2:698-699, 1974.
18. Hutchinson TA, Lane DA: Assessing methods for causality assessment of suspected adverse drug reactions, *J Clin Epidemiol* 42:5-16, 1989.
19. Kessler DA, for the Working Group: Introducing MEDWatch, *JAMA* 269:183-190, 1993.
20. MacMahon SW, Furberg CD, Culter JA: Women as participants in trials of the primary and secondary prevention of cardiovascular disease. Part I. Primary Prevention: The hypertensive trials. In Eaker ED, Packard B, Wenger NK, Clarkson TB, Tyroler HA, eds: *Coronary heart disease in women,* New York, 1987, Haymarket Doyma.
21. McBride WG: Thalidomide and congenital abnormalities (letter to the editor), *Lancet* ii:1358, 1961.
22. Multicentre International Study: Improvement in prognosis of myocardial infarction by long-term beta-adrenoreceptor blockade using practolol, *BMJ* 3:735-740, 1975.
23. Multiple Risk Factor Intervention Trial Research Group: Baseline rest electrocardiographic abnormalities, antihypertensive treatment, and mortality in the Multiple Risk Factor Intervention Trial, *Am J Cardiol* 55:1-15, 1985.
24. Oken MM, Creech RH, Tormey DC et al: Toxicity and response criteria of the Eastern Cooperative Oncology Group, *Am J Clin Oncol (CCT)* 5:649-655, 1982.
25. Ray WA, Griffin MR, Avorn J: Evaluating drugs after their approval for clinical use (Sounding Board), *N Engl J Med* 329:2029-2032, 1993.
26. Report of the Committee of Principal Investigators: WHO cooperative trial on primary prevention of ischaemic heart disease with clofibrate to lower serum cholesterol: final mortality follow-up, *Lancet* ii:600-604, 1984.

27. Riegelman R: Letter to the editor, *Ann Intern Med* 100:455, 1984.
28. Rogers AS, Israel E, Smith CR et al: Physician knowledge, attitudes, and behavior related to reporting adverse drug events, *Arch Intern Med* 148:1596-1600, 1988.
29. Romanowski B, Gourlie B, Gynp P: Biased adverse effects? (letter to the editor), *N Engl J Med* 319:1157-1158, 1988.
30. Simpson RJ, Tiplady B, Skegg DCG: Event recording in a clinical trial of a new medicine, *BMJ* 280: 1133-1134, 1980.
31. Siscovick DS, Raghunathan TE, Psaty BM, et al: Diuretic therapy for hypertension and the risk of primary cardiac arrest, *N Engl J Med* 330:1852-1857, 1994.
32. Systematic Assessment for Treatment of Emergent Events: National Institute of Mental Health, Alcohol, Drug Abuse, and Mental Health Administration, Rockville, MD, 1983.
33. Temple RJ, Jones JK, Crout JR: Adverse effects of newly marketed drugs, *N Engl J Med* 300:1046-1047, 1979 (editorial).
34. Teutsch SM, Herman WH: Surveillance of acute complications of new therapies, *Diabetes Care* 8:(suppl 1):51-53, 1985.
35. The Diabetes Control and Complications Trial Research Group: The effect of intensive treatment of diabetes on the development and progression of long-term complications in insulin-dependent diabetes mellitus, *N Engl J Med* 329:977-986, 1993.
36. Tubert P, Bégaud B, Péré J-C et al: Power and weakness of spontaneous reporting: a probabilistic approach, *J Clin Epidemiol* 45:283-286, 1992.
37. Venning GR: Identification of adverse reactions to new drugs, II. How were 18 important adverse reactions discovered and with what delays? *BMJ* 286:289-292, 365-368, 1983.
38. Woosley RL, Drayer DE, Reidenberg MM et al: Effect of acetylator phenotype on the rate at which procainamide induces antinuclear antibodies and the lupus syndrome, *N Engl J Med* 298:1157-1159, 1978.

CHAPTER 12

Assessment of Health-Related Quality of Life

Michelle J. Naughton, Ph.D.
Sally A. Shumaker, Ph.D.
Guest Contributors

The term *quality of life* is widely used by psychologists, sociologists, economists, policy makers, and others. However, what is meant by quality of life varies greatly depending on the context. In some settings, it may include such components as employment status, income, housing, material possessions, environment, working conditions, or the availability of public services. The kinds of indices that reflect quality of life from a medical or health viewpoint are different and would include those aspects that might be influenced not only by conditions or diseases, but also by medical treatment or other types of interventions. Thus the term *health-related quality of life* (HRQL) is now commonly used to mean the measurement of one's life quality from a health or medical perspective.

Components incorporated under the broad rubric of HRQL have been part of clinical trials before this term was established. Measures of physical functioning and psychological functioning, for instance, depression and anxiety, and a variety of symptoms such as pain, are well-established outcome variables. Negative effects, typically adverse symptoms from various organ systems, are also routinely assessed (see Chapter 11). In addition, some components have for years been among the baseline factors often collected to characterize the study population. However, the introduction of the HRQL concept has provided important additions and refinements in the way clinical trials are designed. A major advance is that more attention is given to the participants and their experiences and perceptions and how these might be affected by the study intervention. The quantification of these measures has become more sophisticated with assistance from investigators trained in measurement theory and psychometrics.

Over the past 20 years, there has been a growing interest in the inclusion of HRQL measures to assess intervention effects in trials of a variety of interventions.* In

---

*References 36, 46–48, 58

response to this interest, methods to assess health status and HRQL have proliferated. As with any new area of research, controversy persists regarding the relative merit of HRQL and adequacy of available measures. For example, questions have been raised about the degree to which current instruments represent the feelings and perceptions of the target groups (e.g., patients) vs. the perceptions of researchers and clinicians.[15] However, a careful review of the process by which the most frequently used HRQL instruments were developed demonstrates that, for the most part, these instruments evolved from the participants' personal perceptions of their life quality and the key factors that are important in defining life quality for the individual.[58] Thus, there are now several valid and reliable instruments available for use in clinical trials that are the culmination of years of research with various populations. These reflect the target populations' perceptions of their health status and HRQL.* In this chapter, we provide a definition of HRQL, examine the uses of HRQL assessment in clinical trials and give several examples, and discuss design considerations and the interpretation of data. In the last section we provide a brief introduction to utility measures and preference scaling that have limited applicability to the typical clinical trials.

FUNDAMENTAL POINT

Assessment of the effects of interventions on participants' HRQL may be an important component of clinical trials, especially those that involve interventions directed at primary or secondary prevention of chronic diseases.

DEFINITIONS

Historically, investigators in the field of quality of life have held various viewpoints on how to define the concept. Recent years, however, have brought greater convergence of opinion with respect to the definitions of HRQL.[8] Several definitions have been proposed, and these have ranged from very broad perspectives, reminiscent of the early definitions of quality of life, to narrower definitions that are more specific to HRQL.[49] We have adopted a definition of HRQL proposed by Wenger and Furberg.[57] Health-related quality of life encompasses: "Those attributes valued by patients, including their resultant comfort or sense of well-being; the extent to which they were able to maintain reasonable physical, emotional, and intellectual function; and the degree to which they retain their ability to participate in valued activities within the family, in the workplace, and in the community." This definition explicitly emphasizes the multidimensional aspect of HRQL, and that actual functional status and the individuals' perceptions regarding "valued activities" are critical to identify (Table 12-1). Although there has been some debate on the definition of HRQL, a

---

*References 6, 31, 44, 50, 60.

Table 12-1 Dimensions of health-related quality of life

Primary dimensions
  Physical functioning
  Psychological functioning
  Social functioning
  Overall life satisfaction/well-being
  Perceptions of health status
Additional Dimensions
  Neuropsychological functioning
  Personal productivity
  Intimacy and sexual functioning
  Sleep disturbance
  Pain
  Symptoms

recent conference composed of an international group of HRQL investigators reached agreement on the fundamental dimensions essential to any HRQL assessment.[8] These primary dimensions include: physical functioning, psychological functioning, social functioning and role activities, and the individuals' overall life satisfaction and perceptions of their health status. Thus it was the general opinion of these investigators that to assert that HRQL has been measured in a particular clinical trial, a minimum of these dimensions should be included. However, there are instances in which fewer dimensions of HRQL may be applicable to a specific intervention or population. For example, it is unlikely that in the examination of the short-term effects of hormone replacement therapy (HRT) on perimenopausal symptoms, the physical functioning of the study participants, women in their mid-40s to early 50s, will be influenced. That is, this cohort of women will not be limited in their physical functioning, and HRT will not alter their status on this dimension of HRQL. Thus the inclusion of this dimension of HRQL in the trial may simply increase participant burden without benefit. In such instances, investigators would report that they had included a subset of HRQL dimensions in their study design. In such cases, it is important for the investigators to establish the rationale for their selection of a subset of HRQL dimensions to avoid the perception of bias, for example, by deleting HRQL dimensions that might make the treatment under study "look bad."

For specific interventions, other commonly assessed dimensions of HRQL may be important. These include cognitive or neuropsychological functioning, personal productivity, and intimacy and sexual functioning. Measures of sleep disturbance, pain, and symptoms that are associated with a condition/illness and the adverse effects of treatment are also often assessed.

Primary HRQL dimensions

Physical functioning refers to an individual's ability to perform daily life activities. These types of activities are often classified as either "activities of daily living," which include basic self-care activities, such as bathing and dressing, or "intermediate activities of daily living," which refer to a higher level of usual activities, such as cooking, performing household tasks, and ambulation.

Social functioning is defined as a person's ability to interact with family, friends, and the community. Instruments measuring social functioning may include such components as the person's participation in activities with family and friends, and the number of individuals in his or her social network. A key aspect of social functioning is the person's ability to maintain social roles and obligations at desired levels. An illness or intervention may be perceived by people as having little or no negative impact on their daily lives if they are able to maintain role functions that are important to them, such as caring for children or grandchildren or engaging in social activities with friends. In contrast, anything that reduces one's ability to participate in desired social activities, even though it may improve clinical status, may reduce the person's general sense of social functioning.

Psychological functioning of a person refers to the individual's emotional well-being. It has been common to assess the negative effects of an illness or intervention, such as levels of anxiety, depression, guilt, and worry. However, the positive emotional states of individuals should not be neglected. Interventions may produce improvements in a person's emotional functioning, and therefore such aspects as joy, vigor, and hopefulness for the future are also important to assess.

Overall life satisfaction represents a person's perception of his or her overall sense of well-being. For example, participants may be asked to indicate a number between 0 (not at all satisfied) and 10 (extremely satisfied) that indicates their general satisfaction with their lives for a defined period (e.g., in the last month).

Perceptions of health status need to be distinguished from actual health. Individuals who are ill and perceive themselves as such, may after a period of adjustment reset their expectations, adapt to their life situation, and thus possess a positive sense of well-being. In contrast, persons in good health may be dissatisfied with their life situation and rate their overall quality of life as poor. Participants may be asked to rate their overall health in the past month, their health compared with others their own age, or their health now compared with 1 year ago. It is interesting to note that perceived health ratings are strongly and independently associated with an increased risk of mortality.[27,33] In other words, health perceptions are important predictors of health outcomes, independent of clinical health status.

Additional HRQL dimensions

Neuropsychological functioning refers to the cognitive abilities of a person, such as memory, recognition, spatial skills, and motor coordination. These abilities are commonly assessed in elderly people, stroke patients, or those who have undergone various surgical procedures, such as coronary artery bypass graft surgery.

Personal productivity is a term used to encompass the range of both paid and unpaid activities in which individuals engage. Measures of this dimension might include paid employment (for instance, date of return to work, hours worked per week); household tasks; and volunteer or community activities.

Intimacy and sexual functioning refer to one's ability to form and maintain close personal relationships. Instruments measuring sexual functioning may include items regarding a person's ability to perform and/or participate in sexual activities, the types of sexual activities in which one engages, the frequency with which such activities occur, and persons' satisfaction with their sexual functioning or level of activity. This dimension of HRQL is particularly important in studies in which the condition's natural history, or its treatment, can directly influence sexual functioning (e.g., antihypertensive therapy, hormone therapy, and tamoxifen and other forms of cancer therapy).

Sleep disturbance has been related to depression and anxiety[14] and diminished levels of energy and vitality. Instruments assessing sleep habits may examine such factors as sleep patterns (e.g., ability to fall asleep at night, number of times awakened during the night, waking up too early in the morning or difficulty in waking up in the morning, number of hours slept during a typical night) and the restorativeness of sleep.

Pain is another commonly assessed dimension of HRQL, particularly in such chronic conditions as arthritis or orthopedic injuries. Assessments of pain may include measures of the degree of pain related to specific physical activities, such as bending, reaching, or walking upstairs and the type of pain, such as throbbing, shooting, and aching.

Symptoms associated with study conditions or interventions are an integral part of most clinical trials but are also one aspect of HRQL. By incorporating symptoms into HRQL assessments more systematically, we now have more sophisticated accounts of the frequency of symptoms, the severity of symptoms, and the degree to which symptoms interfere with daily functioning. Symptom checklists are often tailored to the specific condition or illness being studied and require investigators to have knowledge of common symptoms associated with an illness, the symptoms that may be produced or relieved by an intervention, and the time course in which these symptoms may be expected to occur during the course of the clinical trial.

Although all of the above dimensions of HRQL are the most commonly assessed aspects of HRQL, the specific dimensions relevant for a given clinical trial will depend on the intervention under investigation, the disease or condition being studied, and the study population, which may vary by age of participants, their ethnic identity, or cultural background.[42]

USES OF HRQL

Kaplan argued that for most individuals, there are really only two outcomes that are important when assessing the efficacy of a particular treatment: changes in their life expectancies and the quality of their remaining years.[28] HRQL provides a method of measuring intervention effects as well as the effects of the untreated course of diseases, in a manner that may be helpful to both the individual and the investigator. It is reasonable for individuals to expect that interventions aimed at disease prevention should decrease the probability of developing a chronic condition, but should not, in the process, significantly reduce their current functioning. In terms of chronic conditions where the goal is generally not a cure, it is important to determine how the person's life is influenced by both the disease and its treatment, and whether the effects of treatment are better or worse than the effects of the course of the underlying disease.

HRQL indices as outcome variables

Sugarbaker et al.[51] tested the hypothesis that limb-sparing surgery plus irradiation would profoundly improve quality of life compared with amputation in 26 patients with soft-tissue sarcoma. The data, covering a range of measures of functions (social, daily life, and psychological), failed to reveal substantial group differences. In fact, there were suggestions that the limb-sparing approach was inferior to amputation.

To assess the impact of antihypertensive therapy on blood pressure and quality of life, 242 hypertensive elderly women were randomly assigned to atenolol, enalapril, or diltiazem.[4] All three treatment regimens were effective in lowering diastolic blood pressure at week 16 without significant differences in rates of adverse events. There was a trend toward participants on atenolol to have somewhat worse quality of life scores, but none of these differences were found to be statistically significant.

Kane et al.[26] examined several outcomes of hospice care in 247 terminally ill cancer patients. The control subjects received conventional care. The authors reported no statistical differences in measures of pain, other symptoms, affect, or activities of daily living. However, the hospice patients expressed more satisfaction with the care they received, and the people caring for them showed less anxiety.

The effect of combinations of diet and low-dose pharmacological therapies was investigated in a study of 697 participants with diastolic blood pressure between 90 and 100 mm Hg and weight between 110% and 160% of ideal weight.[55] Participants were assigned to one of three diets (usual, low-sodium, and high potassium weight loss) and one of three therapies (placebo, chlorthalidone, and atenolol). Low-dose chlorthalidone and atenolol produced few side effects, except a diminished level of sexual functioning in men, particularly those assigned to usual diet. The weight loss diet, however, ameliorated this effect. The low-sodium diet with placebo was associated with greater fatigue, and the low-sodium diet with chlorthalidone increased problems with sleep. The weight loss diet benefited quality of life the most by reducing the total number of physical complaints and increasing satisfaction with health. The total number of physical complaints decreased in 57% to 76% of the participants, depending on the drug and diet group, and were markedly decreased by weight loss.

Wiklund et al.[59] examined the effect of transdermal estradiol and placebo therapy on the quality of life of 223 postmenopausal women experiencing climacteric symptoms in a 12-week randomized trial. Quality of life improved in both groups, but HRQL improved significantly more in the transdermal therapy group, especially sleep disturbance, feelings of social isolation, and frequency of HRQL problems. Well-being, sexual problems and dysfunction, and symptom relief were also significantly improved in women receiving estradiol as compared with placebo.

Trials of elderly men with benign prostatic hyperplasia have revealed a marked discrepancy between the measures urologists use to quantify progression (the amount of urine left in the bladder after voiding, the rate of urine flow, estimates of the size of the prostate) and the troublesome symptoms of the patients (frequent urination and difficulty starting urination).[5,34] The poor correlation between the biomedical markers of disease and symptoms patients experience raises important questions regarding selection of outcome variables in a clinical trial of an intervention that may halt or reverse disease progression. Are we treating the patient or the disease markers?

The examples above illustrate that intervention effects may be perceived differently from what is expected, may be subtle and likely to be missed in a clinical setting, can lead to marked subjective improvements, and are not always congruent with the traditional biomedical markers.

HRQL as baseline covariates

In addition to assessing treatment effects, measures of life quality may be predictive of subsequent mortality and morbidity. Ruberman et al.[41] reported that survivors of acute myocardial infarction classified as being socially isolated and unable to cope with high life stress had a more than fourfold risk of death over a 25-month period compared with others with low levels of both isolation and stress, independent of their baseline clinical status. Measurement of such predictive factors at baseline may be relevant to the assessment of comparability between the study groups (Chapter 8).

Idler et al.[23] evaluated the ability of global self-perceptions of health status (excellent, good, fair, and poor) to predict survival in follow-up studies of two samples of elderly, noninstitutionalized adults. In spite of extensive controls for physical health status, sociodemographic characteristics, and health risk behavior at the beginning of the follow-up period, poor self-perceptions of health significantly increased the risk of mortality. Risks of mortality were also observed in a dose-response relationship in participants who reported their health to be "fair" or "good." Self-perceptions of health status appear to be a factor of prospective importance in mortality studies.

METHODOLOGICAL ISSUES

The rationale for a well-designed and conducted randomized clinical trial to assess HRQL measures is the same as for other response variables. Because the data are primarily subjective, special precautions are necessary. A control group allows the investigator to determine which changes can be reasonably attributed to the study intervention. The double-blind design minimizes the effect of investigator and participant bias. The findings will be all the more credible if hypotheses are established a priori in the trial protocol.

The basic principles of data collection (Chapter 10) that ensure that the data are of the highest quality are also applicable. The criteria to be used and methods for assessment must be clearly defined. Training of investigators and staff are advisable. Pretesting of forms and questionnaires may enhance user and participant acceptability, and ensure higher quality data. An ongoing monitoring or surveillance system enables prompt corrective action when errors and other problems are found.

Trial design

Several protocol issues must be considered when using HRQL measures in clinical trials, including the time course of the trial, the frequency of contact with the study participants, the timing of clinical assessments, the complexity of the trial design, the number of participants enrolled, and participant and staff burden.[42] The goal of the HRQL investigation is to incorporate the HRQL measures into the trial protocol without compromising other aspects of the trial design. For example, in the case of a trial design with frequent participant contacts and multiple clinical measures, it may be necessary to focus the assessment of HRQL on a subset of key dimensions to minimize participant and staff burden.

At the same time, however, if a decision to measure HRQL is made, then like other measures, it should be viewed as an important variable in the overall trial design. Reducing its measurement to very brief and potentially less reliable measures, or to only one or two dimensions, may seriously diminish the integrity of the overall study design and yield useless information. For some trials, HRQL will be the primary endpoint, and the focus with respect to staff and patient time should be on the HRQL battery. For example, in comparing two antihypertensive drugs that have comparable efficacy with respect to blood pressure reduction, but different effects on HRQL, HRQL should be the critical outcome variable, and the study measures and staff and patient time should reflect this fact.[52]

Study population

It is critical to specify key population demographics that could influence the choice of instruments, the relevant dimensions of HRQL to be assessed, or the mode of administration.[42] Thus educational level, gender, age range, the language(s) spoken, and cultural diversity should be considered prior to selecting the HRQL battery of measures. For example, a cohort of patients over the age of 70 may have more vision problems than middle-aged persons, making self-administered questionnaires potentially inadvisable. Ethnically diverse groups also require measures that have been validated across different cultures and/or languages.[43]

It is also important to be sensitive to how the disease will progress and affect the HRQL of participants in the control group, as it is to understand the effects of the study intervention. For example, in patients with congestive heart failure assigned to the placebo-control arm of the study, we can expect a worsening of symptoms such as shortness of breath and fatigue, both of which will influence daily functioning. The point is to select instruments covering key dimensions of HRQL that are sufficiently sensitive to detect changes in *both* the intervention and the control group participants. Use of the same instruments for both groups is important for an unbiased and comparable assessment.

Intervention

Three major intervention-related factors are relevant to HRQL: the positive and adverse effects of the intervention, the time course of the effects, and the possible synergism of the treatment with existing medications and conditions.[42] It is important to hypothesize how a proposed intervention could affect the various dimensions of an individual's life quality in both positive and negative ways. For example, some hormone therapies may relieve vasomotor symptoms associated with the perimenopausal phase, such as hot flashes, and at the same time produce symptoms like bloating and breast tenderness.

The time course of an intervention's effects on dimensions of HRQL is also important both in terms of the selection of measures and the timing of when HRQL measures are administered to study participants. For example, in a trial comparing coronary artery bypass graft (CABG) surgery with angioplasty, an assessment of HRQL 1 week postintervention might lead to an interpretation that the surgical arm was more negative than angioplasty for HRQL since the individuals in this arm of the trial would still be recovering from the surgical procedure, and the effects of sore muscles and surgical site discomfort could overwhelm any benefits associated with CABG. However, at 6 months post-intervention, the benefits of CABG surgery such as relief from angina might be more profound than the benefits received from angioplasty. Thus the timing of the HRQL assessment may influence how one interprets the benefits (or negative effects) of the interventions.

Furthermore, it is important to know the current medications the study population is likely to be on prior to randomization to the study intervention, and how these medications might interact with the trial intervention (either a pharmacological or behavioral intervention) to influence dimensions of HRQL.[42]

Selection of HRQL instruments

Measures of HRQL can be classified as either generic (that is, instruments designed to assess HRQL in a broad range of populations), or condition/population-specific (e.g., instruments designed for specific diseases, conditions, age groups, or ethnic groups).[42] Within these two categories of measures are: single questionnaire items; dimension-specific instruments, which assess a single aspect of HRQL; health profiles, which are single instruments measuring several different dimensions of HRQL; and a battery of measures or a group of instruments assessing both single and multiple dimensions of HRQL. In assessing HRQL outcomes the trend has been toward the use of either profiles or batteries of instruments.

Some of the more commonly used generic HRQL instruments are the Sickness Impact Profile (SIP)[7] and the Rand-36 Item Health Status Profile.[22] Frequently used condition-specific instruments include the Spitzer Quality of Life Index (QL)[47] and the European Organization for Research and Treatment of Cancer Quality of Life Questionnaire (EORTC-QLQ),[1,3] both of which are multidimensional measures assessing the HRQL of individuals with cancer. Other condition-specific instruments include the McGill Pain Questionnaire,[32] for the measurement of pain, the Centers for Epidemiological Studies-Depression (CES-D),[37] the General Health Questionnaire (GHQ),[16] and the Psychological General Well-Being Index (PGWB),[11] all of which assess psychological distress and well-being; and the Barthel Index[10,17] to measure physical functioning and independence.

One criticism of current HRQL measures is that although they may reliably assess an individual's functional status within a particular dimension (e.g., physical functioning and mental health), these dimensions are treated as if each is of equal importance to all individuals. Yet, the importance of a particular HRQL dimension for one individual may be different from the importance for another, and the importance of a given dimension may vary over time for the same individual. Also, the perceived importance of a given dimension could influence one's overall HRQL. Although intuitively compelling, data to date do not appear to support this point. In our own research[45] on the development of condition-specific HRQL measures for urinary incontinence and epilepsy, for example, weighting each of the dimensions by perceived importance did not increase the validity, reliability, or sensitivity to change of the measures.

Early versions of the SIP and the Nottingham Health Profile both included weighting schemes that were dropped into later, more refined iterations of these instruments. Thus, for at least these examples, the importance of weighting does not appear to improve the quality of the measures. One hypothesis for this counterintuitive result is that, in the initial rating of functional status within a given HRQL dimension, an individual is implicitly (unconsciously) incorporating an assessment of importance. For example, if physical activity is not a critical part of a person's life, then an individual may rate physical functioning differently than someone for whom this is a central component of their self-image; yet, objectively, both people may perform at a comparable level of functioning. Since the critical factor is not actual performance, however, but the degree to which one's perception of functioning ties into one's overall HRQL, these obtained rating differences are at the core of HRQL measures.

The type of instruments selected for inclusion in a clinical trial will depend on the goals of the intervention. For example, within a given dimension of HRQL such as physical functioning, one can assess the degree to which an individual is able to perform a particular task, the satisfaction with the level of performance, the importance of performing the task, or the frequency with which the task is performed. Thus the aspects of HRQL measured in clinical trials vary depending on the specific research questions of the trial.

Many investigators have made the mistake of adopting a questionnaire developed for another population only to find that the distribution of responses obtained is skewed. In part, this may be because volunteers for a trial often are healthier than people in general with the same conditions. This point underscores the need to pretest any proposed instrument before a trial.

A range of techniques has been used to construct HRQL measures. It is beyond the scope of this chapter to review these techniques, but references regarding scaling procedures and psychometric considerations of instruments (reliability, validity, and the responsiveness of instruments to change) may be consulted.* It is important to note that in selecting HRQL instruments, investigators should be certain of the psychometric integrity of the measures. Fortunately, today there are several measures available that satisfy the standards of traditional measurement theory.

Modes of administration

HRQL data can be collected from interviews (telephone or face-to-face), or from self-administered instruments (in-person or by mail). There is some debate regarding the relative merit of interviewer-administered vs. self-administered instruments. Self-administered instruments are more cost-effective from a staffing perspective and may yield more disclosure on the part of the participant, particularly with the collection of sensitive information. However, self-administered instruments tend to yield more missing and incomplete data and do not allow for clarification. In the long run, and with some populations, they may actually prove to be more expensive than interviewer-administered instruments.

Interviewer-administered instruments usually provide more complete data sets and allow for probes and clarification. However, there may be a reluctance on the part of some participants to discuss openly some HRQL issues (e.g., depression and sexuality), whereas they may be willing to respond to questions about these same

---

*References 21, 31, 44, 50, 60.

issues in a self-administered format. For populations with a relatively high proportion of functional illiteracy, in-person interviewer administration may be required. Interviewer administration may also be the best way to obtain information for culturally diverse populations. Finally, interviewer-administered instruments are subject to interviewer bias and require intensive interviewer training, certification, and repeat training, especially within the context of multi-site clinical trials that may be of a long duration. Thus often they can be considerably more expensive than self-administered instruments. Serious thought must be given at the planning phases of a trial regarding the trade-offs between these two strategies.

In an observational study, Jachuck et al.[24] evaluated the quality of life in 75 people with hypertension controlled by drugs. Their physicians judged that all the patients had improved. These opinions were based on the fact that the blood pressure was controlled, that no clinical deterioration had been observed, and that the patients had not complained to the doctors about any ill effects of the drug treatment. However, relatives reported that three quarters of the patients had suffered moderate or severe impairment in their quality of life after receiving the antihypertensive therapy. The ratings from the relatives showed changes in all four areas of functioning—social, physical, emotional, and cognitive. The patients rated their own quality of life, assigning values intermediate between ratings done by their physicians and their relatives. It has been suggested that patients underreport problems in an attempt to please their physicians.

In practice, clinical trials that include HRQL measures as outcomes usually incorporate a combination of profiles augmented with either generic or population-specific measures of the dimensions most relevant to the study population and intervention.[2] In addition, most HRQL measures are designed to be either interviewer-administered or self-administered, and both modes of administration can be used within single trials.

Frequency of assessment (acute vs. chronic)

The frequency with which HRQL will need to be assessed in a clinical trial will depend on the nature of the condition being investigated (acute vs. chronic), the intervention, and the expected effects (both positive and negative) of treatment. At a minimum, as with all measurements collected in a clinical trial, a baseline and an end-of-study assessment should be completed. In addition, other HRQL assessments should be timed to match expected changes in functioning because of either the intervention or condition itself.

In general, acute conditions resolve themselves in one of four ways: a rapid resolution without a return of the condition or symptoms; a rapid resolution with a subsequent return of the condition after some period of relief (relapse); conversion of the condition to a chronic problem; or death.[9] In the case of rapid resolution, HRQL assessments would likely focus on the participant's symptoms in the short term.

These would allow for comparisons between the side effects of treatment that might assist resolution vs. the relative impact of symptoms on the participant's daily life. With respect to an acute condition where there is a risk of relapse (e.g., gastric ulcer), a longer duration of follow-up is necessary, because relapses can occur frequently and may have a broad impact on the participant's general functioning and well-being.

If the acute problem converts to a chronic condition, the evaluation of adverse symptoms vs. intervention side effects remains important but is complicated by the duration of time and the problem of how to balance health outcomes in making treatment decisions.[9] For example, a cancer patient experiencing acute pain will be treated with narcotics where appropriate, despite their negative side effects. Most patients will gladly accept the negative effects of the drugs (for instance, sedating effect) in exchange for immediate relief from pain. However, if treatment extends for a long period, the cumulative effects of sedation and other side effects must be weighed against the benefit of pain control. Interest in HRQL has been greater in the management of chronic conditions, where there is a growing interest in reducing morbidity, rather than just mortality. In chronic conditions, postponement of onset and treatment of associated symptoms may be the most important factors to assess.

Symptom expression (episodic vs. constant)

Chronic conditions with episodic symptomatic flare-ups (e.g., asthma) can mimic acute conditions.[9] However, a major distinction between the two is that often some interventions for chronic conditions must be administered during the asymptomatic periods. In addition, relief from symptoms from many chronic conditions is not as complete as that for acute conditions which, by definition, resolve in a short period. If the intervention carries side effects or adds to unrelated health risks, HRQL assessments ought to be completed during both latent and symptomatic periods to better characterize the impact of the condition and intervention on the participants.

Functional impact (present vs. absent)

For specific conditions and/or interventions that have little or no adverse effect upon a participant's function, interventions are best evaluated on the basis of their impact on survival.[9] In these situations, HRQL assessments will be of secondary importance. However, when a disease or condition affects functional capacity, treatments for that condition ought to be evaluated for their influence, both positive and negative, upon the participants' level of functioning and well-being. Again, in these situations, the type of HRQL instruments used and the timing of the assessments will depend on the nature of the condition, the intervention, and the expected time course of effects on the participants.

INTERPRETATION

The dimensions composing HRQL are influenced by a broad range of factors. It is important to maintain a distinction between these moderating factors and HRQL. Moderating factors can be divided into three categories: contextual, interpersonal, and intrapersonal.[44] Contextual factors include such variables as the setting (e.g., urban-rural, single dwelling building vs. high rise); the economic structure; and sociocultural variations. Interpersonal factors include such variables as the social support available to individuals, stress, economic pressures, and the occurrence of major life events, such as bereavement and sweepstakes' wins. Intrapersonal factors have to do with factors associated with the individual, such as coping skills, personality traits, or physical health. This distinction between the dimensions that compose HRQL and the factors that moderate HRQL has implications for the selection of HRQL measures in specific trials and data analysis and interpretation.

In addition to these three categories of moderating factors, it is important to realize that any intervention may induce changes, improvements as well as impairments, in a participant's perceived well-being. Changes in the natural course of the disease or condition must be considered, especially in trials of relatively long duration. Concomitant interventions or the regimen of care itself may also affect HRQL. This is particularly likely to happen in trials where the active intervention is considerably different from that for the control group. It is important to consider what effects the intervention will have on the participants' well-being before initiating the trial, to be able to assess the impact of these factors on the HRQL of the participants.

Scoring of HRQL measures

In most clinical trials, HRQL is assessed by several instruments measuring dimensions of HRQL considered to be critical to the intervention. Scores resulting from these measures are usually calculated within dimensions of HRQL, so that, for example, a separate score is calculated for physical functioning or social well-being. Some instruments may also produce an overall HRQL score in addition to separate scores for each dimension (e.g., the Sickness Impact Profile[6]).

Scores resulting from HRQL instruments are used to address specific research questions, most notably, to assess changes in specific HRQL dimensions, throughout the course of the trial; to describe the intervention and control groups at distinct times; and to examine the correspondence between HRQL measures and clinical or physiological measures. Plans for data analysis are tailored to the specific goals and research questions of the clinical trial, and a variety of standard statistical techniques are used to analyze HRQL data.

Determining the significance of HRQL measures

An important issue in evaluating HRQL measures is determining how to interpret score changes or differences between study groups on a given scale.[21] For example, how many points must one increase or decrease on a scale for that change to be considered clinically meaningful? Does the change in score reflect a small, moderate, or large improvement or deterioration in a participant's HRQL? Recent years have seen an increase in research examining the question of clinical significance for HRQL measures. One approach has involved the inclusion of HRQL into Utility Measures and Preference Scales (see next section).

An alternative approach to determining clinical significance has been the direct calibration of HRQL scores. That is, changes in HRQL scores are compared with (or calibrated against) changes in other scores or measures for which the clinical impact is already known. For example, if we know that a change of one half a standard deviation of a physical functioning scale score corresponds to an individual's moving from being able to walk unaided to requiring assistance, clinical significance would be inferred. Also, participants can be asked directly how many points of change on a particular scale (e.g., social functioning) would be required in order for them to feel the decline or improvement was important. Finally, the degree to which a change in a scale score predicts mortality or severe morbidity can be used to calibrate an instrument.

An example of the calibration process for HRQL data comes from the RAND Health Insurance Experiment data that were used to examine the effect of four common negative life events on changes in people's health status.[56] Thus, for example, the average effect of being laid off from work was a -2.3 change in score on the 38-item Mental Health Inventory (comparable to the emotional functioning dimension of HRQL). The impact of being attacked physically, experiencing property damage, or being robbed were associated with decreases of 5.4, 1.4, and 0.6 units, respectively. Similarly, Testa et al.[51] examined changes in general well-being in relation to life events in a study of hypertensive males. Jaeschke et al.[25] present data that suggest that small, medium, or large effects correspond to changes of approximately 0.5, 1.0, and > 1.0 units per question for instruments that present response options on seven-point scales. Investigators used this criterion to interpret a study on the clinical significance of HRQL scores on the use of bronchodilators.[20] That is, bronchodilator use resulted in small, but clinically important, improvements in fatigue, dyspnea, and emotional functioning in patients with chronic airflow limitation.

UTILITY MEASURES AND PREFERENCE SCALING

The types of HRQL instruments discussed in this chapter have been limited to measures that were derived using psychometric methods. These methods examine the reliability, validity, and responsiveness of instruments. Other approaches to measuring quality of life and health states are used, however, and include utility measures and preference scaling. Utility measures are derived from economic and decision theory and incorporate the preferences of individuals for particular treatment interventions and health outcomes.[19] Utility scores reflect a person's preferences and values for specific health states and allow morbidity and mortality improvements to be combined into a single weighted measure, called *quality-adjusted life years* (QALY).[19,40] These measures provide a single summary score representing the net change in the participant's quality of life (the gains from the treatment effect minus the burdens of the side effects of treatment). These scores can be used in cost-utility analyses that combine quality of life and duration of life. For example, ratios of cost per QALY can be used to decide among competing interventions.[12]

In utility approaches, one or more scaling methods are used to assign a numerical value from 0.0 (death) to 1.0 (full health) to indicate an individual's quality of life. The procedure commonly used to generate utilities is the lottery, or standard gamble (most usually, the risk of death that one would be willing to take to improve a state of health).[40] Preferences for health states are generated from the general population, clinicians, or patients using multiattribute scales, visual analogue rating scales, time trade-off (how many months or years of life one would be willing to give up in exchange for a better health state), or other scaling methods.[29,40,53]

Revicki estimated health utilities for antihypertensive therapy and assessed the relationship between psychometrically based HRQL measures and health utility measures.[38] The participants were 180 community-based individuals initially diagnosed with mild to moderate hypertension. A categorical rating scale and standard gamble scaling methods were used to obtain patient health utilities (a value between 0, death, and 1, perfect health). The results indicated that after adjusting for age, race, comorbidity, and duration of hypertension, angiotensin converting enzyme (ACE) inhibitor treatment was associated with higher standard gamble utilities. The health utilities, however, were only moderately correlated with the psychometrically based HRQL measures. The utilities assigned by patients regarding their own health status on antihypertensive medications were also lower than those based on physician judgment.

HRQL measures and utility scores derived by standard gamble and categorical rating methods were also compared in a 48-week trial of 73 chronic renal disease patients with anemia.[39] Standard gamble utility was significantly related to home management, and the categorical rating utility was significantly related to home management, energy, alertness behavior, social interaction, and life satisfaction scale scores. However, only 25% to 27% of the variance in utility scores was explained by the HRQL measures.

Utility measures are useful for determining if the participant has experienced a positive or negative change because of treatment, but they do not indicate in which specific dimensions of HRQL improvement or deterioration occurred. Utility measures may also not be sensitive to small yet meaningful changes in clinical status. Other disadvantages of utility methods include controversy regarding the definition of utilities/preferences and the methods used to derive these values; the cognitive complexity of the measurement task; potential population and contextual effects on utility values; and the issue of how to interpret utility scores.[40] In general, psychometric and utility-based methods measure different components of health. The two approaches result in different yet related and sometimes complementary assessments of health outcomes, and both may be useful in clinical research. For a further review of issues related to utility analyses/preference scaling and the relationship between psychometric and utility-based approaches to the measurement of life quality, additional references may be consulted.*

REFERENCES

1. Aaronson NK, Ahmedzai S, Bullinger M et al: The EORTC core quality-of-life questionnaire: Interim results of an international field study. In Osoba D, ed: *Effect of cancer on quality of life,* Boca Raton, Fla, 1991, CRC Press.
2. Aaronson NK: Quality of life: What is it? How should it be measured? *Oncology* 2:69-74, 1988.
3. Aaronson NK, Ahmedzai S, Bergman B et al: The European Organization for Research and Treatment of Cancer QLQ-C30: A quality-of-life instrument for use in international clinical trials in oncology, *J Natl Cancer Inst* 85:365-376, 1993.
4. Applegate WB, Phillips HL, Schnaper H et al: A randomized controlled trial of the effects of three antihypertensive agents on blood pressure control and quality of life in older women, *Arch Intern Med* 151:1817-1823, 1991.
5. Barry MJ, Cockett ATK, Holtgrewe HL, et al: Relationship of symptoms of prostatism to commonly used physiological and anatomical measures of the severity of benign prostatic hyperplasia, *J Urol* 150:351-358, 1993.
6. Bergner M, Bobbitt RA, Carter WB et al: The Sickness Impact Profile: development and final revision of a health status measure, *Med Care* 19:787-805, 1981.
7. Bergner M, Bobbitt RA, Kressel S et al: The Sickness Impact Profile: conceptual foundation and methodology for the development of a health status measure, *Int J Health Serv* 6:393-415, 1976.
8. Berzon R, Hays RD, Shumaker SA: International use, application and performance of health-related quality of life instruments, *Qual Life Res* 2:367-368, 1993.
9. Cella DF, Wiklund I, Shumaker SA et al: Integrating health-related quality of life into cross-national clinical trials, *Qual Life Res* 2:433-440, 1993.
10. Colin C, Wade DT, Davies S, Horne V: The Barthel ADL Index: a reliability study, *Int Disability Stud* 10: 61-63, 1988.
11. Dupuy HJ: The Psychological General Well-Being (PGWB) Index. In Wenger NK, Mattson ME, Furberg CD, Elinson J, eds: *Assessment of quality of life in clinical trials in cardiovascular therapies,* Washington, DC, 1984, LeJacq.
12. Feeny D, Labell R, Torrance GW: Integrating economic evaluations and quality of life assessments. In Spilker B, ed: *Quality of life assessments,* New York, 1990, Raven Press.
13. Feeny D, Torrance GW: Incorporating utility-based quality of life assessment measures in clinical trials, *Med Care* 27:S190-S204, 1989.
14. Ford DE, Kamerow DB: Epidemiological study of sleep disturbances and psychiatric disorders: an opportunity for prevention? *JAMA* 262:1479-1484, 1989.
15. Gill TM, Feinsten AR: A critical appraisal of the quality of quality-of-life measurements, *JAMA* 272: 619-626, 1994.

*References 12, 13, 19, 29, 30, 35, 38–40, 53, 54.

16. Goldberg DP, Hillier VF: A scaled version of the General Health Questionnaire, *Psychol Med* 9:139-145, 1979.

17. Granger CV, Albrecht GL, Hamilton BB: Outcomes of comprehensive medical rehabilitation: measurement by PULSES Profile and the Barthel Index, *Arch Phys Med Rehab* 60:145-154, 1979.

18. Guyatt GH, Cook DJ: Commentary: health status, quality of life and the individual, *JAMA* 272:630-631, 1994.

19. Guyatt GH, Feeny DH, Patrick DL: Measuring health-related quality of life, *Ann Intern Med* 118:622-629, 1993.

20. Guyatt GH, Townsend M, Pugsley SO et al: Bronchodilators in chronic airflow limitation, effects on airway function, exercise capacity and quality of life, *Am Rev Respir Dis* 135:1069-1074, 1987.

21. Hays RD, Anderson R, Revicki D: Psychometric considerations in evaluating health-related quality of life measures, *Qual Life Res* 2:441-449, 1993.

22. Hays RD, Sherbourne CD, Mazel RM: The Rand 36-item health status survey 1.0, *Health Econ* 2:217-227, 1993.

23. Idler EI, Kasl S: Health perceptions and survival: do global evaluations of health status really predict mortality? *J Gerontol* 46:S55-S65, 1991.

24. Jachuck SJ, Brierly H, Jachuck S, Willcox PM: The effect of hypotensive drugs on the quality of life, *J R Coll Gen Pract* 32:103-105, 1982.

25. Jaeschke R, Singer J, Guyatt G: Measurement of health status: ascertaining the minimal clinically important difference, *Controlled Clin Trials* 12:S266-S269, 1991.

26. Kane RL, Wales J, Bernstein L et al.: A randomised controlled trial of hospice care, *Lancet* i:890-894, 1984.

27. Kaplan GA, Camacho T: Perceived health and mortality: a nine-year follow-up of the human population laboratory cohort, *Am J Epidemiol* 117:292-304, 1983.

28. Kaplan RM: Behavior as the central outcome in health care, *Am Psychol* 45:1211-1220, 1990.

29. Kaplan RM: *Utility assessment for estimating quality-adjusted life years,* LaJolla, Calif, 1993, University of California at San Diego.

30. Kaplan RM, Feeny D, Revicki DA: Methods for assessing relative importance in preference based outcome measures, *Qual Life Res* 2:467-475, 1993.

31. McDowell K, Newell C: *Measuring health: a guide to rating scales and questionnaires,* New York, 1987, Oxford University Press.

32. Melzack R: The McGill pain questionnaire: major properties and scoring methods, *Pain* 1:277-299, 1975.

33. Mossey JM, Shapiro E: Self-rated health: a predictor of mortality among the elderly, *Am J Public Health* 72:800-808, 1982.

34. Neal DE, Styles RA, Ng T, et al: Relationship between voiding pressures, symptoms and urodynamic findings in 253 men undergoing prostatectomy, *Br J Urol* 60:554-559, 1987.

35. Patrick DL, Erickson P: *Health status and health policy: allocating resources to health care,* New York, 1992, Oxford University Press.

36. Quality of Life Assessment in Cancer Clinical Trials: Report of the Workshop on Quality of Life Research in Cancer Clinical Trials, *USDHHS,* Bethesda, Md, 1991.

37. Radloff LS: The CES-D Scale: a self-report depression scale for research in the general population, *Appl Psychol Measures* 1:385-401, 1977.

38. Revicki DA, Weinstein M, Alderman M et al: *Health utility and health status outcomes of antihypertensive treatment.* Washington DC, 1992, Battelle Medical Technology Assessment and Policy Research Center.

39. Revicki DA: Relationship between health utility and psychometric health status measures, *Med Care* 30:MS274-MS282, 1992.

40. Revicki DA, Kaplan RM: Relationship between psychometric and utility-based approaches to the measurement of health-related quality of life, *Qual Life Res* 2:477-487, 1993.

41. Ruberman W, Weinblatt E, Goldberg JD, Chaudhary BS: Psychosocial influences on mortality after myocardial infarction, *N Engl J Med* 311:552-559, 1984.

42. Schron EB, Shumaker SA: The integration of health quality of life in clinical research: experiences from cardiovascular clinical trials, *Prog Cardiovasc Nurs* 7:21-28, 1992.

43. Shumaker SA, Anderson R, Berzon R, Hays R, eds: Special Issue: International use, application and performance of health-related quality of life measures, *Qual Life Res* 2, 1993.
44. Shumaker SA, Anderson R, Czajkowski SM: Psychological aspects of HRQL measurement: tests and scales. In Spilker B, ed: *Quality of life assessment in clinical trials,* New York, 1990, Raven Press.
45. Shumaker SA, Wyman JF, Uebersax JS, et al.: Health-related quality of life measures for women with urinary incontinence: the Incontinence Impact Questionnaire and the Urogenital Distress Inventory. *Qual Life Res* 3:291-306,1994.
46. Spilker B, ed: *Quality of life assessment in clinical trials,* New York, 1990, Raven Press.
47. Spilker B, Molinek FR, Johnston KA, et al: Quality of life bibliography and indexes, *Med Care* 28:DS1-DS77, 1990.
48. Spitzer WO, Dobson AJ, Jall J et al: Measuring the quality of life of cancer patients, *J Chronic Dis* 34:585-597, 1981.
49. Stewart A: Conceptual and methodologic issues in defining quality of life: state of the art, *Prog Cardiovasc Nurs* 7:3-11, 1992.
50. Stewart AL, Ware JE, eds: *Measuring functioning and well-being,* Durham, NC, 1992, Duke University Press.
51. Sugarbaker PH, Barofsky I, Rosenberg SA, Gionola FJ: Quality of life assessment of patients in extremity sarcoma clinical trials, *Surgery* 91:17-23, 1982.
52. Testa MA, Anderson RB, Nackley JF et al: Quality of life and antihypertensive therapy in men: a comparison of captopril and enalapril, *N Engl J Med* 328:901-913, 1993.
53. Torrance GW: Measurement of health state utilities for economic appraisal, *J Health Econ* 5:1-30, 1986.
54. Torrance GW: Utility approach to measuring health-related quality of life, *J Chronic Dis* 40:593-600, 1987.
55. Wassertheil-Smoller S, Blaufox D, Oberman A et al: Effects of antihypertensives on sexual function and quality of life: the TAIM study, *Ann Intern Med* 114:613-620, 1991.
56. Wells KB, Manning WG, Valdez RB: The effects of insurance generosity on the psychological distress and well-being of a general population: results from a randomized trial of insurance, Santa Monica, Calif, RAND, R-3682-NIMH-HCF.
57. Wenger NK, Furberg CD: Cardiovascular disorders. In Spilker B, ed: *Quality of life assessment in clinical trials,* New York, 1990, Raven Press.
58. Wenger NK, Mattson ME, Furberg CD, eds: *Assessment of quality of life in clinical trials of cardiovascular therapies,* Washington, DC, 1984, LeJacq.
59. Wiklund I, Karlberg J, Mattsson L-A: Quality of life of post-menopausal women on a regimen of transdermal estradiol therapy: a double-blind placebo-controlled study, *Am J Obstet Gynecol* 168:824-830, 1993.
60. Wilkin D, Hallam L, Doggett M: *Measures of need and outcome for primary health care,* New York, 1992, Oxford Medical.

CHAPTER 13

Participant Adherence

The terms *compliance* and *adherence* are often used interchangeably. Compliance is defined as the extent to which a person's behavior (in terms of taking medications, following diets, or executing lifestyle changes) coincides with medical or health advice.[20] This book uses the term *adherence* in the same way. For example, an adherer is a participant who meets the standards of adherence as established by the investigator. In a drug trial, he may be a participant who takes at least a minimum predetermined amount, such as 80% of the protocol dose. Ensuring maximum adherence to the intervention regimen and trial procedures involves the collaboration of the investigators and their staffs with the participants.

The optimal study from an adherence viewpoint is one in which the investigator has total control over the participant, the administration of the intervention regimen, which may be a drug, diet, exercise, or other intervention and follow-up. That situation exists only in animal experiments. Any clinical trial that, according to the definition in this text, must involve human beings, is likely to have in practice less than 100% adherence with the intervention and the study procedures. There are several reasons for nonadherence: (1) people experience side effects, (2) they may be unwilling to change their behaviors, (3) they may not understand instructions given to them, (4) they may lack family support, or (5) they may change their minds regarding participation. Therefore even studies of a one-time intervention such as surgery or a single medication dose can suffer from nonadherence. In fact, surgical procedures have been reversed. In addition, the participant's condition may deteriorate and thus require termination of the study treatment or a switch from control to intervention. For example, in a clinical trial of medical vs. surgical intervention, a participant's status may so change that it is in the best interest of that participant, if assigned to the medical group, to undergo surgery. In the Coronary Artery Surgery Study, an average of 4.7% of participants assigned to medical intervention had bypass surgery every year.[6]

Obviously, trial results can be affected by nonadherence with the intervention. Nonadherence leads to underestimating possible therapeutic and toxic effects and can undermine even a properly designed study. A 20% reduction in drug adherence may result in the need for a greater-than-50% increase in sample size.[8]

Monitoring adherence is important in a clinical trial for two reasons: first, to identify any problems so steps to enhance adherence can be taken; second, to be able to relate the trial findings to the level of adherence. This chapter will discuss what can be done before enrollment to reduce future adherence problems, how to maintain good adherence during a study, and how to monitor adherence. Readers interested in a more detailed discussion of various issues are referred to two excellent texts.[20,50] Vander Stichele[51] recently reviewed the literature on adherence and provides an extensive bibliography. Most of the available information on adherence is obtained from the clinical therapeutic situation rather than from the clinical trial setting. Although the difference between patients and volunteer participants may be important, tending to minimize nonadherence in trials, it is assumed that the basic principles apply to both.

FUNDAMENTAL POINT

Many potential adherence problems can be prevented or minimized before participant enrollment. Once a participant is enrolled, taking measures to enhance and monitor participant adherence is essential.

Because nonadherence with the intervention has a major impact on the power of a trial, realistic estimates of crossovers, drop-ins, and drop-outs must be used in calculating the sample size. A *crossover* is a participant who, although assigned to the control group, follows the intervention regimen; or a participant who, assigned to an intervention group, follows either the control regimen or the regimen of another intervention group when more than one intervention is being evaluated. A *drop-in* is a special kind of crossover. In particular, the drop-in is unidirectional, referring to a person who was assigned to the control group but begins following the intervention regimen. A *drop-out* is a person assigned to an intervention group who fails to comply with the intervention regimen. If the control group is either on placebo or on no standard intervention or therapy, the drop-out is equivalent to a crossover. However, if the control group is assigned to an alternative therapy, then a drop-out from an intervention group does not necessarily begin following the control regimen. Rather, he takes on some characteristics of a person outside the trial. Moreover, in this circumstance, there may be a drop-out from the control group. Participants who are unwilling or unable to return for follow-up visits represent another type of nonadherence, sometimes also referred to as *drop-outs*. Because of the possible confusion in meanings, this text will limit the term *drop-out* to mean the previously defined behavior. See Chapter 7 for further discussion of the sample size implications of nonadherence.

CONSIDERATIONS BEFORE PARTICIPANT ENROLLMENT

Before enrollment, several steps can be taken to minimize adherence problems. Study design is a key aspect. The shorter the study, the more likely participants are to adhere to the intervention regimen.[47] A study started and completed in 1 day or during a hospital stay has great advantages over longer trials. Studies in which the participants are under supervision, such as hospital-based trials, tend to have fewer problems of nonadherence.[18] However, there is a difference between special hospital wards and clinics with trained attendants who are familiar with research requirements, and general medical or surgical wards and clinics, where research experience might not be common or protocol requirements might not be appreciated. Regular hospital staff have many other duties that compete for their attention, and they perhaps have little understanding of the need for precisely following a study protocol. In the latter case, explaining the various aspects of a trial to everyone who may become involved in the study is especially important.

Whenever the study involves participants who will be living at home, the chances for nonadherence increase. Studies of interventions that require changing a habit are particularly susceptible to this hazard.[7,33] In dietary studies, when the participant's food source comes only from the hospital kitchen, he is more likely to adhere to the study regimen than when he buys and cooks his own food. Using a special commissary to supply the food is one possible approach to dietary intervention for people who are living at home. It also allows for blinded design.[36]

Simplicity of intervention is important. Single-daily-dose drug regimens are preferable to multiple-daily-dose regimens.[3,42] When on a three- or four-times-a-day regimen, many people forget to take every dose at exactly the right time. Adding multiple types of drugs, perhaps with different dosage schedules, increases the possibility of confusion and results in mistakes. Complying with multiple interventions simultaneously poses special difficulties. For example, quitting smoking, losing weight, and reducing the intake of saturated fat at the same time require dedicated participants. Unlike on-going interventions such as drugs, diet, or exercise, surgery and vaccination generally have the design advantage, with few exceptions, of enforcing adherence to the intervention.

An important factor in preventing adherence problems before enrollment is selection of appropriate participants. Ideally, only those people likely to follow the study protocol should be enrolled. This may, however, influence the ability to generalize the findings. (See Chapter 4 for a discussion of generalization.) It has been concluded that "there is convincing evidence that noncompliers are substantially different from compliers in ways that are quite independent of the effects of the treatment prescribed."[10] Numerous studies[3,19,20] have been conducted in an effort to determine what factors distinguish good from poor adherers. Sociodemographic, psychological, disease-related, therapy-related, and investigator-related factors are among the many variables that have been studied. Only a limited number have generally been shown to be associated with future adherence. One factor is the participant's belief in his susceptibility to the consequences of the condition or disease being studied and his general feelings of vulnerability.[3,19] Related to feelings of

susceptibility and vulnerability is the participant's perception of the possible reper-
cussions of an illness. If the consequences are serious, adherence to therapy may be
increased. An additional factor is the benefit that the participant thinks is probable
from the intervention. Higher level of education has been reported to correlate with
good adherence.[49] Clinic site in a multicenter trial has also been noted to influence
adherence.[15]

It is usually advisable to exclude certain types of people from participation in a
trial. These include persons addicted to drugs or alcohol (unless the treatment of
drug or alcohol addiction is being studied), persons who live too far away, and
those who are likely to move before the scheduled termination of the trial. Travel-
ing long distances may be an undue burden on disabled people. Those with concomitant disease sometimes may be less adherent because they have other medicines to take or are participating in other trials. Furthermore, there is the potential
for contamination of the study results by these other medicines or trials.

A truly informed participant appears to be a better adherer.[3,16] Therefore, for scientific and ethical concerns the participant (or, in special circumstances, his
guardian) in any trial should be clearly instructed about the study and told what is
expected from him. Sufficient time should be spent with a candidate. He should be
encouraged to consult with his family or private physician. A brochure with information concerning the study is often helpful. As an example, the text of a pamphlet
used in the NIH-sponsored Women's Health Initiative trial is shown in Box 13-1.

Where feasible, a run-in period before actual randomization ought to be considered to identify those likely to become poor adherers and exclude them from the
trial. During the run-in, potential participants may be given either active medication
or placebo over several weeks or months. This approach was successfully employed
in a trial of aspirin and beta-carotene in U.S. physicians.[26,28] By excluding physicians
who reported taking less than 50% of the study pills, the investigators were able to
randomize excellent adherers. After 5 years of follow-up, more than 90% of those
allocated to aspirin were still taking this drug.

The use of the active study drug during the run-in has the advantage of detecting
drug intolerance that may require discontinuation of treatment. An additional goal
of the run-in is to stabilize potential trial participants on specific treatment regimens
or to wash-out the effects of discontinued medications. A MEDLINE search for a 6
month period in 1988 yielded 26 trials that used a run-in phase.[26] Knipschild et al.
summarized these and other benefits of a run-in.[25] Though the number of participants eliminated by the run-in period is usually small (5% to 10%), it can be important, as even this level of nonadherence affects study power.[38,39] A potential disadvantage of such run-in is that participants may notice a change in their medication
following randomization, thereby influencing the blindness of assignment. It also
delays entry of participants into a trial.[27] Brittain and Wittes[5] argue that in the
absence of a specific reason, the low rejection rate in most run-in periods and the

---

Box 13-1 **Women's Health Initiative Brochure**

What is the Women's Health Initiative?

The Women's Health Initiative (WHI) is a major research study of women and their health. It will help decide how diet, hormone therapy, and calcium and vitamin D might prevent heart disease, cancer, and bone fractures. This is the first such study to examine the health of a very large number of women over a long period of time. About 160,000 women of various racial and ethnic backgrounds from 45 communities across the United States will take part in the study.

Who can join the WHI?

You may be able to join if you are:
- a woman 50–79 years old
- past menopause or the "change of life"
- planning to live in the same area for at least 3 years

Why is this study important?

Few studies have focused on health concerns unique to women. Being a part of this important project will help you learn more about your own health. You will also help doctors develop better ways to treat all women. This study may help us learn how to prevent the major causes of death and poor health in women: heart disease, cancer, and bone fractures.

What will I be asked to do?

If you agree to join us, you will be scheduled for several study visits. These visits will include questions on your medical history and general health habits, a brief physical exam, and some blood tests. Based on your result, you may be able to join at least one of the following programs:

- **Dietary:** In this program you are asked to follow either your usual eating pattern or a low-fat eating program.

- **Hormone:** In this program you are asked to either take hormone pills or inactive pills (placebos). If you are on hormones now, you would need to talk with your doctor about joining this program.

- **Calcium and Vitamin D:** In this program you are asked to either take calcium and vitamin D pills or inactive pills. Only women in the Dietary or Hormone programs may join this program.

- **Health Tracking:** If you are not able to join the other programs, your medical history and health habits will be followed during the study.

How long will the study last?

You will be in the study for a total of 8 to 12 years, depending on what year you enter the study. This period of time is necessary to study the long-term effects of the programs.

How will I benefit?

If you join the study, your health will be followed by the staff at our center. Certain routine tests will be provided, although these are not meant to replace your usual health care. Depending on which program you join, you may receive other health-care services, such as study pills and dietary sessions. You will not have to pay for any study visits, tests, or pills.

You will also have the personal satisfaction of knowing that results from the WHI may help improve your health and the health of women for generations to come.

possibility of misclassification may be counterproductive to the efficiency of the trial. We suggest that if a run-in can be implemented without important delay to the actual trial, and if at least 8% to 10% of potential participants are excluded, the run-in should be strongly considered.

In another approach, the investigator may instruct prospective participants to refrain from taking the active agent and then evaluate how well his request was followed. In the Aspirin Myocardial Infarction Study, for instance, urinary salicylates were monitored before enrollment, and very few participants were excluded because of a positive urine test.

Hunninghake[22] summarized the relationship between the recruitment process and adherence. In addition to the many approaches discussed above, he points to the importance of staff selection, continuity of care, careful selection of recruitment sources and participants, and clinic organization.

Modification of health beliefs is another approach that is based on the observed relationship between health belief and adherence.[3,10] Perceived susceptibility is a predictor of adherence but the strength of this association appears to vary with timing of assessment, the population, and type of health behavior studied.[10] The associations between perceived severity of illness and perceived benefits and medication adherence are also weak. The most frequently used techniques to achieve adherence involve fear-arousal. This appears to work in participants who have health concerns and who believe that treatment will be beneficial. Also, fear arousal early in a trial may influence individuals if recommendations can be followed easily and quickly.

More thorough delivery of the intervention appears to be another feasible and worthwhile approach to enhance adherence in clinical trials.[3] This approach often entails involving various health care providers in providing instructions and reinforcement and answering questions. Use of nurses[32] and pharmacists[48] in efforts to improve adherence has been shown to be effective. Contracting with the participants is another potential technique. It is a behavioral method that offers participants a written outline of the expected behavior, involves them in the decision-making process, provides them with opportunities to discuss problems and solutions, expects a formal commitment to the program by the participants and, in return, offers various types of rewards for achieving goals.

Efforts to optimize participants' experiences at clinic visits also have a beneficial effect on adherence. This approach covers the spectrum from warm and friendly interactions with investigators and staff, to adequate time to discuss complaints, showing of sincere concern and sympathy when called for, convenient clinic environment, and short waiting times. Satisfied participants are better adherers.

Family support has emerged as a major determinant of adherence. The family can assist, encourage, and supervise. Not only spouses or other family members, but also friends, can be helpful during the enrollment and follow-up phases of trials.

MAINTAINING GOOD PARTICIPANT ADHERENCE

The framework for understanding adherence behavior[3,17] has led to several adherence-enhancing strategies for both adherence with medications and appointment keeping.

A combination of counseling, use of a special medication container and mailed reminders, and self-recording of medication intake and seizures markedly improved adherence measured by plasma anticonvulsant levels, prescription refill frequency, and seizure frequency in outpatients with epilepsy.[37] Adherence to a 10-day antibiotic regimen for children with otitis media improved as a result of an intervention consisting of an educational handout about ear infections, a self-monitoring calendar, and a mid-regimen telephone reminder.[12] Two forms of so-called health belief model intervention enhanced adherence to referral appointments among patients with urinary tract infection who presented to an emergency department.[24] A quantitative meta-analysis concluded that adherence to appointments can be accomplished by any of the following strategies: mailed reminders, telephone prompts, "orientation statements," "contracting" with patients, and prompts from physicians.[30] The excellent visit adherence in the Beta-Blocker Heart Attack Trial has been attributed to a series of adherence-enhancing efforts described by Bell et al.[4]

The difficult task in any trial is dealing with poor adherers. Probstfield et al.[40,41] developed and implemented a remarkable recovery program. Through counseling, the investigators succeeded in inducing 90% of the 36 participants who had stopped coming for clinic visits to resume such visits. Even more notable was the virtual absence of recidivism over the remaining 5 years of intervention. Approximately 70% resumed taking their study medication, though typically at a lower dose than specified in the protocol.

After enrollment, several steps can be taken to maintain good adherence. These steps have evolved over the years and are used by experienced clinic staff. They are particularly important in studies of long duration. Experienced investigators and staff stay in close contact with the participants early after randomization to get participants involved and, later, to keep them interested when their initial enthusiasm may have worn off. Between scheduled visits, clinic staff may make frequent use of the telephone and mail. Sending cards on special occasions such as birthdays and holidays is a helpful gesture. Visiting the participant if he is hospitalized shows concern. The investigator may make notes of what the participant tells him about his family, hobbies, and work so that in subsequent visits the investigator can show interest and involvement.

Clinic staff typically remind the participant of upcoming clinic visits or study procedures. Sending out postcards or calling a few days before a scheduled visit can help. A telephone call has the obvious advantage that immediate feedback is obtained and a visit can be rescheduled if necessary—a process that reduces the number of participants who fail to keep appointments. Telephoning also helps to identify a participant who is ambivalent regarding his continued participation. To preclude the clinic staff's imposing on a participant, it helps to ask in advance if the participant objects to being called periodically. Asking a participant about the best time to contact him is usually appreciated. Reminders can then be scheduled accordingly. In cases where participants are reluctant to come to clinics, more than one staff person might contact the participant. For example, the lead investigator could have more influence with the participant than the staff member who usually schedules visits. In summary, the quantity and quality of interaction between an investigator and the participant seems to be important for adherence.

Many investigators routinely involve the participant's spouse or other family member in the study. Informed family members can be effective supporters of the study.[21] They frequently make sure that visits are kept and drugs are taken on schedule. In addition, staff who are trying to alter the diet of a participant find it useful to have good rapport with the person who does the cooking. In the Multiple Risk Factor Intervention Trial,[31] which tried to reduce cholesterol by dietary means, many clinics conducted sessions during which the families of the participants could discuss meal planning and learn new recipes.

Educating participants about the intervention is an integral part of clinical trials, because of the possibility of improving adherence, with little chance of reducing it. Clearly, participants are likely to follow dietary or exercise regimens better when they understand their relation to the disease and the rationale behind the intervention. Brochures, newsletters with articles addressing these issues, and group sessions for all study participants and spouses can be worthwhile, particularly in long-term trials.

Many investigators try to maintain continuity of care. Trial experience suggests that whenever possible, the same investigator and staff should see the participant throughout the study. Participants often express preference to see the same clinic staff and investigators.

Making clinic visits pleasant is also common sense. Providing such things as parking facilities, free transportation, and comfortable waiting room facilities, and minimizing waiting time will make the participant more willing to come. Participants who have problems getting to clinic during usual working hours might find evening or weekend sessions helpful. Home visits by staff can also be attempted. For participants who have moved, the investigator might be able to arrange for follow-up in other cities.

For drug studies, special pill dispensers help the participant keep track of when he has taken his medication.[34] Special reminders such as noticeable stickers in the bathroom or on the refrigerator door or watches have been used. Placing the pill bottles on the kitchen table or nightstand is another suggestion from participants.

A special brochure that contains essential information and reminders may be helpful in maintaining good participant adherence (Box 13-2). The phone number where the investigator or staff can be reached should be included in the brochure.

Box 13-2 **Aspirin Myocardial Infarction Study Brochure**

Text of brochure used to promote participant adherence in the Aspirin Myocardial Infarction Study. DHEW Publication No. (NIH) 76-1080.

1. **Your Participation in the Aspirin Myocardial Infarction Study (AMIS) is Appreciated!** AMIS, a collaborative study supported by the National Heart and Lung Institute, is being undertaken at thirty clinics throughout the United States and involves over 4000 volunteers. As you know, this study is trying to determine whether aspirin will decrease the risk of recurrent heart attacks. It is hoped that you will personally benefit from your participating in the study and that many other people with coronary heart disease may also greatly benefit from your contribution.

2. **Your Full Cooperation is Very Important to the Study.** We hope that you will follow all clinic recommendations contained in this brochure, so that working together, we may obtain the most accurate results. If anything is not clear, please ask your AMIS Clinic Physician or Coordinator to clarify it for you. *Do not hesitate to ask questions.*

3. **Keep Appointments.** The periodic follow-up examinations are very important. If you are not able to keep a scheduled appointment, call the clinic coordinator as soon as possible and make a new appointment. It is also important that the dietary instructions you have received, be followed carefully on the day that blood samples are drawn. At the annual visit you must be *fasting.* At the non-annual visits you are allowed to have a *fat-free diet.* Follow the directions on your Dietary Instruction Sheet. *Don't forget to take your study medication as usual on the day of your visit.*

4. **Change in Residence.** If you are moving within the Clinic area, please let the Clinic Coordinator know of your change of address and telephone number as soon as possible. If you are moving away from the Clinic area, every effort will be made to arrange for continued follow-up here or at another participating AMIS Clinic.

   Long Vacations. If you are planning to leave your Cinic area for an extended period of time, let the Clinic Coordinator know so that you can be provided with sufficient study medication. Also give the Clinic Coordinator your address and telephone number so that you can be reached if necessary.

5. **New Drugs.** During your participation in AMIS you have agreed not to use non-study prescribed aspirin or aspirin-containing drugs. Therefore, please call the Clinic Coordinator before starting any new drug as it might interfere with study results. At least 400 drugs contain aspirin, among them cold and cough medicines, pain relievers, ointments and salves, as well as many prescribed drugs. Many of these medications may not be labeled as to whether or not they contain aspirin or aspirin-related components. To be sure, give the Clinic Coordinator a call.

6. **Aspirin-Free Medication.** Your Clinic will give you aspirin-free medication for headaches, other pains and fever at no cost. The following two types may be provided:

   • Acetaminophen. The effects of this drug on headaches, pain and fever resemble those of aspirin. The recommended dose is 1-2 tablets every 6 hours as needed or as recommended by your Clinic Physician.

   • Propoxyphene hydrochloride. The drug has an aspirin-like effect on pain only and cannot be used for the control of fever. The recommended dose is 1-2 capsules every 6 hours as needed or as recommended by your Clinic Physician.

continued

7. **Study Medication.** You will be receiving study medication from your Clinic. You are to take two capsules each day unless prescribed otherwise. Should you forget to take your morning capsule, take it later during the day. Should you forget the evening dose, you can take it at bedtime with a glass of water or milk. The general rule is: *Do not take more than 2 capsules a day.*

8. **Under Certain Circumstances It Will Be Necessary to Stop Taking the Study Medication:**
   - If you are hospitalized, stop taking the medication for the period of time you are in the hospital. Let the Clinic Coordinator know. After you leave the hospital, a schedule will be established for resuming medication, if it is appropriate to do so.

   - If you are scheduled for surgery, we recommend that you stop taking your study medication 7 days prior to the day of the operation. This is because aspirin may, on rare occasions, lead to increased bleeding during surgery. In case you learn of the plans for surgery less than 7 days before it is scheduled, we recommend that you stop the study medication as soon as possible. And again please let the clinic coordinator know. After you leave the hospital, a schedule will be established for resuming medication, if it is appropriate to do so.

   - If you are prescribed non-study aspirin or drugs containing aspirin by your private physician, stop taking the study medication. Study medication will be resumed when these drugs are discontinued. Let the Clinic Coordinator know.

   - If you are prescribed anti-coagulants (blood thinners), discontinue study medication and let your Clinic Coordinator know.

   - If you have any adverse side effects which you think might be due to the study medication, stop taking it and call the Clinic Coordinator immediately.

9. **Study-Related Problems or Questions**. Should you, your spouse, or anyone in your family have any questions about your participation in AMIS, your Clinic will be happy to answer them. The clinic would like you or anyone in your family to call if you have any side effects that you suspect are caused by your study medication and also if there is any change in your medical status, for example, should you be hospitalized.

10. **Your Clinic Phone Number Is on the Back of This Brochure. Please Keep This Brochure as a Reference Until the End of the Study.**

ADHERENCE MONITORING

Monitoring adherence is critical, as the interpretation of study results will be influenced by knowledge of adherence with the intervention (see Chapter 16). To the extent that the control group is not truly a control and the intervention group is not being treated as intended, group differences are diluted and generally lead to an underestimate of both the therapeutic effect and the adverse effects. Feinstein[11] points out that differential adherence to two equally effective regimens can lead to possibly erroneous conclusions about the effects of the intervention.

In some studies, measuring adherence is relatively easy. This is true for trials in which one group receives surgery and the other group does not, or for trials requiring only a one-time intervention. Most of the time, however, assessment of adherence is more complex. No single measure of adherence gives a complete picture, and all are subject to possible inaccuracies and varying interpretations. Furthermore, there is no widely accepted definition or criterion for either good or poor adherence.[9,43]

In monitoring adherence for a long-term trial, the investigator may also be interested in changes over time. When reductions in adherence are noted, corrective action should be taken, if possible. Monitoring could be by calendar time (e.g., current 6 months vs. previous 6 months) or by clinic visit (e.g., follow-up visit number four vs. previous visits). In multicenter trials, adherence to the intervention also can be examined by clinic. In all studies, it is important for clinic staff to receive feedback about level of adherence. In double-blind trials where data by study group generally should not be disclosed, the adherence data can be combined for the study groups. In non–double-blind trials, adherence tables, by intervention assignment, can be reviewed with the clinic staff.

Frequent determinations obviously have more value than infrequent ones. A better indication of true adherence can be obtained. Moreover, when the participant is aware that adherence is being monitored, frequent measures may encourage him to adhere.

In drug trials, pill or capsule count is the easiest and most commonly used method of evaluating participant adherence. Since this assumes that the participant has ingested all medication not returned to the clinic, the validity of pill count is debated.[9,43,46] For example, if the participant returns the appropriate number of leftover pills at a follow-up visit, did he in fact take what he was supposed to, or did he take only some and throw the rest out? Drug dispensers have been devised that indicate whether each dose was removed in a regular manner or all at one time.[34] However, the method is expensive and cumbersome. Furthermore, taking the drug out of the dispenser does not ensure that the drug is ingested. In general, good rapport with the participants will encourage cooperation and lead to a more accurate pill count.

Pill count is possible only as long as the pills are available to be counted. Participants may neglect to bring their pills to the clinic to be counted. In such circumstances, the investigator may ask the participant to count the pills himself at home and to notify the investigator of the result by telephone. Obviously, these data may be less reliable. The frequency with which data on pill counts are missing gives an estimate of the reliability of pill count as an adherence monitoring tool.

In monitoring pill count, investigators ought to anticipate questions of interest to readers of the trial report when published. What was the overall adherence to the protocol prescription? If overall adherence with the intervention was reduced, what was the main reason for the reduction? Were participants prescribed a reduced dose of the medication, or did they not follow the investigator's prescription? Was there any difference between the study groups with regard to overall adherence to protocol dosage, adherence to investigator prescription, or participant adherence to the prescribed dosage? What was the reason for reduced participant adherence? Was it because of specific side effects, or was it simply forgetfulness? The answers to these questions may increase the understanding of the trial results.

When discussing adherence assessed by pill count, the investigator has to keep in mind that these data may be inflated and misleading, because they obviously do not include information from participants who omit a visit. Those who miss one or more visits are often poor adherers. Therefore the adherence data should be viewed within the framework of all participants who should have been seen at a particular visit. Tables 13-1 and 13-2 address several of the questions raised above and illustrate ways of presenting adherence data.

Laboratory determinations are also sometimes used to monitor adherence to medications. Tests done on either blood or urine can detect the presence of active drugs or metabolites. A limitation in measuring substances in urine or blood is the short half-life of most drugs. Therefore laboratory determinations usually indicate

Table 13-1   Average number of tablets prescribed, average adherence to prescription, and average adherence to protocol, by clinic, study groups combined

Clinic	Average no. of tablets prescribed per day	Average no. of tablets taken per day	Average adherence to prescription[*]	Average adherence to protocol[†]
A	1.97	1.92	97.5%	96.0%
B	1.83	1.67	91.3%	83.5%
C	1.96	1.88	95.9%	94.0%
Total	1.92	1.82	94.9%	91.0%

Table used in Aspirin Myocardial Infarction Study: Coordinating Center, University of Maryland

[*]Average adherence to prescription is average number of tablets taken per day divided by average number of tablets prescribed per day.

[†]Average adherence to protocol is average number of tablets taken per day divided by daily protocol dosage (in this case, two tablets per day).

Table 13-2   Average number of tablets prescribed, average adherence to prescription, and average adherence to protocol, by follow-up visit and study group

Visit	Average no. of tablets prescribed per day		Average no. of tablets taken per day		Average adherence to prescription[*]		Average adherence to protocol[†]	
	Group A	Group B	Group A	Group B	Group A	Group B	Group A	Group B
1	1.95	1.94	1.91	1.89	97.9%	97.4%	95.5%	94.5%
2	1.93	1.90	1.82	1.78	94.3%	93.7%	91.0%	89.0%
3	1.92	1.89	1.83	1.80	95.3%	95.2%	91.5%	90.0%

[*] Average adherence to prescription is average number of tablets taken per day divided by average number of tablets prescribed per day.

[†]Average adherence to protocol is average number of tablets taken per day divided by daily protocol dosage (in this case, two tablets per day).

only what has happened in the preceding day or two. A control participant who takes the active drug (obtained from a source outside the trial) until the day prior to a clinic visit or a participant in the intervention group who takes the active drug only on the day of the visit might not be detected as being a poor adherer. Moreover, drug adherence in participants taking an inert placebo tablet cannot be assessed by any laboratory determination. Adding a specific chemical substance such as riboflavin can serve as a marker in cases where the placebo, the drug, or its metabolites are difficult to measure. However, the same drawbacks apply to markers as to masking substances; the risk of toxicity in long-term use may outweigh benefits. The clinical requirements, the chemical and pharmacological properties, and costs for ideal markers have been proposed.[23]

Tables 13-3 and 13-4 illustrate how adherence based on a laboratory determination can be monitored. The examples are from a placebo-control trial of aspirin[2] in which the salicylate level in urine was used as an indicator of drug adherence. The tables were designed to provide information on both drop-outs (participants in the aspirin group not taking aspirin) and drop-ins (participants in the placebo group taking aspirin). Ideally, the percentages in Table 13-3 ought to be 100 and 0 for group A and group B, respectively, but they very rarely are. The investigator should determine in advance, preferably in a pretest, the definition of an indicator of positive adherence. The selection of the cut-off may affect the estimates of adherence. If the investigator chooses a high level of urine salicylate and accepts only values over that cut-off as being positive, he will probably have a high drop-out rate, because a proportion of participants who faithfully take aspirin may have low levels of urine salicylate. The interval between the time the last tablet was taken and the time the urine specimen was obtained might be long enough for most of the salicylate to be excreted. When the cut-off level is low, the investigator runs the risk of finding what appears to be a high drop-in rate. In fact, for selected tests, these drop-ins may be attributable to imprecision of the method at low values. In addition, there may be false-positive results. For example, a urine salicylate determination is not specific for aspirin. Products that contain methyl salicylate can also give measurable levels of salicylate in the urine. Again, caution is necessary in a double-blind trial when adherence tables based on laboratory determinations of the active drug or metabolite are shared with the clinic staff. Combining data from the study groups as shown in Table 13-4 is one way of overcoming the problem of unblinding.

Laboratory tests obtained on occasions not associated with clinic visits may give a better picture of regular adherence. Thus the participant may be instructed, at certain intervals, to send to the clinic a vial of urine. Such a technique is of value only as long as the participant does not associate it with an adherence-monitoring procedure. In at least one study,[2] information obtained in this manner contributed no additional information to laboratory results done at scheduled visits, except perhaps as a confirmation of such results.

Table 13-3   Percentage of participants with positive urine salicylate by visit and study group

Visit	Group A		Group B	
	Participants completing visits	Percentage of participants with positive test	Participants completing visits	Percentage of participants with positive test
1	260	88.5	264	3.0
2	251	86.1	250	4.4
3	242	86.8	237	4.2

Table 13-4   Percent of participants adhering to protocol as defined by urine salicylate tests, by clinic and follow-up visit, study groups combined

Visit	Follow-up visit 1		Follow-up visit 2	
	Participants completing visits	Percentage of adherers	Participants completing visits	Percentage of adherers
A	173	92.5	165	90.9
B	145	90.3	141	87.9
C	206	94.7	195	92.8
Total	524	92.7	501	90.8

Measurement of physiological response variables can be helpful. Cholesterol reduction by drug or diet is unlikely to occur in 1 or 2 days. Therefore a participant in the intervention group cannot suddenly adhere to the regimen the day before a clinic visit and expect to go undetected. Similarly, the cholesterol level of a nonadherent control participant is unlikely to rise in the 1 day before a visit if he skips his lipid-lowering drug. Other physiological response variables that might be monitored are blood pressure in an antihypertensive study, carbon monoxide in a smoking study, platelet aggregation in an aspirin study, and graded exercise in an exercise study. In all these cases, the indicated response variable would not be the primary response variable but merely an intermediate indicator of adherence to the intervention regimen. Unfortunately, some measures, such as triglyceride levels, are highly variable; indications of nonadherence of individual participants using these measures are not easily interpreted. Group data, however, may be useful.

Other adherence-monitoring techniques fall under the category of interview or record keeping. A diet study might use a 24-hour recall or a 7-day food record. Exercise studies might use diaries or charts to indicate frequency and kind of exercise. Studies of people with angina pectoris might record frequency of attacks of pain and nitroglycerine administration. The techniques mentioned depend greatly on participant recall (even diaries require participants to remember to make entries) and are subjective. As a result, interpretations of adherence in individual participants can be misleading. Group data, again, are more reliable. Interviews of the participants have been proposed as a useful method of measuring participant adherence to the intervention.[13] However, others[45] feel that an interview alone is an unreliable indicator. Most participants tend to overestimate their adherence either in an effort to please the investigator or because of faulty memory.[9] In the Multiple Risk Factor Intervention Trial, the investigators measured serum thiocyanate to adjust for participants' claims of quitting smoking.[35] As seen in Table 13-5, a substantial correction was made in the Special Intervention group, particularly at year 1.

Investigator ratings of adherence have been used. It is probably the least reliable of the various techniques and tends to overestimate adherence.[9,45]

The kinds of adherence monitoring and the uses to which they can be put depend on whether the study is blinded. In a double-blind study, laboratory measurements and physiological response variables on individual participants must be kept from the examining investigator. They can be used only in evaluating total study results and not in ongoing maintenance of good adherence. For this purpose, the investigator must rely on pill count. In single-blind and unblinded studies, all of the techniques mentioned above can be used to encourage good participant adherence.

Another aspect of monitoring deals with participant adherence to study procedures such as attendance at scheduled visits. One of the purposes of these visits is to collect response variable data. The data will be better if they are more complete. Thus completeness of data in itself can be a measure of the quality of a clinical trial. Studies with even a moderate amount of missing data or participants lost to follow-up could give misleading results and should be interpreted with caution. By reviewing the reasons why participants missed scheduled clinic visits, the investigator can identify factors that can be corrected or improved. Having the participants come in for study visits facilitates and encourages adherence to study medication. Study drugs are dispensed at these visits, and the dose is adjusted when necessary. Tables 13-6 and 13-7 show ways of monitoring missed visits.

From a statistical viewpoint, every randomized participant should be included in the analysis (Chapters 5 and 16). Consequently, the investigator must keep trying to

Table 13-5   Reported and thiocyanate-adjusted cigarette smoking quit rate (%) by group in the Multiple Risk Factor Intervention Trial

Year	Special Intervention		Usual Care	
	Reported	Adjusted	Reported	Adjusted
1	43	31	14	12
6	50	46	29	29

get all participants back for scheduled visits until the trial is over. Even if a partici-pant is taken off his study medication by an investigator or if he stops taking it on his own, he should be encouraged to come in for his regular study visits. Complete follow-up data on the response variables are critical. In addition, participants do change their minds. For a long time, they may want to have nothing to do with the trial and later may agree to come back for visits and even resume taking their assigned intervention regimen. Special attention to each participant's problems and an emphasis on potential contribution to the trial can lead to successful retrieval of a large proportion.[30] Inasmuch as the participant will be counted in the analysis, leaving open the option for the participant to return to active participation in the study is worthwhile.

SPECIAL POPULATIONS

Although approaches to dealing with prevention of nonadherence and mainte-nance of high adherence are applicable to people in general, there are factors that need specific consideration when dealing with special populations. For example, health-seeking behaviors and utilization of health care differ between Caucasians and African-Americans.[29] Available resources, ways of dealing with stress and adver-sity, and the positive influence of the family and community are especially meaning-ful factors that apply to African-Americans. Children and adolescents also require special attention,[1] as they are legally dependent on parents or guardians. Motivation

Table 13-6   Missed visits by study group and follow-up visit

Visit	Group A Possible visits	No. missed visits	Percentage missed visits	Group B Possible visits	No. missed visits	Percentage missed visits
1	270	10	3.7	272	8	2.9
2	263	12	4.6	258	8	3.1
3	257	15	5.8	251	14	5.6
Total	790	37	4.7	781	30	3.8

Table 13-7   Missed visits by clinic and follow-up visit, study groups combined

Clinic	Follow-up visit 1 Possible visits	No. missed visits	Percentage missed visits	Follow-up visit 2 Possible visits	No. missed visits	Percentage missed visits
A	177	4	2.3	170	5	2.9
B	153	8	5.2	148	7	4.7
C	212	6	2.8	203	8	3.9
Total	542	18	3.3	521	20	3.8

to adhere to an intervention can be difficult to promote in persons who are not cognitively and emotionally developed. Elderly individuals represent another special population.[44] Since metabolism and physiology change with age, finding the proper dose of an intervention represents a challenge. Polypharmacy and sometimes complex or inadequate instructions can lead to failure to take the medication or to an overdose of medication. Drug interactions are another concern, even with over-the-counter drugs. In addition, elderly participants typically have more complaints than their younger counterparts. Assessment of intervention-related adverse reactions is another challenge. Data from a hypertension trial showed that elderly participants are good medication adherers, but adherence levels may be lower in participants after the age of 80.[14]

REFERENCES

1. Aledort LM, Weiss H, Parker CT et al: Life-style interventions in the young. In Shumaker SA, Schron EB, Ockene JK, eds.: *Health behavior changes,* New York, 1990, Springer.
2. Aspirin Myocardial Infarction Study Research Group: A randomized, controlled trial of aspirin in persons recovered from myocardial infarction, *JAMA* 243:661-669, 1980.
3. Becker MH: Theoretical models of adherence and strategies for improving adherence. In Shumaker SA, Schron EB, Ockene JK, eds: *Health behavior changes,* New York, 1990, Springer.
4. Bell RL, Curb JD, Friedman LM et al: Enhancement of visit adherence in the national Beta-Blocker Heart Attack Trial, *Controlled Clin Trials* 6:89-101, 1985.
5. Brittain E, Wittes J: The run-in period in clinical trials. The effect of misclassification on efficiency, *Controlled Clin Trials* 11:327-338, 1990.
6. CASS Principal Investigators and Their Associates: Coronary Artery Surgery Study (CASS): a randomized trial of coronary artery bypass surgery. Survival data, *Circulation* 68:939-950, 1983.
7. Coates TJ, Vander Martin R, Gerbert B et al: Physician and dentist compliance with smoking cessation counseling. In Shumaker SA, Schron EB, Ockene JK eds: *Health behavior changes,* New York, 1990, Springer.
8. Davis CE: Prerandomization compliance screening: a statistician's view. In Shumaker SA, Schron EB, Ockene, JK eds: *Health behavior changes,* New York, 1990, Springer.
9. Dunbar J: Adherence measures and their utility, *Controlled Clin Trials* 5:515-521, 1984.
10. Dunbar J: Predictors of patient adherence: patient characteristics. In Shumaker SA, Schron EB, Ockene JK, eds: *Health behavior changes,* New York, 1990, Springer.
11. Feinstein A: Clinical biostatistics. XXX. Biostatistical problems in "compliance bias," *Clin Pharmacol Ther* 16:846-857, 1974.
12. Finney JW, Friman PC, Rapoff MA, Christophersen ER: Improving compliance with antibiotic regimens of otitis media. Randomized clinical trial in a pediatric clinic, *AJDC* 139:89-95, 1985.
13. Fletcher SW, Pappius EM, Harper SJ: Measurement of medication compliance in a clinical setting, *Arch Intern Med* 139:635-638, 1979.
14. Furberg CD, Black DM: The systolic hypertension in the elderly pilot program: methodological issues, *Eur Heart J* 9:223-227, 1988.
15. Goldman AI, Holcomb R, Perry HM Jr et al: Can dropout and other noncompliance be minimized in a clinical trial? Report from the Veterans Administration-National Heart, Lung, and Blood Institute cooperative study on antihypertensive therapy: mild hypertension, *Controlled Clin Trials* 3:75-89, 1982.
16. Green LW: Educational strategies to improve compliance with therapeutic and preventive regimens: the recent evidence. In Haynes RB, Taylor DW, Sackett DL, eds: *Compliance in health care,* Baltimore, 1979, Johns Hopkins University Press.
17. Gritz ER, DiMatteo MR, Hays RD: Methodological issues in adherence to cancer control regimens, *Prev Med* 18:711-720, 1989.

18. Harkapaa K, Jarvikoski A, Mellin G, Hurri H: A controlled study of the outcome of inpatient and outpatient treatment of low back pain. Part I. Pain, disability, compliance, and reported treatment benefits three months after treatment, *Scand J Rehab Med* 21:81-89, 1989.
19. Haynes RB, Dantes R: Patient compliance and the conduct and interpretation of therapeutic trials, *Controlled Clin Trials* 8:12-19, 1987.
20. Haynes RB, Taylor DW, Sackett DL, eds: *Compliance in health care,* Baltimore, 1979, Johns Hopkins University Press.
21. Hogue CC: Nursing and compliance. In Haynes RB, Taylor DW, Sackett DL, eds: *Compliance in health care,* Baltimore, 1979, Johns Hopkins University Press.
22. Hunninghake DB: The interaction of the recruitment process with adherence. In Shumaker SA, Schron EB, Ockene JK, eds: *Health behavior changes,* New York, 1990, Springer.
23. Insull W Jr: Workshop summary, *Controlled Clin Trials* 5:451-558, 1985.
24. Jones PK, Jones SL, Katz J: A randomized trial to improve compliance in urinary tract infection patients in the emergency department, *Ann Emerg Med* 19:16- 20, 1990.
25. Knipschild P, Leffers P, Feinstein AR: The qualification period, *J Clin Epidemiol* 44:461-464, 1991.
26. Lang JM: The use of a run-in to enhance compliance, *Stat Med* 9:87-95, 1990.
27. Lang JM: No free lunch, *J Clin Epidemiol* 45:563-565, 1992 (letter to the editor).
28. Lang JM, Buring JE, Rosner B et al: Estimating the effect of the run-in on the power of the Physicians' Health Study, *Stat Med* 10:1585-1593, 1991.
29. Lewis D, Belgrave FZ, Scott RB: Patient adherence in minority populations. In Shumaker SA, Schron EB, Ockene JK, eds: *Health behavior changes,* New York, 1990, Springer.
30. Macharia WM, Leon G, Rowe BH et al: An overview of interventions to improve compliance with appointment keeping for medical services, *JAMA* 267:1813-1817, 1992.
31. Mandriota R, Bunkers B, Wilcox ME: Nutrition intervention strategies in the Multiple Risk Factor Intervention Trial (MRFIT), *J Am Diet Assoc* 77:138-140, 1980.
32. Marston MW: Nursing management of compliance with medical regimens. In Barofsky I, ed: *Medication compliance: a behavioral management approach,* Thorofore, NJ, 1977, Slack.
33. McCann BS, Retzlaff BM, Walden CE, Knopp RH: Dietary intervention for coronary heart disease prevention. In Shumaker SA, Schron EB, Ockene JK, eds: *Health behavior changes,* New York, 1990, Springer.
34. Moulding TS: The unrealized potential of the medication monitor, *Clin Pharmacol Ther* 25:131-136, 1979.
35. Multiple Risk Factor Intervention Trial Research Group: Multiple Risk Factor Intervention Trial. Risk factor changes and mortality results, *JAMA* 248:1465-1477, 1982.
36. National Diet-Heart Study Research Group: Diet Heart Study. Final report, *Circulation* 37(suppl I):I-1-I-428, 1968.
37. Peterson GM, McLean S, Millingen KS: A randomised trial of strategies to improve patient compliance with anticonvulsant therapy, *Epilepsia* 25:412-417, 1984.
38. Probstfield JL: Adherence and its management in clinical trials: implications for arthritis treatment trials, *Arthritis Rheum* 2:S48-S57, 1989.
39. Probstfield JL: Clinical trial prerandomization compliance (adherence) screen. In Cramer JA and Spilker B, eds.: *Patient compliance in medical practice and clinical trials,* New York, 1991, Raven Press.
40. Probstfield JL, Russell ML, Henske JC et al: Successful program for recovery of dropouts to a clinical trial, *Am J Med* 80:777-784, 1986.
41. Probstfield JL, Russell ML, Insull W Jr, Yusuf S: Dropouts from a clinical trial, their recovery and characterization: a basis for dropout management and prevention. In Shumaker SA, Schron EB, Ockene JK, eds: *Health behavior changes,* New York, 1990, Springer.
42. Pullar T, Kumar S, Feely M: Compliance in clinical trials, *Ann Rheum Dis* 48:871-875, 1989.
43. Rand CS: Issues in the measurement of adherence. In Shumaker SA, Schron EB, Ockene JK, eds: *Health behavior changes,* New York, 1990, Springer.
44. Roth HP: Problems with adherence in the elderly. In Shumaker SA, Schron EB, Ockene JK, eds: *Health behavior changes,* New York, 1990, Springer.

45. Roth HP, Caron HS: Accuracy of doctors' estimates and patients' statements on adherence to a drug regimen, *Clin Pharmacol Ther* 23:361-370, 1978.
46. Rudd P, Byyny RL, Zachary V et al.: The natural history of medication compliance in a drug trial: limitations of pill counts, *Clin Pharmacol Ther* 46:169-176, 1989.
47. Sackett DL, Snow JC: The magnitude of compliance and non-compliance. In Haynes RB, Taylor DW, Sackett DL, eds: *Compliance in health care,* Baltimore, 1979, Johns Hopkins University Press.
48. Schwartz MA: The role of the pharmacist in the patient-health team relationship. In Lasagna L, ed: *Patient compliance,* Mount Kisco, New York, 1976, Futura.
49. Shulman N, Cutter G, Daugherty R et al.: Correlates of attendance and compliance in the Hypertension Detection and Follow-up Program, *Controlled Clin Trials* 3:13-27, 1982.
50. Shumaker SA, Schron EB, Ockene JK, eds: *Health behavior change,* New York, 1990, Springer.
51. Vander Stichele R: Measurement of patient compliance and the interpretation of randomized clinical trials, *Eur J Clin Pharmacol* 41:27-35, 1991.

CHAPTER 14

Survival Analysis

This chapter reviews some of the fundamental concepts and basic methods in survival analysis. Frequently, event rates such as mortality or frequency of nonfatal myocardial infarction are selected as primary response variables. The analysis of such event rates in two groups could employ the chi-square statistic or equivalent normal statistic for the comparison of two proportions. However, since the length of observation is often different for each participant, estimating an event rate is more complicated. Furthermore, simple comparison of event rates between two groups is not necessarily the most informative type of analysis. For example, the 5-year survival for two groups may be nearly identical, but the survival rates may be quite different at various times during the 5 years. This is illustrated by the survival curves in Fig. 14-1. This figure shows survival probability on the vertical axis and time on the horizontal axis. For group *A*, the survival rate (or one minus the mortality rate) declines steadily over the 5 years of observation. For group *B*, however, the decline in the survival rate is rapid during the first year and then levels off. Obviously, the survival experience of the two groups is not the same, although the mortality rate at 5 years is nearly the same. If only the 5-year survival rate, instead of the 5-year survival experience, is considered, group *A* and group *B* appear equivalent. Curves such as these might reasonably be expected in a trial of surgical vs. medical intervention, where surgery might carry a high initial operative mortality.

FUNDAMENTAL POINT

Survival analysis methods are important in trials where participants are entered over a period of time and have various lengths of follow-up. These methods permit the comparison of the entire survival experience during the follow-up and may be used for the analysis of time to any dichotomous response variable such as a nonfatal event or an adverse effect.

A review of the basic techniques of survival analysis can be found in some elementary statistical textbooks[*] and overview papers.[13] A more complete and technical

---

[*]References 1, 2, 6, 8, 17, 46.

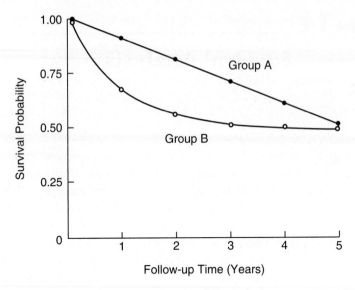

Fig. 14-1 Survival experience for two groups (*A* and *B*).

review is in other texts.[11,18,23,30] Many methodological advances in the field have occurred in recent years, and this book will not be able to cover all developments. The following discussion will concern two basic aspects: first, estimation of the survival experience or survival curve for a group of participants in a clinical trial and second, comparison of two survival curves to test whether the survival experience is significantly different. Although the term *survival analysis* is used, the methods are applicable more widely than to just survival. The methods can be used for any dichotomous response variable in a clinical trial when the time from enrollment to the time of the event, not just the fact of its occurrence, is an important consideration. For ease of communication, we shall use the term *event,* unless death is specifically the event.

ESTIMATION OF THE SURVIVAL CURVE

The graphical presentation of the total survival experience during the period of observation is called the survival curve, and the tabular presentation is called the lifetable. In the sample size discussion (Chapter 7), we used a parametric model to represent a survival curve, denoted $S(t)$, where t is the time of follow-up. A classic parametric form for $S(t)$ is to assume an exponential distribution $S(t) = e^{-\lambda t}$, where λ is the hazard rate.[30] If we estimate λ, we have an estimate for $S(t)$. One possible estimate for the hazard ratio is the number of observed events divided by the total exposure time of the person at risk of the event (G). Other estimates are also available and described later. While this estimate is not difficult to obtain, the hazard rate may not be constant during the trial. If λ is not constant but rather a function of time, we can define a hazard rate $\lambda(t)$, but now the definition is more complicated. Specifically, $S(t) = \exp [\int_{0}^{t} \lambda(s) ds]$; that is, the exponential of the area under the hazard function curve from time 0 to time t. Furthermore, we cannot always be guaranteed that the observed survival data will be described well by the exponential model, even though we often make this assumption for computing sample size. Thus, biostatisticians have relied on parameter-free or nonparametric ways to estimate the survival curve.

This chapter will cover two similar nonparametric methods, the Kaplan-Meier method[24] and the Cutler-Ederer method[14] for estimating the true survival curve or lifetable. Before a review of these specific methods, however, it is necessary to explain how survival experience is typically obtained in a clinical trial and to define some of the associated terminology.

The clinical trial design may, in a simple case, require that all participants be observed for T years. This is referred to as the follow-up time or exposure time. If all the participants are entered as a single cohort at the same time, the actual period of follow-up is the same for all participants. If, however, as in most clinical trials, the entry of participants is staggered over some recruitment period, then the T year period of follow-up may be a different actual or calendar time for each participant, as illustrated in Fig. 14-2.

During the course of follow-up, a participant may have an event. The event time is the accumulated time from entry into the study to the event. The interest is not in the actual calendar date when the event took place but rather the interval of time from entry into the trial until the event. Figures 14-3 and 14-4 illustrate the way the actual survival experience for staggered entry of participants is translated for the

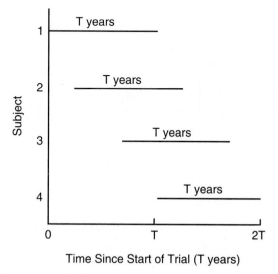

Fig. 14-2 *T* year follow-up time for four participants with staggered entry.

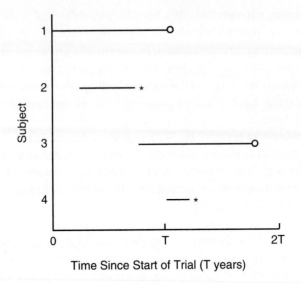

Fig. 14.3 Follow-up experience of four participants with staggered entry: two participants with observed events (*) and two participants followed for time *T* without events (o).

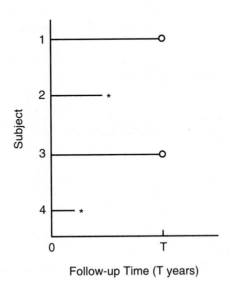

Fig. 14.4 Follow-up experience of four participants with staggered entry converted to a common starting time: two participants with observed events (*) and two participants followed for time *T* without events (o).

analysis. In Fig. 14-3, participants 2 and 4 have an event while participants 1 and 3 do not during the follow-up time. Since, for each participant, only the time interval from entry to the end of the scheduled follow-up period or until an event is of interest, the time of entry can be considered as time zero for each participant. Figure 14-4 illustrates the same survival experience as Fig. 14-3, but the time of entry is considered as time zero.

In most clinical trials, the investigator may be unable to assess the occurrence of the event in some participants. The follow-up time or exposure time for these participants is said to be censored; that is, the investigator does not know what happened to these participants after they stopped participating in the trial. Another example of censoring is when participants are entered in a staggered fashion, and the study is terminated at a common date before all participants have had at least their complete T years of follow-up. These participants are also considered as losses, but the reason for censoring is administrative. Administrative censoring could also occur if a trial is terminated prior to the scheduled time because of early benefits or harmful effects of the intervention. In all cases, censoring is assumed to be independent of occurrence of events.

Figure 14-5 illustrates several of the possibilities for observations during follow-up. Note that in this example the investigator has planned to follow all participants to a common termination time, with each participant being followed for at least T years. The first three participants were randomized at the start of the study. The first participant was observed for the entire duration of the trial with no event, and her survival time was censored because of study termination. The second participant had an event before the end of follow-up. The third participant was lost to follow-up. The second group of three participants was randomized later during the course of the trial with experiences similar to the first group of three. Participants 7 through 11 were randomized late in the study and were not able to be followed for at least T years because the study was terminated early. Participant 7 was lost to follow-up, and participant 8 had an event before T years of follow-up time had elapsed and before the study was terminated. Participant 9 was administratively censored but theoretically would have been lost to follow-up had the trial continued. Participant 10 was also censored because of early study termination, although he had an event afterward that would have been observed had the trial continued to its scheduled end. Finally, the last participant who was censored would have survived for at least T years had the study lasted as long as first planned. The survival experiences illustrated in Fig. 14-5 would all be shifted to have a common starting time equal to zero as in Fig. 14-4. The follow-up time, or the time elapsed from calendar time of entry to calendar time of an event or censoring, could then be analyzed.

In summary, the investigator needs to record for each participant the time of entry and the time of an event, the time of loss to follow-up, or whether the participant was

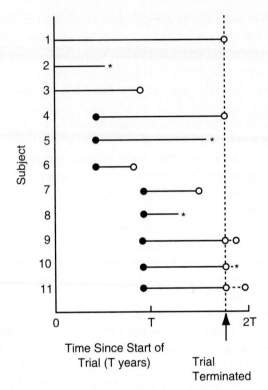

Fig. 14-5 Follow-up experience of 11 participants for staggered entry and a common termination time, with observed events (*) and censoring (o). Follow-up experience beyond the termination time is shown for participants 9 through 11.

still being followed without having had an event when the study is terminated. These data will allow her to compute the survival curve.

Kaplan-Meier estimate

In a clinical trial with staggered entry of participants and censored observations, survival data will be of varying degrees of completeness. As a very simple example, suppose that 100 participants were entered into a study and followed for 2 years. One year after the first group was started, a second group of 100 participants was entered and followed for the remaining year of the study. Assuming no losses to follow-up, the results might be as shown in Table 14-1. For group I, 20 participants died during the first year, and of the 80 survivors, 20 more died during the second year. For group II, which was followed for only 1 year, 25 participants died. Now suppose the investigator wants to estimate the 2-year survival rate. The only group of participants followed for 2 years was group I. One estimate of 2-year survival, $p(2)$, would be $p(2) = 60/100$ or 0.60. Note that the first-year survival experience of

Table 14-1   Participants entered at two points in time (groups I and II) and followed to a common termination time

Years of follow-up		Group	
		I	II
1	Participants entered	100	100
	First-year deaths	20	25
	First-year survivors	80	75
2	Participants entered	80	
	Second-year deaths	20	
	Second-year survivors	60	

After Kaplan and Meier.[24]

group II is ignored in this estimate. If the investigator wants to estimate 1-year survival rate, $p(1)$, she would observe that a total of 200 participants were followed for at least 1 year. Of those, 155 (80 + 75) survived the first year. Thus $p(1) = 155/200$ or 0.775. If each group were evaluated separately, the survival rates would be 0.80 and 0.75. In estimating the 1-year survival rate, all the available information was used, but for the 2-year survival rate the 1-year survival experience of group II was ignored.

Another procedure for estimating survival rates is to use a conditional probability. For this example, the probability of 2-year survival, $p(2)$, is equal to the probability of 1-year survival, $p(1)$, times the probability of surviving the second year, given that the participant survived the first year, $p(2 \mid 1)$. That is, $p(2) = p(1)\, p(2 \mid 1)$. In this example, $p(1) = 0.775$. The estimate for $p(2 \mid 1)$ is $60/80 = 0.75$ since 60 of the 80 participants who survived the first year also survived the second year. Thus the estimate for $p(2) = 0.775 \times 0.75$ or 0.58, which is slightly different from the previously calculated estimate of 0.60.

Kaplan and Meier[24] described how this conditional probability strategy could be used to estimate survival curves in clinical trials with censored observations. Their procedure is usually referred to as the Kaplan-Meier estimate, or sometimes the product-limit estimate, since the product of conditional probabilities leads to the survival estimate. This procedure assumes that the exact time of entry into the trial is known and that the exact time of the event or loss of follow-up is also known. For some applications, time to the nearest month may be sufficient, while for other applications the nearest day or hour may be necessary. Kaplan and Meier assumed that a death and loss of follow-up would not occur at the same time. If a death and loss to follow-up are recorded as having occurred at the same time, this tie is broken on the assumption that the death occurred slightly before the loss to follow-up.

In this method, the follow-up period is divided into intervals of time so that no interval contains both deaths and losses. Let p_j be equal to the probability of surviving the jth interval, given that the participant has survived the previous interval. For the rest of this chapter, lower-case p refers to the conditional probability of surviving a particular interval. Upper-case P refers to the cumulative probability of surviving up through a specific interval. For intervals labeled j with deaths only, the estimate for p_j, which is $\hat{p}_j$, is equal to the number of participants alive at the beginning of the jth interval, n_j, minus those who died during the interval, δ_j, with this difference being divided by the number alive at the beginning of the interval, that is $\hat{p}_j = (n_j - \delta_j)/n_j$. For an interval j with only l_j losses, the estimate $\hat{p}_j$ is one. Such conditional probabilities for an interval with only losses would not alter the product. This means that an interval with only losses and no deaths may be combined with the previous interval.

As a simple example, suppose 20 participants are followed for a period of 1 year, and to the nearest tenth of a month, deaths were observed at the following times: 0.5, 1.5, 1.5, 3.0, 4.8, 6.2, and 10.5 months. In addition, losses to follow-up were recorded at: 0.6, 2.0, 3.5, 4.0, 8.5, and 9.0 months. It is convenient for illustrative purposes to list the deaths and losses together in ascending time with the losses indicated in parentheses. Thus the following sequence is obtained: 0.5, (0.6), 1.5, 1.5, (2.0), 3.0, (3.5), (4.0), 4.8, 6.2, (8.5), (9.0), 10.5. The remaining seven participants were all censored at 12 months because of termination of the study.

Table 14-2 presents the survival experience for this example as a lifetable. Each row in the lifetable indicates the time at which a death or an event occurred. One or more deaths may have occurred at the same time, and they are included in the same row in the lifetable. In the interval between two consecutive times of death, losses to follow-up may have occurred. Hence, a row in the table actually represents an interval of time, beginning with the time of a death, up to but not including the time of the next death. In this case, the first interval is defined by the death at 0.5 months up to the time of the next death at 1.5 months. The columns labeled n_j, δ_j, and l_j corre-

Table 14-2   Kaplan-Meier lifetable for 20 participants followed for 1 year

Interval	Interval number	Time of death	n_j	δ_j	l_j	$\hat{p}_j$	$\hat{P}(t)$	$V[\hat{P}(t)]$
[0.5,1.5)	1	0.5	20	1	1	0.95	0.95	0.0024
[1.5,3.0)	2	1.5	18	2	1	0.89	0.85	0.0068
[3.0,4.8)	3	3.0	15	1	2	0.93	0.79	0.0089
[4.8,6.2)	4	4.8	12	1	0	0.92	0.72	0.0114
[6.2,10.5)	5	6.2	11	1	2	0.91	0.66	0.0133
[10.5, ∞)	6	10.5	8	1	7*	0.88	0.58	0.0161

*Censored due to termination of study.

  n_j = Number of participants alive at the beginning of the jth interval
  δ_j = Number of participants who died during the jth interval
  l_j = Number of participants who were lost or censored during the jth interval
  $\hat{p}_j$ = Estimate for p_j, the probability of surviving the jth interval given that the participant has
       survived the previous intervals
  $\hat{P}(t)$ = Estimated survival curve
$V[\hat{P}(t)]$ = Variance of $\hat{P}(t)$

spond to the definitions given above and contain the information from the example. In the first interval, all 20 participants were initially at risk, one died at 0.5 months, and later in the interval (at 0.6 months) one participant was lost to follow-up. In the second interval, from 1.5 months up to 3.0 months, 18 participants were still at risk initially, two deaths were recorded at 1.5 months, and one participant was lost at 2.0 months. The remaining intervals are defined similarly. The column labeled $\hat{p}_j$ is the conditional probability of surviving the interval j and is computed as $(n_j - \delta_j)/n_j$ or $(20 - 1)/20 = 0.95$, $(18 - 2)/18 = 0.89$, etc. The column labeled $\hat{P}(t)$ is the estimated survival curve and is computed as the accumulated product of the p_j ($0.85 = 0.95 \times 0.89$, $0.79 = 0.95 \times 0.89 \times 0.93$, etc.).

The graphical display of the next-to-last column of Table 14-2, $\hat{P}(t)$, is given in Fig. 14-6. The step function appearance of the graph is because the estimate of $P(t)$, $\hat{P}(t)$, is constant during an interval and changes only at the time of a death. With very large sample sizes and more observed deaths, the step function has smaller steps and looks more like the usually visualized smooth survival curve. If no censoring occurs, this method simplifies to the number of survivors divided by the total number of participants who entered the trial.

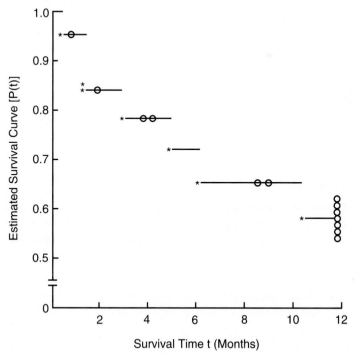

Fig. 14-6 Kaplan-Meier estimate of a survival curve, $\hat{P}(t)$, from a 1-year study of 20 participants, with observed events (*) and censoring (o).

Since $\hat{P}(t)$ is an estimate of $P(t)$, the true survival curve, the estimate will have some variation because of the sample selected. Greenwood[20] derived a formula for estimating the variance of an estimated survival function that is applicable to the Kaplan-Meier method. The formula for the variance of $\hat{P}(t)$, denoted $V[\hat{P}(t)]$, is given by:

$$V\left[\hat{P}(t)\right] = \hat{P}^2(t) \sum_{j=1}^{K} \frac{\delta_j}{n_j\left(n_j - \delta_j\right)}$$

where n_j and δ_j are defined as before, and K = the number of intervals. In Table 14-2, the last column labeled $V[\hat{P}(t)]$ represents the estimated variances for the estimates of $P(t)$ during the six intervals. Note that the variance increases as one moves down the column. When fewer participants are at risk, the ability to estimate the survival experience is diminished.

Other examples of this procedure and a more detailed discussion of some of the statistical properties of this estimate are provided by Kaplan and Meier.[24] Computer programs are available[44] so that survival curves can be obtained quickly, even for very large sets of data.

The Kaplan-Meier curve can also be used to estimate the hazard rate, λ, if the survival curve is exponential. For example, if the median survival time is estimated as t_μ, then $0.5 = S(T_m) = e^{-\lambda T_\mu}$ and thus $\lambda = ln\ (0.5)/T_M$. Then the estimate for $S(t)$ would be $e^{-\lambda t}$. In comparison with the Kaplan-Meier, another parametric estimate for $S(t)$ at time t_j, described by Nelson,[31] is

$$\hat{S}\left(t_j\right) = \exp\left\{-\sum_{j=1}^{J} \delta_i / n_i\right\}$$

where δ_i is the number of events in the ith interval and n_i is the number at risk for the event. While this is a straightforward estimate, the Kaplan-Meier does not assume an underlying exponential distribution and thus is used more than this type of estimator.

Cutler-Ederer estimate

In the Kaplan-Meier estimate, it was required that the exact time of death or loss be known so that the observations could be ranked, or at least grouped approximately, into intervals with deaths preceding losses. For some studies, all that is known is that within an interval of time from t_{j-1} to t_j, denoted $(t_{j-1} - t_j)$, δ_j deaths and l_j losses occurred among the n_j participants at risk. Within the interval the order in which the events and losses occurred is unknown. In the Kaplan-Meier procedure, the intervals were chosen so that all deaths preceded all losses in any interval.

In the Cutler-Ederer or actuarial estimate,[14] the assumption is made that the deaths and losses are uniformly distributed over an interval. On the average, this means that one half the losses will occur during the first half of the interval. The estimate for the probability of surviving the jth interval, given that the previous intervals were survived, is $\hat{p}_j$, where

$$\hat{p}_j = \frac{n_j - \delta_j - 0.5\lambda_j}{n_j - 0.5\lambda_j}$$

Notice the similarity to the Kaplan-Meier definition. The modification is that the λ_j losses are assumed to be at risk, on the average, one half the time and thus should be counted as such. These conditional probabilities, $\hat{p}_j$, are then multiplied together as in the Kaplan-Meier procedure to obtain an estimate $\hat{P}_t$ of the survival function $P(t)$. The estimated variance for $\hat{P}_t$ in this case is given by

$$V\,[\hat{p}] = \hat{P}^2(t) \sum_{j=1}^{K} \frac{\delta_j}{(n_j - 0.5\lambda_j)(n_j - 0.5\lambda_j - \delta_j)}$$

Specific applications of this method are described by Cutler and Ederer.[14] The parallel to the example shown in Table 14-2 would require recomputing the $\hat{p}_j$, $\hat{p}(t)$ and $V[\hat{P}(t)]$.

COMPARISON OF TWO SURVIVAL CURVES

We have just discussed how to estimate the survival curve in a clinical trial for a single group. For two groups, the survival curve would be estimated for each group separately. The question is whether the two survival curves $P_C(t)$ and $P_I(t)$, for the control and intervention groups, respectively, are different based on the estimates $\hat{P}_C(t)$ and $\hat{P}_I(t)$.

Point-by-point comparison

One possible comparison between groups is to specify a time t^* for which survival estimates have been computed using the Kaplan-Meier[24] or Cutler-Ederer[14] method. At time t^*, one can compare the survival estimates $\hat{P}_C(t^*)$ and $\hat{P}_I(t^*)$ using the statistic

$$Z(t^*) = \frac{\hat{P}_C(t^*) - \hat{P}_I(t^*)}{\left\{V\left[\hat{P}_C(t^*)\right]\right\} + \left\{V\left[\hat{P}_I(t^*)\right]\right\}^{1/2}}$$

where $V[\hat{P}_C(t^*)]$ and $V[\hat{P}_I(t^*)]$ are the Greenwood estimates of variance. The statistic $Z(t^*)$ has approximately a normal distribution with mean zero and variance one under the null hypothesis that $\hat{P}_C(t^*) = \hat{P}_I(t^*)$. The problem with this approach is the multiple looks issue described in Chapter 15. Another problem exists in interpretation. For example, what conclusions should be drawn if two survival curves are judged significantly different at time t^* but not at any other points? The issue then becomes, what point in the survival curve is most important.

For some studies with a T year follow-up, the T year mortality rates are considered important and should be tested in the manner just suggested. Annual rates might also be considered important and, therefore, compared. One criticism of this suggestion is that the specific points may have been selected to yield the largest difference based on the observed data. One can easily visualize two survival curves for which significant differences are found at a few points. However, when survival curves are compared, the large differences indicated by these few points are not supported by the overall survival experience. Therefore point-by-point comparisons are not recommended unless a few points can be justified prior to data analysis and are specified in the protocol.

Comparison of median survival times

One summary measure of survival experience is the time at which 50% of the cohort has had the event. One common and easy way to estimate the median survival time is from the Kaplan-Meier curve. (See, for example, Altman.[1]) This assumes that the cohort has been followed long enough so that more than one half of the individuals have had the event. Confidence intervals may be computed for the median survival times. If this is the case, we can compare the median survival times for intervention and control M_I and M_C, respectively. This is most easily done by estimating the ratio of the estimates M_I/M_C. A ratio larger than unity implies that the intervention group has a larger median survival and thus a better survival experience. A ratio less than unity would indicate the opposite.

We can estimate 95% confidence intervals for M_I/M_C by

$$\left(M_I/M_C\right)e^{-1.96S}, \left(M_I/M_C\right)e^{+1.96S}$$

where the standard deviation, S, of M_I/M_C is computed as

$$S = \sqrt{1/O_I + 1/O_C}$$

for cases where the survival curves are approximately exponential, and O_I = total number of events in the intervention group (i.e., $\Sigma \, \delta_i$), and O_C = the total number of events in the control group.

Total curve comparison

Because of the limitations of comparison of point-by-point estimates, Gehan[19] and Mantel[27] originally proposed statistical methods to assess the overall survival experience. These two methods were important steps in the development of analytical methods for survival data. They both assume that the hypothesis being tested is whether two survival curves are equal, or whether one is consistently different from the other. If the two survival curves cross, these methods should be interpreted cautiously. Since these two original methods were proposed, an enormous literature has developed on comparison of survival curves and is summarized in several texts.[11,18,23,30] The basic methods described here provide the fundamental concepts used in survival analysis.

Mantel[27] proposed the use of the procedure described by Cochran[9] and Mantel and Haenszel[29] for combining a series of 2-by-2 tables. In this procedure, each time, t_j, a death occurs in either group, a 2-by-2 table is formed as follows:

	Death at time t_j	Survivors at time t_j	At risk prior to time t_j
Intervention	a_j	b_j	$a_j + b_j$
Control	c_j	d_j	$c_j + d_j$
	$a_j + c_j$	$b_j + d_j$	n_j

The entry a_j represents the observed number of deaths at time t_j in the intervention group and c_j represents the observed number of deaths at time t, in the control group. At least a_j or c_j must be nonzero. One could create a table at other time periods (that is, when a_j and c_j are zero), but this table would not make any contribution to the statistic. Of the n_j participants at risk just prior to time t_j, $a_j + b_j$ were in the intervention group and $c_j + d_j$ were in the control group. The expected number of deaths in the intervention group, denoted $E(a_j)$, can be shown to be:

$$E(a_j) = (a_j + c_j)(a_j + b_j)/n_j$$

and the variance of the observed number of deaths in the intervention group, denoted as $V(a_j)$ is given by:

$$V(a_j) = \frac{(a_j + c_j)(b_j + d_j)(a_j + b_j)(c_j + d_j)}{n_j^2(n_j - 1)}$$

These expressions are the same as those given for combining 2-by-2 tables in the Appendix of Chapter 16. The Mantel-Haenszel (*MH*) statistic is given by:

$$MH = \left(\sum_{j=1}^{K} a_j - E(a_j) \right)^2 \bigg/ \sum_{j=1}^{K} V(a_j)$$

and has approximately a chi-square distribution with one degree of freedom, where K is the number of distinct event times in the combined intervention and control groups. The square root of *MH*, $Z_{mn} = \sqrt{HM}$, has asymptotically a standard normal distribution.[12,34]

Application of this procedure is straightforward. First, the times of events and losses in both groups are ranked in ascending order. Second, the time of each event, the total number of participants in each group who were at risk just before the death ($a_j + b_j$, $c_j + d_j$), and the number of events in each group (a_j, c_j) are determined. With this information, the appropriate 2-by-2 tables can be formed.

Example

Assume that the data in the example shown in Table 14-2 represents the data from the control group. Among the 20 participants in the intervention group, two deaths occurred at 1.0 and 4.5 months, with losses at 1.6, 2.4, 4.2, 5.8, 7.0, and 11.0 months. The observations, with parentheses indicating losses, can be summarized as follows:

Intervention: 1.0, (1.6), (2.4), (4.2), 4.5, (5.8), (7.0), (11.0)
Control: 0.5, (0.6), 1.5, 1.5, (2.0), 3.0, (3.5), (4.0), 4.8, 6.2, (8.5), (9.0), 10.5.

Using the data described above with remaining observations being censored at 12 months, Table 14-3 shows the eight distinct times of death, (t_j), the number in each group at risk prior to the death $(a_j + b_j, c_j + d_j)$, the number of deaths at time t_j, (a_j, c_j), and the number of participants lost to follow-up in the subsequent interval (l_j). The entries in this table are similar to those given for the Kaplan-Meier lifetable shown in Table 14-2. Note in Table 14-3, however, that the observations from two groups have been combined with the net result being more intervals. The entries in Table 14-3 labeled $a_j + b_j$, $c_j + d_j$, $a_j + c_j$, and $b_j + d_j$ become the entries in the eight 2-by-2 tables shown in Table 14-4.

The Mantel-Haenszel statistic can be computed from these eight 2-by-2 tables (Table 14-4) or directly from Table 14-3. The term $\sum_{j=1}^{8} E(a_j) = 2$ since there are only

Table 14-3 Comparison of survival data for a control group and an intervention group using the Mantel-Haenszel procedures

Rank	Event times	Intervention			Control			Total	
j	t_j	$a_j + b_j$	a_j	b_j	$c_j + d_j$	c_j	d_j	$a_j + c_j$	$b_j + d_j$
1	0.5	20	0	0	20	1	1	1	39
2	1.0	20	1	0	18	0	0	1	37
3	4.5	19	0	2	18	1	1	2	35
4	3.0	14	0	1	15	2	2	1	31
5	4.5	16	1	0	12	0	0	1	27
6	4.8	15	0	1	12	0	0	1	26
7	6.2	14	0	1	11	2	2	1	24
8	10.5	13	0	13	8	7	7	1	20

$a_j + b_j$ = Number of participants at risk in the intervention group prior to the death at time t_j
$c_j + d_j$ = Number of participants at risk in the control group prior to the death at time t_j
a_j = Number of participants in the intervention group who died at time t_j
c_j = Number of participants in the control group who died at time t_j
l_j = Number of participants who were lost or censored between time t_j and t_{j+1}
$a_j + c_j$ = Number of participants in both groups who died at time t_j
$b_j + d_j$ = Number of participants in both groups who are alive minus the number who died at time t_j

Table 14-4   Eight 2-by-2 tables corresponding to the event times used in the Mantel-Haen-szel statistic comparison of intervention (*I*) and control (*C*) groups

1. (0.5 mo)*		D†	A‡	R§	5. (4.5 mo)		D	A	R
	I	0	20	20		*I*	1	15	16
	C	1	19	20		*C*	0	12	12
		1	39	40			1	27	28
2. (1 mo)		D	A	R	6. (4.8 mo)		D	A	R
	I	1	19	20		*I*	0	15	15
	C	0	18	18		*C*	1	11	12
		1	37	38			1	26	27
3. (1.5 mo)		D	A	R	7. (6.2 mo)		D	A	R
	I	0	19	19		*I*	0	14	14
	C	2	16	18		*C*	1	10	11
		2	35	37			1	24	25
4. (3 mo)		D	A	R	8. (10.5 mo)		D	A	R
	I	0	17	17		*I*	0	13	13
	C	1	14	15		*C*	1	7	8
		1	31	32			1	20	21

*Number in parentheses indicates time, t_j, of a death in either group.
†D = Number of participants who died at time t_j.
‡A = Number of participants who are alive between time t_j and time t_{j+1}.
§R = Number of participants who were at risk before death at time t_j ($R = D + A$).

two deaths in the intervention group. Evaluation of the term $\Sigma_{j=1}^{8} E(a_j) = 20/40 + 20/38 + 2 \times 19/37 + 17/32 + 16/28 + 15/27 + 14/25 + 13/21$ or $\Sigma_{j=1}^{8} E(a_j) = 4.89$. The value of $\Sigma_{j=1}^{8} V(a_j)$ is computed as:

$$\sum_{j=1}^{8} V(a_j) = \frac{(1)(39)(20)(20)}{(40)^2(39)} + \frac{(1)(37)(20)(18)}{(38)^2(37)} + \ldots$$

This term is equal to 2.21. The computed statistic is $MH = (2 - 4.89)^2 / 2.21 = 3.78$. This is not significant at the 0.05 significance level for a chi-square statistic with one degree of freedom. The *MH* statistic can also be used when the precise time of death is unknown. If death is known to have occurred within an interval, 2-by-2 tables can be created for each interval and the method applied. For small samples, the *MH* statis-tic using a continuity correction is sometimes used. The modified numerator is:

$$\left(\left| \sum_{j=1}^{K} \left[a_j - E(a_j) \right] \right| - 0.5 \right)^2$$

where the vertical bars denote the absolute value. For this example, applying the continuity correction reduces the *MH* statistics from 3.76 to 2.59.

Gehan[19] developed another procedure for comparing the survival experience of two groups of participants by generalizing the Wilcoxon rank statistic. The Gehan statistic is based on the ranks of the observed survival times. The null hypothesis, $P_I(t) = P_C(t)$, is tested. The procedure, as originally developed, involved a complicated calculation to obtain the variance of the test statistic. Mantel[28] proposed a simpler version of the variance calculation, which is most often used.

The N_I observations from the intervention group and N_C observations from the control group must be combined into a sequence of $N_C + N_I$ observations and ranked in ascending order. Each observation is compared with the remaining $N_C + N_I - 1$ observations and given a score U_i, which is defined as follows:

> U_i = (number of observations ranked definitely less than the ith observation) – (number of observations ranked definitely greater than the ith observation).

The survival outcome for the ith participant will certainly be larger than that for participants who died earlier. For censored participants, it cannot be determined whether survival time would have been less than, or greater than, the ith observation. This is true whether the ith observation is a death or loss. Thus the first part of the score U_i assesses how many deaths definitely preceded the ith observation. The second part of the U_i score considers whether the current, ith, observation is a death or loss. If it is a death, it definitely precedes all later ranked observations regardless of whether the observations correspond to a death or a loss. If the ith observation is a

Table 14-5   Example of Gehan statistics scores U_i for intervention (I) and control (C) groups

Observation i	Ranked observed time	Group	Definitely less	Definitely more	U_i
1	0.5	C	0	39	–39
2	(0.6)*	C	1	0	1
3	1.0	I	1	37	–36
4	1.5	C	2	35	–33
5	1.5	C	2	35	–33
6	(1.6)	I	4	0	4
7	(2.0)	C	4	0	4
8	(2.4)	I	4	0	4
9	3.0	C	4	31	–27
10	(3.5)	C	5	0	5
11	(4.0)	C	5	0	5
12	(4.2)	I	5	0	5
13	4.5	I	5	27	–22
14	4.8	C	6	26	–20
15	(5.8)	I	7	0	7
16	6.2	C	7	24	–17
17	(7.0)	I	8	0	8
18	(8.5)	C	8	0	8
19	(9.0)	C	8	0	8
20	10.5	C	8	20	–12
21	(11.0)	I	9	0	9
22–40	(12.0)	12I,7C	9	0	9

* Parentheses indicate censored observations.

loss, it cannot be determined whether the actual survival time will be less than or greater than any succeeding ranked observation, since there was no opportunity to observe the ith participant completely.

Table 14-5 ranks the 40 combined observations (N_C = 20, N_I = 20) from the example used in the discussion of the Mantel-Haenszel statistic. The last 19 observations were all censored at 12 months of follow-up, 7 in the control group and 12 in the intervention group. The score U_1 is equal to the zero observations definitely less than 0.5 months, minus the 39 observations that are definitely greater than 0.5 months, or U_1 = −39. The score U_2 is equal to the one observation definitely less than the loss at 0.6 months, minus none of the observations which will be definitely greater, since at 0.6 months the observation was a loss, or U_2 = 1. U_3 is equal to the one observation (0.5 months) definitely less than 1.0 month minus the 37 observations definitely greater than 1.0 month giving U_3 = −36. The last 19 observations will have scores of 9 reflecting the nine deaths that definitely precede censored observations at 12.0 months.

The Gehan statistic, G, involves the scores U_i and is defined as:

$$G = W^2/V(W)$$

where $W = \Sigma\, U_i$, (U_i's in control group only) and

$$V(W) = \frac{N_C\, N_I}{(N_C + N_I)(N_C + N_I - 1)} \sum_{i=1}^{N_C + N_I} \left(U_i^2\right)$$

The G statistic has approximately a chi-square distribution with one degree of freedom.[19,28] Therefore the critical value is 3.84 at the 5% significance level and 6.63 at the 1% level. In the example, W = −87 and the variance $V(W)$ = 2314.35. Thus G = $(-87)^2/2314.35 = (87)^2/2314.35$ or 3.27 for which the p value is equal to 0.071. This is compared with the p value of 0.052 obtained using the Mantel-Haenszel statistic.

The Gehan statistic assumes the censoring pattern to be equal in the two groups. Breslow[3] considered the case in which censoring patterns are not equal and used the same statistic G with a modified variance. This modified version should be used if the censoring patterns are radically different in the two groups. Peto and Peto[33] also proposed a version of a censored Wilcoxon test. The concepts are similar to what has been described for Gehan's approach. However, most software packages now use the Breslow[3] or Peto and Peto[33] versions.

Generalizations

This general methodology of comparing two survival curves has been further evaluated.* These two tests by Mantel-Haenszel and Gehan can be viewed as a

---

*References 21, 26, 32, 36, 40, 43.

weighted sum of the difference between observed number of events and the expected number at each unique event time.[13,43] Consider the previous equation for the log rank test and rewrite the numerator as:

$$W = \sum_{j=1}^{K} w_j \left[a_j - E(a_j) \right]$$

where

$$V(W) = \sum_{j=1}^{K} w_j^2 \, \frac{(a_j + c_j)(b_j + d_j)(a_j + b_j)(c_j + d_j)}{n_j^2 (n_j - 1)}$$

and w_j is a weighting factor. The test statistic $W^2/V(W)$ has approximately a chi-square distribution with one degree of freedom, or equivalently $W/\sqrt{V(W)}$ has approximately a standard normal distribution. If $w_i = 1$, we obtain the Mantel-Haenszel or log rank test. If $w_i = n_j/(N + 1)$, where $N = N_C + N_I$ or the combined sample size, we obtain the Gehan version of the Wilcoxon test. Tarone and Ware[43] pointed out that the Mantel-Haenszel and Gehan are only two possible statistical tests. They suggested a general weight function $w_i = n_j/(N + 1)]^\theta$ where $0 \le \theta \le 1$. In particular, they suggested that $\theta = 0.5$. Prentice[36] suggested a weight $w_i = \prod_{j=1}^{i} n_j/(n_j + d_j)$ where $d_j = (a_j + c_j)$, which is related to the product limit estimator at t_j as suggested by Peto and Peto.[33] Harrington and Fleming[21] generalize this further by suggesting weights $w_j = \{\prod_{j=1}^{i} [n_j/n_j + d_j)]\}^\rho$ for $\rho \ge 0$.

All of these methods give different weights to the various parts of the survival curve. The Mantel-Haenszel or log rank statistic is more powerful for survival distributions of the exponential form where $\lambda_I(t) = \theta \lambda_C(t)$ or $S_I(t) = \{S_C(t)\}^\theta$ where $\theta \ne 1$.[28] The Gehan-type statistic,[19] on the other hand, is more powerful for survival distributions of the logistic form $S(t,\theta) = e^{t+\theta}/(1 + e^{t+\theta})$. In actual practice, however, the distribution of the survival curve of the study population is not known. When the null hypothesis is not true, the Gehan-type statistic gives more weight to the early survival experience, whereas the Mantel-Haenszel weighs the later experience more. Tarone and Ware[43] indicate other possible weighting schemes could be proposed that are intermediate to these two statistics. Thus, when survival analysis is done, it is certainly possible to obtain different results using different weighting schemes depending on where the survival curves separate, if they indeed do so. The log rank test is the standard in many fields such as cancer and heart disease. The condition $\lambda_I(t) = \theta \lambda_C(t)$ says that risk of the event being studied in the intervention is a constant multiple of the hazard $\lambda_C(t)$. That is, the hazard rate in one arm is proportional to the other, and so the log rank test is best for testing proportional hazards. This idea is appealing and is approximately true for many studies.

There has been considerable interest in asymptotic (large sample) properties of rank tests[32,40] and comparisons of the various analytic methods.[26] While there exists an enormous literature on survival analysis, the basic concepts of rank tests can still be appreciated by the methods previously described.

Earlier, we discussed using an exponential model to summarize a survival curve where the hazard rate λ determines the survival curve. If we can assume that the hazard rate λ is reasonably constant during the period of follow-up for the intervention and the control group, then comparison of hazard rates is a comparison of survival curves.[1] The most commonly used comparison is the ratio of the hazards, $R = \lambda_I/\lambda_C$. If the ratio is unity, the survival curves are identical. If $R > 1$, the intervention hazard is greater than control so the intervention survival curve falls below the control curve. That is, the intervention is worse. On the other hand, if $R < 1$, the control group hazard is larger, the control group survival curve falls below the intervention curve, and intervention is better.

We can estimate the hazard ratio by comparing the ratio of total observed events (O) divided by expected number of events (E) in each group; that is, the estimate of R can be expressed as:

$$\hat{R} = \frac{O_I/E_I}{O_C/E_C}.$$

That is, $O_I = \Sigma a_i$, $O_C = \Sigma b_i$, $E_I = \Sigma E(a_i)$, and $E_C = \Sigma E(b_i)$. Confidence intervals for the odds ratio R are most easily determined by constructing confidence intervals for the log of the odds ratio $\ln R$.[41] The 95% confidence interval for $\ln R$ is $K - 1.96/\sqrt{V}$ to $K + 1.96/\sqrt{V}$ where $K = (O_I - E_I)/V$ and V is the variance as defined in the logrank or Mantel-Haenszel statistics. That is, $V = \Sigma V(a_i)$ We then convert confidence intervals for $\ln R$ to confidence intervals for R by taking antilogs of the upper and lower limit. If the confidence interval excludes unity, we could claim superiority of either intervention or control depending on the direction. Hazard ratios not included in the interval can be excluded as likely outcome summaries of the intervention. If the survival curves have relatively constant hazard rates, this method provides a nice summary and complements the Kaplan-Meier estimates of the survival curves.

Covariate adjusted analysis

Previous chapters have discussed the rationale for taking stratification into account. If differences in important covariates or prognostic variables exist at entry between the intervention and control groups, an investigator might be concerned that the analysis of the survival experience is influenced by that difference. To adjust for these differences in prognostic variables, the investigator could do a stratified analysis or a covariance type of survival analysis. If these differences are not important in the analysis, the adjusted analysis will give approximately the same results as the unadjusted.

Three basic techniques for stratified survival analysis are of interest. The first compares the survival experience between the study groups within each stratum, using the methods described in the previous section. By comparing the results from each stratum, the investigator can get some indication of the consistency of results across strata and the possible interaction between strata and intervention.

The second and third methods are basically adaptations of the Mantel-Haenszel and Gehan statistics and allow the results to be accumulated over the strata. The Mantel-Haenszel stratified analysis involves dividing the population into S strata and within each stratum j, forming a series of 2-by-2 tables for each K_j event, where K_j is the number of events in stratum j. The table for the ith event in the jth stratum would be as follows:

	Event	Alive	
Intervention	a_{ij}	b_{ij}	$a_{ij} + b_{ij}$
Control	c_{ij}	d_{ij}	$c_{ij} + d_{ij}$
	$a_{ij} + c_{ij}$	$b_{ij} + d_{ij}$	n_{ij}

The entries a_{ij}, b_{ij}, c_{ij}, and d_{ij} are defined as before and

$$E\left(a_{ij}\right) = \left(a_{ij} + c_{ij}\right)\left(a_{ij} + b_{ij}\right) / n_{ij}$$

$$V\left(a_{ij}\right) = \frac{\left(a_{ij} + c_{ij}\right)\left(b_{ij} + d_{ij}\right)\left(a_{ij} + b_{ij}\right)\left(c_{ij} + d_{ij}\right)}{n_{ij}^2\left(n_{ij} - 1\right)}$$

Similar to the nonstratified case, the Mantel-Haenszel statistic is:

$$MH = \left\{ \sum_{j=1}^{S} \sum_{i=1}^{Kj} a_{ij} - E\left(a_{ij}\right) \right\}^2 / \sum_{j=i}^{S} \sum_{i=1}^{Kj} V\left(a_{ij}\right)$$

which has a chi-square distribution with one degree of freedom. Analogous to the Mantel-Haenszel statistic for stratified analysis, one could compute a Gehan statistic W_j and $V(W_j)$ within each stratum. Then an overall stratified Gehan statistic is computed as:

$$G = \left\{ \sum_{j=1}^{S} W_j \right\}^2 / \sum_{j=1}^{S} V\left(W_j\right)$$

which also has a chi-square statistic with one degree of freedom.

If there are many covariates, each with several levels, the number of strata can quickly become large, with few participants in each. Moreover, if a covariate is continuous, it must be divided into intervals and each interval assigned a score or rank before it can be used in a stratified analysis. Cox[10] proposed a regression model that allows for analysis of censored survival data adjusting for continuous and discrete covariates, thus avoiding these two problems.

One way to understand the Cox regression model is to again consider a simpler parametric model. If one expresses the probability of survival to time t, denoted $S(t)$, as an exponential model, then $S(t) = e^{-\lambda t}$ where the parameter, λ, is called the force of mortality or the hazard rate as described earlier. The larger the value of λ, the faster the survival curve decreases. Some models allow the hazard rate to change with time, that is $\lambda = \lambda(t)$. Models have been proposed[16,38,47] that attempt to incorporate the hazard rate as a linear function of several baseline covariates, X_1, X_2, ..., X_p, that is, $\lambda(X_1, X_2, ..., X_p) = b_1X_1 + b_2X_2 + ... + b_pX_p$. One of the covariates, say X_1, might represent the intervention, and the others, for example, might represent age, sex, performance status, or prior medical history. The coefficient, b_1, then would indicate whether intervention is a significant prognostic factor, that is, remains effective after adjustment for the other factors. Cox[10] suggested that the hazard rate could be modeled as a function of both time and covariates, denoted $\lambda(t, X_1, X_2, ..., X_p)$. Moreover, this hazard rate could be represented as the product of two terms, the first representing an unadjusted force of mortality $\lambda_0(t)$ and the second the adjustment for the linear combination of a particular covariate profile. More specifically, the Cox proportional hazard model assumes that:

$$\lambda\left(t, x_1, x_2, ... x_p\right) = \lambda_0\left(t\right)\exp\left(b_1X_1 + b_2X_2 + ... + b_pX_p\right)$$

That is, the hazard $\lambda(t, X_1, X_2, ..., X_n)$ is proportional to an underlying hazard function $\lambda_0(t)$ by the specific factor $\exp(b_1X_1 + b_2X_2 ...)$. From this model, we can estimate an underlying survival curve $S_0(t)$ as a function of $\lambda_0(t)$. The survival curve for participants with a particular set of covariates X, $S(t,x)$ can be obtained as $S(t,x) = [S_0(t)]^{\exp(b1\ x1 + b2\ x2 + ...)}$. Other summary test statistics from this model are also used. The estimation of the regression coefficients $b_1, b_2, ..., b_p$ is complex, requiring nonlinear regression methods, and goes beyond the scope of this text. Many elementary texts on biostatistics[1,6,17] or review articles[13] present further details. A more advanced discussion may be found in Kalbfleisch and Prentice[23] or Fleming and Harrington.[18] However, programs exist in many statistical computing packages that provide these estimates and summary statistics to evaluate survival curve comparisons. Despite the complexity of the parameter estimation, this method is widely applied and has been studied extensively.* Pocock, Gore, and Kerr[35] demonstrate the value of some of these methods with cancer data. For the special case where group assignment is the only covariate, the Cox model is essentially equivalent to the Mantel-Haenszel statistic.

The techniques described in this chapter and the extensions or generalizations referenced are powerful tools in the analysis of survival data. Perhaps none is exactly correct for any given set of data, but experience indicates they are fairly robust and quite useful.

REFERENCES

1. Altman DG: *Practical statistics for medical research,* New York, 1991, Chapman & Hall, p. 383-392.
2. Armitage P: *Statistical methods in medical research,* New York, 1977, John Wiley & Sons.

---

*References 4, 5, 15, 22, 25, 35, 37, 39, 42, 45.

3. Breslow N: A generalized Kruskal-Wallis test for comparing K samples subject to unequal patterns of censorship, *Biometrika* 57:579-594, 1970.
4. Breslow N: Covariance analysis of censored survival data, *Biometrics* 30:89-99, 1974.
5. Breslow N: Analysis of survival data under the proportional hazards model, *Int Stat Rev* 43:45-58, 1975.
6. Breslow N: Comparison of survival curves. In Buyse B, Staquet M, Sylvester R, eds: *The practice of clinical trials in cancer,* Oxford, 1982, Oxford University Press.
7. Brookmeyer R, Crowley J: A confidence interval for the median survival time, *Biometrics* 38:29-42, 1982.
8. Brown BW, Hollander M: *Statistics: a biomedical introducion,* New York, 1977, John Wiley & Sons.
9. Cochran W: Some methods for strengthening the common χ^2 tests, *Biometrics* 10:417-451, 1954.
10. Cox DR: Regression models and lifetables, *J R Stat Soc Ser B* 34:187-202, 1972.
11. Cox DR, Oakes D: *The Analysis of survival data,* New York, 1984, Chapman & Hall.
12. Crowley J, Breslow N: Remarks on the conservatism of $\Sigma(0-E)^2/E$ in survival data, *Biometrics* 31:957-961, 1975.
13. Crowley J, Breslow N: Statistical analysis of survival data, *Ann Rev Public Health* 5:385-411, 1984.
14. Cutler, S, Ederer F: Maximum utilization of the lifetable method in analyzing survival, *J Chronic Dis* 8:699-712, 1958.
15. Efron B: The efficiency of Cox's likelihood function for censored data, *J Am Stat Assoc* 72:557-565, 1977.
16. Feigl P, Zelen M: Estimation of exponential survival probabilities with concomitant information, *Biometrics* 21:826-838, 1965.
17. Fisher L, VanBelle G: *Biostatistics: a methodology for the health sciences,* New York, 1993, John Wiley & Sons.
18. Fleming T, Harrington D: *Counting processes and survival analysis,* New York, 1991, John Wiley & Sons.
19. Gehan E: A generalized Wilcoxon test for comparing arbitrarily single censored samples, *Biometrika* 52:203-223, 1965.
20. Greenwood M: The natural duration of cancer, *Rep Public Health Med Subjects*, London, Her Majesty's Stationary Office 33:1-26, 1926.
21. Harrington DP, Fleming TR: A class of rank test procedures for censored survival data, *Biometrika* 69:553-566, 1982.
22. Kalbfleisch JD, Prentice RL: Marginal likelihoods based on Cox's regression and life model, *Biometrika* 60:267-278, 1973.
23. Kalbfleisch JD, Prentice RL: *The statistical analysis of failure time data,* New York, 1980, John Wiley & Sons.
24. Kaplan E, Meier P: Nonparametric estimation from incomplete observations, *J Am Stat Assoc* 53:457-481, 1958.
25. Kay R: Proportional hazard regression models and the analysis of censored survival data, *J R Stat Soc Ser C* 26:227-237, 1977.
26. Leurgans SL: Three classes of censored data rank tests: strengths and weakness under censoring, *Biometrika* 70:651-658, 1983.
27. Mantel N: Evaluation of survival data and two new rank order statistics arising in its consideration, *Cancer Chemother Rep* 50:163-170, 1966.
28. Mantel N: Ranking procedures for arbitrarily restricted observations, *Biometrics* 23:65-78, 1967.
29. Mantel N, Haenszel W: Statistical aspects of the analysis of data from retrospective studies of disease, *J Natl Cancer Inst* 22:719-748, 1959.
30. Miller RG Jr: *Survival analysis,* New York, 1981, John Wiley & Sons.
31. Nelson W: Hazard plotting for incomplete failure data, *J Qual Technol* 1:27-52, 1969.
32. Oakes D: The asymptotic information in censored survival data, *Biometrika* 64:441-448, 1977.
33. Peto R, Peto J: Asymptotically efficient rank invariant test procedures, *J R Stat Soc Ser A* 135:185-207, 1972.
34. Peto R, Pike MC: Conservatism in the approximation $\Sigma(0-E)^2/E$ in the logrank test for survival data or tumor incidence data, *Biometrics* 29:579-584, 1973.

35. Pocock SJ, Gore SM, Kerr GR: Long term survival analysis: the curability of breast cancer, *Stat Med* 1:93-104, 1982.
36. Prentice RL: Linear rank tests with right censored data, *Biometrika* 65:167-179, 1978.
37. Prentice RL, Gloeckler LA: Regression analysis of grouped survival data with application to breast cancer, *Biometrics* 34:57-67, 1978.
38. Prentice RL, Kalbfleisch JD: Hazard rate models with covariates, *Biometrics* 35:25-39, 1979.
39. Schoenfeld D: Chi-squared goodness-of-fit tests for the proportional hazards regression model, *Biometrika* 67:145-153, 1980.
40. Schoenfeld D: The asymptotic properties of non-parametric tests for comparing survival distributions, *Biometrika* 68:316-319, 1981.
41. Simon R: Confidence intervals for reporting results of clinical trials, *Ann Intern Med* 105:429-435, 1986.
42. Storer BE, Crowley J: Diagnostics for Cox regression and general conditional likelihoods, *J Am Stat Assoc* 80:139-147, 1985.
43. Tarone R, Ware J: On distribution-free tests for equality of survival distributions, *Biometrika* 64:156-160, 1977.
44. Thomas DG, Breslow N, Gart J: Trend and homogeneity analysis of proportions and life table data, *Computers Biomed Res* 10:373-381, 1977.
45. Tsiatis AA: A large sample study of Cox's regression model, *Annals Stat* 9:93-108, 1981.
46. Woolson R: *Statistical methods for the analysis of biomedical data,* New York, 1987, John Wiley & Sons.
47. Zelen M: Application of exponential models to problems in cancer research, *J R Stat Soc Ser A* 129: 368-398, 1966.

CHAPTER 15

Monitoring Response Variables

The investigator's ethical responsibility to the study participants demands that results in terms of safety and clinical benefit be monitored during the trial. If data partway through the trial indicate that the intervention is harmful to the participants, early termination of the trial should be considered. If these data demonstrate a clear benefit from the intervention, the trial may also be stopped early because to continue would be unethical. In addition, if differences in primary, and possibly secondary, response variables are so unimpressive that the prospect of a clear result is extremely unlikely, it may not be justifiable in terms of time, money, and effort to continue the trial. Also, monitoring of response variables can identify the need to collect additional data to clarify questions of benefit or toxicity that may arise during the trial. Finally, monitoring may reveal logistical problems or issues involving poor data quality that need to be promptly addressed. Thus there are ethical, scientific, and economic reasons for interim evaluation of a trial.[15,20,61,92,170] To fulfill the monitoring function, the data must be collected and processed in a timely fashion as the trial progresses. Data monitoring would be of limited value if conducted only at a time when all or most of the data had been collected. The specific issues related to monitoring of recruitment, adherence, and quality control are covered in other chapters and will not be discussed here. One of the earliest discussions of the basic rationale for data monitoring was included in an NIH committee report, chaired by Bernard Greenberg.[92] This Greenberg report outlined a clinical trial model that has been implemented widely by the various institutes of the NIH, the pharmaceutical industry, and others. Many of the experiences have been described.*

FUNDAMENTAL POINT

During the trial, response variables need to be monitored for early dramatic benefits or potential harmful effects. Preferably, monitoring should be done by a person or group independent of the investigators. Although many techniques are available to assist in monitoring, none of them should be used as the sole basis for the decision to stop or continue the trial.

---

*References 8, 12, 13, 16, 34, 42, 65, 70, 79, 80, 111, 135, 142, 146, 151, 156, 165, 166, 173, 177, 180, 184, 203.

246

DATA MONITORING COMMITTEE

Keeping in mind the scientific, ethical, and economic rationale, data monitoring is not simply a matter of looking at tables or results of statistical analysis of the primary outcome. Rather, it is an active process in which additional tabulations and analysis are suggested and developed as a result of ongoing review. Data monitoring also involves an interaction between the individuals responsible for collating and analyzing the data and those reviewing and interpreting the results. For single-center studies, the monitoring responsibility could, in principle, be assumed by the investigator. However, he may find himself in a difficult situation. While monitoring the data, he may discover that the results trend in one direction while participants are still being enrolled. Presumably, he recruits participants to enter a trial on the basis that he favors neither intervention nor control, a state of clinical equipoise.[67] Knowing that a trend exists may make it difficult for him to continue enrolling participants. It is also difficult for the investigator to follow, evaluate, and care for the participants in an unbiased manner knowing that a trend exists. Furthermore, the credibility of the trial is enhanced if independent persons monitor the response variable data. Because of these considerations we, and others,[15,20,61,170] recommend that the individuals who monitor a clinical trial have no formal involvement with the participants or the investigators, although some disagree.[89]

Except for small, short-term studies, when one or two knowledgeable individuals may suffice, the responsibility for monitoring response variable data is usually placed with an independent group with expertise in various disciplines.[*] The independence protects the members of the monitoring committee from being influenced in the decision-making process by investigators, participants, or sponsors. The committee would usually include experts in the relevant clinical fields or specialities, individuals with experience in the conduct of clinical trials, epidemiologists, and biostatisticians knowledgeable in design and analysis. While we will describe statistical procedures that are often helpful in evaluating interim results, the decision process to continue, terminate a trial early, or modify the design is invariably complex, and no single statistical procedure can address all these complexities. Furthermore, no single individual is likely to have all the experience and expertise to deal with these issues. Thus as was recommended in the Greenberg Report,[92] we suggest that the independent data monitoring committee have a multidisciplinary membership.

The independence of the data monitoring committee is critical for the model to be effective.[†] The priority of the data monitoring committee must first be to ensure the safety of the participants in the trial. The second priority is to the investigators,

---

*References 35, 43, 55, 64, 84, 93, 147, 194, 204.
†References 42, 61, 64, 70, 92, 142, 184, 194.

who place an enormous trust in the data monitoring committee both to protect their participants from harm and to ensure the integrity of the trial. Third, the data monitoring committee has a responsibility to the sponsor of the trial, whether it be federal or private. Finally, the data monitoring committee provides a service to the drug or device regulatory agency, especially for trials that are using drugs, biologics, or devices that still have investigational status.

Although many formats for data monitoring committee meetings have been used, one that seems to be very workable allows for exchange of information by all relevant parties and allows for the appropriate confidential and independent review.[43,70] The format uses an open session, a closed session, and an executive session. The open session allows for interaction between investigator representatives such as the study principal investigator or chair, the sponsor, the statistical center, regulatory agencies, the relevant industrial participants, and the data monitoring committee. At this session, issues of participant recruitment, data quality, general adherence and toxicity issues and any other logistical matter that may affect either the conduct or the outcome of the trial are considered. After a thorough discussion, the data monitoring committee may go into a closed session, where analyses of the blinded outcome data are reviewed by members of the committee and the statistical analysis center. This review would include comparison by intervention groups of baseline variables, primary or secondary variables, safety or adverse outcome variables, and adherence measures for the entire group, and examinations of any relevant subgroups. After this review, the meeting would move into an executive session of only the data monitoring committee where decisions about continuation, termination, or protocol modification are made. These different sessions may be formally or informally divided, depending on who attends the data monitoring committee meetings. Regardless of how formal, most data monitoring committee meetings have such components. This particular model, for example, has been used extensively in NIH-sponsored AIDS trials.[43]

Before a trial begins and a data monitoring committee meeting is scheduled, it must be decided very specifically who attends the various sessions, as outlined above. In general, attendance should be limited to those who are essential for proper monitoring. As noted, it is common for the study principal investigator or chair, sponsor representatives, industry representatives, and perhaps regulatory agency representatives to attend the open session. If the study chair or principal investigator does not care for participants in the trial, that individual may attend the closed session, although there is variation in that practice. If the study is not industry sponsored, the industry representative typically does not attend the closed session. Even if the study is sponsored by industry, independence and credibility of the study may be best served by limited attendance. Industry-sponsored trials that are also managed by industry require a biostatistician from the sponsor to attend the data monitoring committee meeting. Regulatory agency representatives usually do not attend the closed session because being involved in the monitoring decision may affect their regulatory role, should the product be submitted for subsequent approval. An executive session may involve only the voting members of the data monitoring committee and the senior study biostatistician, though the study sponsor representative may also attend. There are many variations of this general outline, including a merger of the closed and executive session since attendance may be by the same individuals.

Most data monitoring committees evaluate one, or perhaps two, clinical trials. When a trial is completed, the data monitoring committee is dissolved. However, as exemplified by cancer and AIDS research, standing networks of clinical centers conduct many trials concurrently.* Cancer trial cooperative groups may conduct trials across several cancer sites, such as breast, colon, lung, or head and neck, at any given time, and even multiple trials for a given site depending on the stage of the cancer or other risk factors. The AIDS trial networks in the United States have likewise conducted trials simultaneously in AIDS participants with differing stages of the disease. In these areas, data monitoring committees may follow the progress of several trials. In such instances, a very disciplined agenda and a standardized format of the data report enhance the efficiency of the review. Regardless of the model, the goals and procedures are similar.

Another factor that needs to be resolved before the start of the trial is how the intervention or treatment comparisons will be presented to the data monitoring committee. In some trials, the data monitoring committee knows the identity of the interventions in each table or figure of the report. In other trials, the data monitoring committee is blinded throughout the interim monitoring. To achieve this, data reports have complex labeling schemes such as A vs. B for baseline tables, C vs. D for primary outcomes, E vs. F for toxicity, and G vs. H for various laboratory results. While this degree of blinding may enhance objectivity, it may conflict with the data monitoring committee's primary purpose of protecting the participants in the trial from harm or unnecessary continuation. To assess best the progress of the trial, the risk and benefit profile of the intervention must be well understood and the possible tradeoffs weighed. If each group of tables is labeled by a different code, the committee cannot easily assess the overall risk/benefit profile of the intervention and thus may put participants at unnecessary risk or continue a trial beyond the point at which benefit outweighs risks. A reasonable compromise is to label all tables consistently, such as arm A and B, or at most by two codes, with the understanding that the committee can become unblinded. Thus if there are no trends in either benefit or harm, which is likely to be the case early in a trial, there is no overwhelming reason to know the identity of groups A and B. When trends begin to emerge in either direction, the data monitoring committee should have full knowledge of the group identities.

---

*References 12, 13, 16, 35, 43, 64, 80, 84, 146, 173, 203.

No simple formula can be given for how often a monitoring committee should meet. The frequency may vary depending on the phase of the trial.[42,61,70,129,156] Participant recruitment, follow-up, and closeout phases require different activity levels. Meetings should not be so frequent that little new data are accumulated in the interim, given the time and expense of convening a committee. If potential toxicity of one of the interventions becomes an issue during the trial, special meetings may be needed. In many long-term clinical trials, the monitoring committees have met regularly at 4- to 6-month intervals, with additional meetings as needed. In some circumstances, an annual review may be sufficient. However, less frequent review is not recommended since too much time may elapse before a serious adverse effect is uncovered. As described later, another strategy is to schedule data monitoring committee meetings when approximately 10%, 25%, 50%, 75%, and 100% of the primary outcomes have been observed, or some similar pattern. Thus there might be an early analysis to check for serious immediate adverse effects with later analyses to evaluate evidence of treatment benefit or harm. Other approaches provide for additional analyses at intervals if strong but as yet nonsignificant trends emerge. Patterns such as those suggested capture most of the opportunity or need for early termination. Between committee meetings, the person or persons responsible for collating, tabulating, and analyzing the data assume the responsibility for monitoring unusual situations that may need to be brought to the attention of the data monitoring committee.

REPEATED TESTING FOR SIGNIFICANCE

In the discussion on sample size (Chapter 7) the issue of testing several hypotheses was raised and referred to as the "multiple testing" problem. Similarly, while repeated significance testing of accumulating data is essential to the monitoring function, it does have statistical implications.* If the null hypothesis, H_0, of no difference between two groups is, in fact, true, and repeated tests of that hypothesis are made at the same level of significance using accumulating data, the probability that, at some time, the test will be called significant by chance alone will be larger than the significance level selected. That is, the rate of incorrectly rejecting the null hypothesis will be larger than what is normally considered to be acceptable. Trends may emerge and disappear, especially early in the trial, and caution must be used. Here, we shall present the issue from a classical frequentist viewpoint, although other statistical approaches exist, such as the Bayesian methods that will be discussed at the end of this chapter.

In a clinical trial in which the participant response is known relatively soon after entry, the difference in rates between two groups may be compared repeatedly as more participants are added to the study. The usual test statistic for comparing two

---

*References 3, 4, 6, 151, 163, 164, 190.

proportions used is the chi-square test or the equivalent normal test statistic. The null hypothesis is that the true response rates or proportions are equal. If a significance level of 5% is selected and the null hypothesis, H_0, is tested only once, the probability of rejecting H_0 if it is true is 5% by definition. However, if H_0 is tested twice, first when one half of the data are known and then when all the data are available, the probability of incorrectly rejecting H_0 is increased from 5% to 8%.[6] If the hypothesis is tested five times, with one fifth of the participants added between tests, the probability of finding a significant result if the usual statistic for the 5% significance level is used becomes 14%. For 10 tests, this probability is almost 20%. In a clinical trial in which long-term survival experience is the primary outcome, repeated tests might be done as more information becomes known about the enrolled participants. Canner[15] performed computer simulations of such a clinical trial in which both the control group and intervention group event rates were assumed to be 30% at the end of the study. He performed 2000 replications of this simulated experiment. He found that if 20 tests of significance are done within a trial, the chance of crossing the 5% significance level boundaries ($Z = \pm 1.96$) is, on the average, 35%. Thus, in either of the situations described, repeated testing of accumulating data without taking into account the number of tests increases the overall probability of incorrectly rejecting H_0 to levels that could be unacceptable. If the repeated testing continues indefinitely, the null hypothesis is certain to be rejected eventually. Although it is unlikely that a large number of repeated tests will be done, even 5 or 10 can lead to a misinterpretation of the trial results when the multiple testing issue is ignored.

A classic illustration of the repeated testing problem is provided by the Coronary Drug Project (CDP)[34] for the clofibrate vs. placebo mortality comparison, shown in Fig. 15-1. This figure presents the standardized mortality comparisons over the follow-up or calendar time of the trial. The upper and lower horizontal lines indicate the conventional value of the test statistic, corresponding to a two-sided 0.05 significance level, used to judge statistical significance for studies where the comparison is made only once. It is evident that the trends in this mortality comparison emerged and weakened throughout, touching the conventional critical values on five occasions. However, as shown in Fig. 15-2, the mortality curves at the end of the trial are nearly identical, corresponding to the very small standardized statistic at the end of Fig. 15-1. The data monitoring committee for this trial took into consideration the repeated testing problem and did not terminate this trial early because the conventional values were exceeded. If this arm of the CDP had been terminated early at any of these crossings, the longer-term outcome would not have been known.

For ethical, scientific, and economic reasons, trials must be monitored so as not to expose participants unnecessarily to harmful or ineffective interventions, waste precious fiscal and human resources, or miss opportunities to correct flaws in the design.[34,42,61] However, in the process of evaluating interim results to meet these

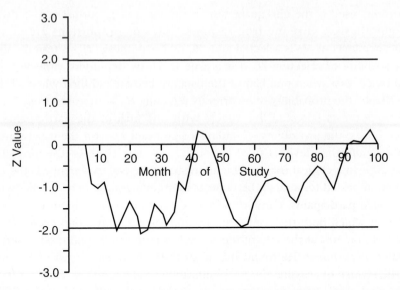

Fig. 15-1 Interim survival analyses comparing mortality in clofibrate- and placebo-treated participants in the Coronary Drug Project. A positive Z value favors placebo.[34] Reprinted by permission of Elsevier Science.

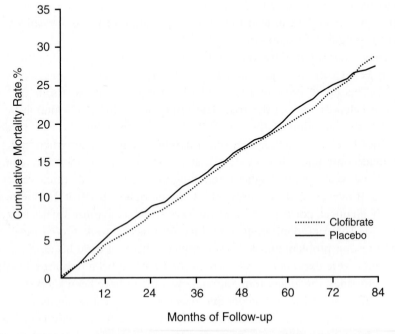

Fig. 15-2 Cumulative mortality curves comparing clofibrate- and placebo-treated participants in the Coronary Drug Project.[34] Reprinted by permission of Elsevier Science.

responsibilities, incorrect conclusions can be drawn by overreacting to emerging or nonemerging trends in primary, secondary, or adverse effect outcomes. In general, the solution to multiple testing is to adjust the critical value used in each single analysis so that the overall significance level for the trial remains at the desired level. It has been suggested that a trial should not be terminated early unless the difference is highly significant for beneficial effects.[151] More formal monitoring techniques are reviewed later in this chapter. They include the group sequential methods and stochastic curtailed sampling procedures.

DECISION FOR EARLY TERMINATION

There are four major reasons for terminating a trial earlier than scheduled.[16,34,42,61] The trial may show serious adverse effects in the entire intervention group or in a dominating subgroup. In addition, the trial may indicate greater-than-expected beneficial effects. Third, it may become clear that a statistically significant difference by the end of the study is improbable. Finally, logistical or data-quality problems may be so severe that correction is not feasible. For a variety of reasons, a decision to terminate a study early must be made with much caution and in the context of all pertinent data. Several issues or factors must be considered thoroughly as part of the decision process.*

1. Possible differences in prognostic factors between the two groups at baseline should be explored and necessary adjustments made in the analysis.
2. Any chance of bias in the assessment of response variables must be considered, especially when the trial is not double-blind.
3. The possible impact of missing data should be evaluated. For example, could the conclusions be reversed if the experience of participants with missing data from one group were different from the experience with missing data from the other group?
4. Differential concomitant intervention and levels of participant adherence should be evaluated for their possible impact.
5. Potential side effects and outcomes of secondary response variables should be considered in addition to the outcome of the primary response variable.
6. Internal consistency should be examined. Are the results consistent across subgroups and the various primary and secondary outcome measures? In a multicenter trial, the monitoring committee should assess whether the results are consistent across centers. Before stopping, the committee should make certain that the outcome is not because of unusual experience in only one or two centers.
7. In long-term trials, the experience of the study groups over time should be explored. Survival analysis techniques (Chapter 14) partly address this issue.

---

*References 16, 34, 38, 42, 61, 85, 155.

8. The outcomes of similar trials should be reviewed.
9. The impact of early termination on the credibility and acceptibility of the results is an important factor.

Some trials request the chair of the data monitoring committee to review frequently serious adverse events, by intervention, to protect the safety of the participants. While such frequent informal, or even formal, review of the data is also subject to the problems of repeated testing or analyses, the adjustment methods presented are typically not applied. Also, safety may be measured by many response variables. Rather than rely on a single outcome showing a worrisome trend, a profile of safety measures might be required. Thus, the decision to stop a trial for safety reasons can be quite complex.

The early termination of a clinical trial can be difficult,* not only because the issues involved may be complex and the study complicated, but because the final decision often lies with the consensus of a committee. The statistical methods discussed in this chapter are useful guides in this process but should not be viewed as absolute rules. The published literature provides examples[†] of trials that stopped early. A few examples are described here to illustrate several key points.

One of the earlier clinical trials conducted in the United States illustrates how controversial the decision for early termination may be. The University Group Diabetes Program (UGDP)[112,162,191,192] was a placebo-control, randomized, double-blind trial designed to test the effectiveness of four interventions used in diabetes treatment. The primary measure of efficacy was the degree of retinal damage. The four interventions were: a fixed dose of insulin, a variable dose of insulin, tolbutamide, and phenformin. The tolbutamide group was stopped early because the monitoring committee felt the drug could be harmful and did not appear to have any benefit.[191] An excess in cardiovascular mortality was observed in the tolbutamide group as compared with the placebo group (12.7% vs. 4.9%), and the total mortality was in the same direction (14.7% vs. 10.2%). Analysis of the distribution of the baseline factors known to be associated with cardiovascular mortality revealed an imbalance, with participants in the tolbutamide group being at higher risk. This, plus questions about the classification of cause of death, drew considerable criticism. Later, the phenformin group was also stopped because of excess mortality compared with the control group (15.2% vs. 9.4%).[192] The controversy led to a review of the data by an independent group of statisticians. Although they basically concurred with the decisions made by the UGDP monitoring committee,[162] the debate over the study and its conclusions continued.[112]

---

*References 16, 34, 38, 42, 61, 111, 135, 155, 180.
[†]References 7, 9, 17-19, 24, 29-33, 46, 50-54, 71, 72, 97, 98, 112, 136, 138, 140, 148, 149, 162, 182, 183, 191, 192.

The decision-making process during the course of the CDP,[31] a long-term randomized, double-blind, multicenter study that compared the effect on total mortality of several lipid-lowering drugs (high- and low-dose estrogen, dextrothyroxine, clofibrate, and nicotinic acid) against placebo, has been reviewed.* Three of the drug interventions were terminated early because of potential side effects and no apparent benefit. One of the issues in the discontinuation of the high-dose estrogen and dextrothyroxine interventions[29,30] concerned subgroups of participants. In some, the interventions appeared to cause increased mortality, in addition to having several adverse effects. In others, the adverse effects were present, but mortality was only slightly reduced or unchanged. After considerable debate, both treatment groups were discontinued. The adverse effects were felt to more than outweigh the minimal benefit in selected subgroups. Also, positive subgroup trends in the dextrothyroxine arm were not maintained over time. The low-dose estrogen intervention[32] was discontinued because there was the question of major toxicity. Furthermore, it was extremely improbable that a significant difference favoring estrogen could have been obtained had the study continued to its scheduled termination. Using the data available at the time, the number of future deaths in the control group was projected. This indicated that there had to be almost no further deaths in the intervention group for the remainder of the trial for a significance level of 5% to be reached.

The CDP experience also warns against the dangers of stopping too soon.[33,34] In the early months of the study, clofibrate appeared to be beneficial, with the significance level exceeding 5% on five occasions (Fig. 15-1). However, because of the repeated testing issue described earlier in this chapter, the decision was made to continue the study and closely monitor the results. The early difference was not maintained, and at the end of the trial the drug showed no benefit over the placebo. It is notable that the mortality curves shown in Fig. 15-2 do not suggest the wide swings observed in the interim analyses shown in Fig. 15-1. The fact that participants were entered over a period and thus had various lengths of follow-up at any given interim analysis explains the difference between the two types of analyses. (See Chapter 14 for a discussion of survival analysis.)

The Nocturnal Oxygen Therapy Trial was a randomized, multicenter clinical trial comparing two levels of oxygen therapy in people with advanced chronic obstructive lung disease.[50,140] While mortality was not considered as the primary outcome in the design, a strong mortality difference emerged during the trial, notably in one particular subgroup. Before any decision was made, the participating clinical centers were surveyed to ensure that the mortality data were as current as possible. A delay in reporting mortality was discovered. When all the deaths were considered, the trend disappeared. The earlier results were an artifact caused by incomplete

---

*References 15, 34, 29, 30, 32, 33.

mortality data. Although a significant mortality difference ultimately emerged, the results were similar across subgroups.

Early termination of a subgroup can be especially error prone if not done carefully. Peto[98] et al. illustrated the danger of subgroup analysis by reporting that treatment benefit in ISIS-2 did not apply to individuals born during a certain astrologic sign. Nevertheless, treatment benefits may be observed in subgroups that may be compelling. An AIDS trial conducted by the AIDS Clinical Trial Research Group (ACTG), ACTG-019[42,43,61] indicated that zidovudine (AZT) led to improved status in AIDS participants who had a low level of CD4 cell counts (under 500 per mm³), which is a measure of poor immune response. The results were not significant for participants with a higher CD4 value. Given previous experience with this drug, and given the unfavorable prognosis for untreated AIDS participants, the trial was stopped early in those with the low CD4 cell count and continued in the rest of the participants.

A scientific and ethical issue was raised in the Diabetic Retinopathy Study, a randomized trial of 1758 participants with proliferative retinopathy.[53] Each participant had one eye randomized to photocoagulation and the other to standard care. After 2 years of a planned 5-year follow-up, a highly significant difference in the incidence of blindness was observed (16.3% vs. 6.4%) in favor of photocoagulation.[51] Since the long-term efficacy of this new therapy was not known, the early benefit could possibly have been negated by subsequent adverse reactions. After much debate, the data monitoring committee decided to continue the trial, publish the early results, and allow any untreated eye at high risk of blindness to receive photocoagulation therapy.[52,54] In the end, the early treatment benefit was sustained over a longer follow-up, despite the fact that some of the eyes randomized to control received photocoagulation. Furthermore, no significant long-term adverse effect was observed.

The Beta-Blocker Heart Attack Trial[9,46] provided another example of early termination. This randomized placebo-controlled trial enrolled more than 3800 participants with a recent myocardial infarction to evaluate the effectiveness of propranolol in reducing mortality. After an average of 2 years of a planned 3-year follow-up, a mortality difference was observed, as shown in Fig. 15-3. The results were statistically significant, allowing for repeated testing, and would, with high probability, not be reversed during the next year.[46] The data monitoring committee debated whether the additional year of follow-up would add valuable information. It was argued that there would be too few events in the last year of the trial to provide a good estimate of the effect of propranolol treatment in the third and fourth year of therapy. Thus the committee decided that prompt publication of the observed benefit was more important than waiting for the marginal information yet to be obtained.

Some trials are also stopped early because of adverse or harmful effects although interventions may already be in widespread use. One example comes from the treatment of arrhythmias after a heart attack. Epidemiological data suggest an association between the presence of irregular ventricular heartbeats or arrhythmias and the

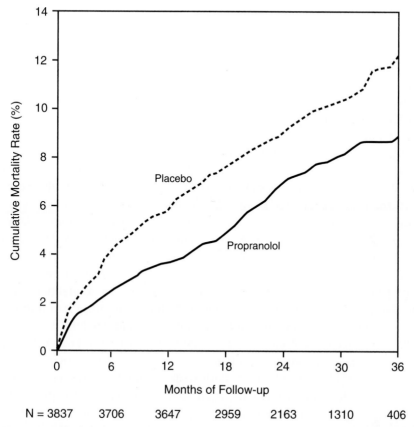

Fig. 15-3 Cumulative mortality curves comparing propranolol and placebo in the Beta-Blocker Heart Attack Trial. Reproduced with permission of Beta-Blocker Heart Attack Study Group.[9]

incidence of sudden death, presumably because of serious arrhythmias.[17] Drugs have been developed that suppress arrhythmias and have become widely used after approval by the drug regulatory agencies for that indication. The Cardiac Arrhythmia Suppression Trial (CAST)[17] was a multicenter randomized double-blind placebo-controlled trial evaluating three such drugs (encainide, flecainide, and moricizine) in the effect on total mortality and sudden death. However, the encainide and flecainide arms of the trial were terminated with only 15% of the expected mortality event observed because of an adverse experience (55 vs. 26 total deaths).

At the first data monitoring committee review, the mortality trend began to appear, but the number of events was relatively small.[71] Since the data monitoring committee decided no definitive conclusion could be reached on the basis of so few events, it elected to remain blinded to the treatment assignment. However, before the next scheduled meeting, the statistical center alerted the committee that the trends continued and were now nearing the CAST monitoring criteria for stopping. In a conference-call meeting, the data monitoring committee became unblinded and learned that the trends were in the unexpected direction, that is, toward harm from the active treatment. Several confirmatory and exploratory analyses were requested by the data monitoring committee, and a meeting was held a few weeks later to discuss and evaluate fully these unexpected results. After a thorough review, the data monitoring committee recommended immediate termination of the encainide and flecainide portions of the trial.[17] Results were consistent across outcome variables and participant subgroups, and no biases could be identified that would explain these results. The third arm (moricizine) continued since there were no convincing trends at that time, but it too was eventually stopped because of adverse experiences.[18] The CAST experience points out that data monitoring committees must be prepared for the unexpected and that large trends may emerge quickly. Even with this dramatic result, the decision was not simple or straightforward. Many of the issues discussed earlier were covered thoroughly before a decision was reached.[71]

Not all negative trends emerge as dramatically as in the CAST. Two other examples are provided by trials in congestive heart failure. Yearly mortality from severe congestive heart failure is approximately 40%. Inotropic drugs can improve the exercise tolerance of such participants. The PROMISE and PROFILE[144,145] trials evaluated inotropic agents (milrinone and flosequinone) that were known to improve exercise tolerance. PROMISE and PROFILE were randomized, placebo-controlled trials comparing survival outcomes. Both trials terminated early with statistically significant harmful mortality results, even after adjusting for repeated testing of these data. In both cases, the results were again unexpected since these drugs had been approved for use on the basis of the improved exercise tolerance, a surrogate response. Because the disease has a high mortality rate and the drugs were already in use, it is difficult to decide how much evidence is needed to decide that this therapy is harmful rather than helpful. In both trials, the data monitoring committees allowed results to achieve statistical significance since a negative but nonsignificant trend might have been viewed by some as evidence consistent with no effect on mortality. In this case, given the improved exercise tolerance, these drugs may have continued to have widespread use.

The PROMISE and PROFILE experiences illustrate the most difficult of the monitoring scenarios, the emerging negative trend. If negative trends persist but are nonsignificant, the trial may still have no real chance of reversing trends and showing a treatment benefit. In some circumstances, that condition may be sufficient to abandon the trial since if a result falls short of establishing benefit, the intervention would not be used unless it has other indications. For example, a new expensive or invasive intervention would likely need to be more effective than a standard intervention to be used. In other circumstances, a neutral result may be important, so a small negative trend, still consistent with a neutral result, would argue for continuation. If a treatment is already in clinical use on the basis of other indications, as in the case of the drugs used in PROMISE and PROFILE, an emerging negative trend may not be sufficient evidence for termination. If a trial terminates early without resolving convincingly the harmful effects of an intervention, that intervention may still continue to be used. This practice would put future participants at risk, and perhaps even participants in the trial as they return to their usual health care system. In that case, the investment of participants, investigators, and sponsors would not have resolved an important question. There is a serious and delicate balance between the responsibility toward safeguarding the participants in the trial and the responsibility for all current and future participants.

Trials may continue to their scheduled termination even though interim results are very positive and persuasive[97] or so similar that almost surely no significant results will emerge.[7,19,138] In one case, early significant results did not override the need for getting long-term experience with an intensive intervention strategy.[97] Another trial[138] involved altering smoking and cholesterol levels and drug therapy for altering blood pressure to reduce the risk of heart disease. Although early results showed no trends, it was also not clear how long intervention needed to be continued before the applied risk factor modifications would take effect. It was argued that late favorable results could still emerge. In another trial, which compared medical and surgical treatment of coronary artery atherosclerosis, the medical care group had such a favorable survival experience that there was little room for improvement by immediate coronary artery bypass graft intervention.[19]

In all of these studies, the decisions were difficult and involved many analyses, thorough review of the literature, and an understanding of the biological processes. As previously described, several questions must be answered before serious consideration should be given to early termination. As noted elsewhere, the relationship between clinical trials and practice is very complex, and this complexity is evident in the data monitoring process.[130,143]

DECISION TO EXTEND A TRIAL

The issue about extending a trial beyond the original sample size or planned period of follow-up may arise.[180] Suppose the mortality rate over a 2-year period in the control group is assumed to be 40%. (This estimate may be based on data from another study involving a similar population.) Also specified is that the sample size should be large enough to detect a 25% relative reduction because of the intervention, with a two-sided significance level of 5% and a power of 90%. The total sample size is, therefore, approximately 960. However, say that early in the study, the mortality rate in the control group appears somewhat lower than anticipated, closer to 30%. This difference may result from a change in the study population, selection factors in the trial, or new concomitant therapies. If no design changes are made, the intervention would have to be more effective (30% reduction rather than 25%) for the difference between groups to be detected with the same power. Alternatively, the investigator would have to be satisfied with approximately 75% power of detecting the originally anticipated 25% reduction in mortality. If it is unreasonable to expect a 30% benefit, and if a 75% power is unacceptable, the design needs modification. Given the lower control-group mortality rate, approximately 1450 participants would be required to detect a 25% reduction in mortality because of intervention, while maintaining a power of 90%. Another possible option is to extend the length of follow-up, which would increase the overall event rate. A combination of these two approaches can also be tried.

In a trial of antenatal steroid administration,[24] the incidence of infant respiratory distress in the control group was much less than anticipated. Early in the study, the investigators decided to increase the sample size by extending the recruitment phase. In another trial, the protocol specifically called for increasing the sample size if the control group event rate was less than assumed.[136]

Another approach that has been used[144,145] is to fix the target of the trial to be a specified number of events in the control group that provides the specified power. If event rates are low, it may take longer follow-up per participant, more participants, or both to observe the required number of control-group events. In any case, the target is the fixed number of events. In the above situations, only data from the control group are used. No knowledge of what is happening in the intervention group is needed. However, if the intervention group results are not used in the recalculations, then an increase in sample size could be recommended when the observed difference between the intervention and control groups is actually larger than originally expected. Thus, in the hypothetical example, if early data really did show a 30% benefit from intervention, an increased sample size might not be needed to maintain the desired power of 90%. For this reason, one would not like to make a recommendation about extension without also considering the observed effect of intervention. Computing conditional power is one way of incorporating these results. Conditional power is the probability that the test statistic will be larger than the critical value, given that a portion of the statistic is already known from the observed data. As in other power calculations, the assumed true difference in response variables between groups must be specified. When the early intervention experience is better than expected, the conditional power will be large. When the intervention is doing worse than anticipated, the conditional power will be small unless the sample size is increased. The conditional power concept uses knowledge of outcome in both the intervention and control groups and is, therefore, controversial. Nevertheless, the concept attempts to aid in the decision to extend.

Toward the scheduled end of the study, the investigator may find that he has nearly statistically significant results. He may be tempted to extend or expand the trial in an effort to make the test statistic significant. Such a practice is not recommended. A strategy of extending assumes that the observed relative differences in rates of response will continue. The observed differences that are projected for a larger sample may not hold. In addition, because of the multiple testing issue and the design change, the significance level should be adjusted to a smaller value. However, appropriate adjustments in the significance level to account for the design changes may not easily be determined. Since a more extreme significance level should be employed, and since future responses are uncertain, extension may leave the investigator without the expected benefits.

Adjustments made to either sample size or the length of follow-up should be done as early in the trial as possible. Early adjustments would diminish the criticism that the investigator or the monitoring committee waited until the last minute to see whether the results would achieve some prespecified significance level before changing the study design.

STATISTICAL METHODS USED IN MONITORING

In this section, some statistical methods currently available for monitoring the accumulating data in a clinical trial will be reviewed. The methods address whether the trial should be terminated early or continued to its planned termination. No single statistical test or monitoring procedure ought to be used as a strict rule for decision-making, but rather as one piece of evidence to be integrated with other evidence.[15,38,42,61,184] Most methods are very specific in their applications. Therefore it is difficult to make a single recommendation about which should be used. However, the following methods, when applied appropriately, can be useful guides in the decision-making process.

Classical sequential methods, a modification generally referred to as group sequential methods, and curtailed testing procedures for data monitoring are discussed in the following section. Other approaches are also briefly considered. Classical sequential methods are given more mathematical attention in several articles and texts.[*]

Classical sequential methods

The aim of the classical sequential design is to minimize the number of participants that must be entered into a study. The decision to continue to enroll participants depends on results from those already entered. Most of these sequential methods assume that the response variable outcome is known in a short time relative to the duration of the trial. Therefore, for many trials involving acute illness, these methods are applicable. For studies involving chronic diseases, classical sequential

---

[*]References 4, 5, 11, 27, 39, 73, 74, 174, 193, 196, 200, 202.

methods have not been as useful. Although the sequential approaches have design implications, we have delayed discussing any details until this chapter because they really focus on monitoring accumulating data. Even if, during the design of the trial, consideration were not given to sequential methods, they could still be used to assist in the data monitoring or the decision-making process. Detailed discussions of classical sequential methods are given, for example, by Armitage,[5] Whitehead,[196] and Wald.[193]

The sequential analysis method as originally developed by Wald[193] and applied to the clinical trial by others such as Armitage[4,5] involves repeated testing of data in a single experiment. This method assumes that the only decision to be made is whether the trial should continue or be terminated because one of the groups is responding significantly better, or worse, than the other. This classical sequential decision rule is called an "open plan" by Armitage[5] because there is no guarantee of when a decision to terminate will be reached. Strict adherence to the "open plan" would mean that the study could not have a fixed sample size. Very few clinical trials use the "open" or classical sequential design because there is no certainty of ever reaching a point at which the trial would be stopped. The method also requires data to be paired, one observation from each group. In many instances, the pairing of participants is not appealing because the paired participants may be very different and may not be "well matched" in important prognostic variables. If stratification is attempted to obtain better matched pairs, each stratum with an odd number of participants would have one unpaired participant. Furthermore, the requirement to monitor the data after every pair may be impossible or unnecessary for many clinical trials. Silverman et al.[172] used an open plan in a trial of the effects of humidity on survival in infants with low birth weight. At the end of 36 months, 181 pairs of infants had been enrolled; 52 of the pairs had a discrepant outcome. Nine infants were excluded because they were unmatched, and 16 pairs were excluded because of a mismatch. The study had to be terminated without a clear decision because it was no longer feasible to continue the trial. This study illustrates the difficulties inherent in the classical sequential design.

Armitage[4] introduced the restricted or "closed" sequential design to assure that a maximum limit is imposed on the number of participants ($2N$) to be enrolled. As with the open plan, the data must be paired using one observation from each study group. Criteria for early termination and rejection of no treatment effect are determined so that the design has specified levels of significance and power (α and $1 - \beta$). The restricted plan was used in a comparison of two interventions in participants with ulcerative colitis.[185] In that trial, the criteria for no treatment effect was exceeded, demonstrating short-term clinical benefit of corticosteroids over sulphasalazine therapy.

Another solution to the repeated testing problem, called "repeated significance tests," was proposed by McPherson and Armitage[134] and is also described by Armitage.[5]

Although different theoretical assumptions are used, this approach has features similar to the restricted sequential model. That is, the observed data must be paired, and the maximum number of pairs to be considered can be fixed. Other modifications to the Armitage restricted plan[36,201,202] have also been proposed.

The methods described above can in some circumstances be applied to interim analyses of censored survival data.* If participants simultaneously enter a clinical trial and there is no loss to follow-up, information on interim analyses is said to be "progressively censored." Sequential methods for this situation have been developed using, for example, modified rank statistics. In fact, most participants are not entered into a trial simultaneously, but in a staggered fashion. The log rank statistic may also be used in this situation.

The classical sequential approach has not been widely used, even in clinical trials where the time to the event is known almost immediately. One major reason perhaps is the requirement of analysis after every pair of outcomes or events. For many clinical trials, this is not necessary or even feasible if the data are monitored by a committee that has regularly scheduled meetings. In addition, classical sequential boundaries require an alternative hypothesis to be specified, a feature not demanded by conventional statistical tests for the rejection of the null hypothesis.

Group sequential methods

Because of limitations with classical sequential methods, other approaches to the repeated testing problem have been proposed.† Ad hoc rules have been suggested that attempt to ensure a conservative interpretation of interim results. One ad hoc method is to use a critical value of 2.6 at each interim look and in the final analyses.[7] Another approach[91,151] referred to here as the Haybittle-Peto procedure, favors using a large critical value, such as $Z_i = \pm 3.0$, for all interim tests $(i < K)$. Then any adjustment for repeated testing at the final test $(i = K)$ is negligible, and the conventional critical value can be used. These methods are "ad hoc" in the sense that no precise type-I error level is guaranteed. They might, however, be viewed as precursors of the more formal procedures to be described below.

Pocock[152-154] modified the repeated testing methods of McPherson and Armitage[134] and developed a group sequential method for clinical trials that avoids many of the limitations of classical methods. He discusses two cases of special interest; one for comparing two proportions and another for comparing mean levels of response. Pocock's method divides the participants into a series of K equal-sized groups with $2n$ participants in each, n assigned to intervention and n to control. K is the number of times that data will be monitored during the course of the trial. The total expected sample size is $2nK$. The test statistic used to compare control

---

*References 10, 14, 22, 37, 102–104, 113, 137, 139, 169, 200, 201.
†References 41, 59, 66, 68, 91, 101, 114, 141, 152–154, 160.

and intervention is computed as soon as data for the first group of $2n$ participants are available, and recomputed when data from each successive group become known. Under the null hypothesis, the distribution of the test statistic, Z_i, is assumed to be approximately normal with zero mean and unit variance, where i indicates the number of groups $(i \leq K)$ that have completed data. This statistic Z_i is compared with the stopping boundaries, $\pm Z'_K$, where Z'_K has been determined so that for up to K repeated tests, the overall significance level for the trial will be α. For example, if $K = 5$ and $\alpha = 0.05$ (two-sided), $Z'_K = 2.413$. This critical value is larger than the critical value of 1.96 used in a single test of hypothesis with $\alpha = 0.05$. If the statistic Z_i falls outside the boundaries on the ith repeated test, the trial should be terminated, rejecting the null hypothesis. If the statistic falls inside the boundaries, the trial should be continued until $i = K$ (the maximum number of tests). When $i = K$ and $-Z'_K < Z_K < Z'_K$, the trial would stop and the investigator would "accept" H_0.

O'Brien and Fleming[141] also discuss a group sequential procedure. Using the above notation, their stopping rule compares the statistic Z_i with $Z^*\sqrt{K/i}$ where Z^* is determined so as to achieve the desired significance level. For example, if $K = 5$ and $\alpha = 0.05$, $Z^* = 2.04$. If $K \leq 5$, Z^* may be approximated by the usual critical values for the normal distribution. One attractive feature is that the critical value used at the last test $(i = K)$ is approximately the same as that used if a single test were done.

In Fig. 15-4, boundaries for the three methods described are given for $K = 5$ and $\alpha = 0.05$. If for $i < 5$ the test statistic falls outside the boundaries, the trial is terminated and the null hypothesis rejected. Otherwise, the trial is continued until $i = 5$, at which time the null hypothesis is either rejected or accepted. The three boundaries have different early stopping properties. The O'Brien-Fleming model is unlikely to lead to stopping in the early stages. Later on, however, this procedure leads to a greater chance of stopping prior to the end of the study than the other two. Both the Haybittle-Peto and the O'Brien Fleming boundaries avoid the awkward situation of accepting the null hypothesis when the observed statistic at the end of the trial is much larger than the conventional critical value (i.e., 1.96 for a two-sided 5% significance level). If the observed statistic in Fig. 15-4 is 2.3 when $i = 5$, the result would not be significant using the Pocock boundary. The large critical values used at the first few analyses for the O'Brien-Fleming boundary can be adjusted to some less extreme values (e.g., 3.5) without noticeably changing the critical values used later on, including the final value.

Many data monitoring committees wish to be somewhat conservative in their interpretation of early results because of the uncertainties discussed earlier and because a few additional events can alter the results dramatically. Yet, most would like to use conventional critical values in the final analyses. This means that conventional fixed sample methods for determining sample size can be applied with essentially no adjustments. With that in mind, the O'Brien-Fleming model has considerable appeal, perhaps with the adjusted or modified boundary as described. The group sequential methods have an advantage over the classical methods in that the data do not have to be continuously tested and individual participants do not have to be paired. This concept suits the data review activity of most large clinical trials where monitoring committees meet periodically. Furthermore, in many trials constant consideration of early stopping is unnecessary. Pocock[152-154] discusses the benefits of the group sequential approach in more detail.

The group sequential methods were developed for clinical trials where results are obtained relatively quickly on a group of $2n$ participants before another group of $2n$ participants are entered. The hypothesis being tested could be a comparison of the proportion of successes in each group or the mean level of response. In many trials, however, participants are entered over a period and followed for a relatively long period. Frequently, the primary outcome is time to some event. Instead of

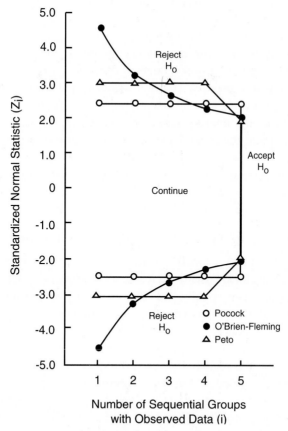

Fig. 15-4 Three group sequential stopping boundaries for the standardized normal statistic (Z_i) for up to five sequential groups with two-sided significance level of 0.05.

adding participants between interim analyses, new events are added. As discussed in Chapter 14, survival analysis methods could be used to compare the experience of the intervention and the control arms. Given their general appeal, it would be desirable to use the group sequential methods in combination with survival analyses. It has been established* for large studies that the log rank or Mantel-Haenszel statistic can be used. Furthermore, even for small studies, the log rank procedure is still quite robust.[75] The Gehan, or modified Wilcoxon test,[77,175] as defined in Chapter 14 cannot be applied directly to the group sequential procedures. A generalization of the Wilcoxon procedure[150] for survival data, though, is appropriate,[188] and the survival methods of analyses can in general terms be applied in group sequential monitoring. Instead of looking at equal-sized participant groups, the group sequential methods described strictly require that interim analyses should be done after an additional equal number of events have been observed. Since data monitoring committees usually meet at fixed calendar times, the condition of equal number of events might not be met exactly. However, the methods applied under these circumstances are approximately correct[44] if the increments are not too disparate. Extensions have been proposed for multiarmed studies.[158]

Interim log rank tests in the Beta-Blocker Heart Attack Trial[46] were evaluated using the O'Brien-Fleming[141] group sequential procedure. Seven meetings had been scheduled to review interim data. The trial was designed for a two-sided 5% significance level. These specifications produce the group sequential boundary shown in Fig. 15-5. In addition, the interim results of the log rank statistic are shown for the first six meetings. From the second analysis on, the conventional significance value of 1.96 was exceeded. Nevertheless, the trial was continued. At the sixth meeting, when the O'Brien-Fleming boundary was crossed, a decision was made to terminate the trial with mortality curves as seen in Fig. 15-3. It should be emphasized that crossing the boundary was only one factor in this decision.

Flexible group sequential procedures—Alpha-spending functions

While the group sequential methods described are an important advance in data monitoring, the Beta-Blocker Heart Attack Trial[46] experience suggested two limitations. One is the need to specify the number K of planned interim analyses in advance. The second is the requirement for equal numbers of either participants or events between each analysis. This also means that the exact time of the interim analysis is specified. As indicated in the Beta-Blocker Heart Attack Trial example, the number of deaths between analyses were not equal, and exactly seven analyses of the data had been specified. If the data monitoring committee had requested an additional analysis between the fifth and sixth scheduled meetings, the O'Brien-Fleming group sequential procedure would not have directly accommodated such a

---

*References 44, 75, 77, 81, 90, 106, 110, 133, 150, 175, 186–188, 198.

modification. Yet such a request could easily have happened. To accommodate unequal numbers of participants or events between analyses and the possibility of larger or fewer numbers of interim analyses than prespecified, Lan and DeMets[48,115,118] developed a flexible procedure that eliminated those restrictions. They proposed a so-called alpha-spending function that allows investigators to determine how they want to "spend" the type-I error or alpha during the course of the trial. The alpha-spending function guarantees that at the end of the trial, the overall type-I error will be the prespecified value of α. As will be described, this approach is a general-ization of the previous group sequential methods† so that Pocock[152] and O'Brien-Fleming[141] monitoring procedures become special cases.

We must first distinguish between calendar time and information fraction.[117] At any particular calendar time t in the study, a certain fraction t^* of the total informa-tion is observed. That may be approximated by the fraction of participants random-ized at that point, n, divided by the total number expected N, or in survival studies, by the number of events observed already, d, divided by the total number

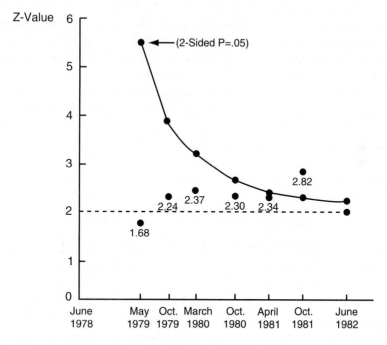

Fig. 15-5 Six interim log rank statistics plotted for the time of data monitoring committee meet-ings with a two-sided O'Brien-Fleming significance level boundary in the Beta-Blocker Heart Attack Trial. Dashed line represents $Z = 1.96$.[46] Reproduced by permission of Elsevier Science.

---

†References 48, 60, 78, 95, 96, 108, 115–118, 121, 124, 159, 160.

expected, D. Thus the value for t^* must be between 0 and 1. The information fraction is more generally defined in terms of the ratio of the inverse of the variance of the test statistic at the particular interim analysis and the final analysis. The alpha-spending function, $\alpha(t^*)$, determines how the prespecified α is allocated at each interim analysis as a function of the information fraction. At the beginning of a trial, $t^* = 0$ and $\alpha(t^*) = 0$ while at the end of the trial, $t^* = 1$ and $\alpha(t^*) = \alpha$. Alpha-spending functions that correspond to the Pocock and O'Brien-Fleming boundaries shown in Fig. 15-4 are indicated in Fig. 15-6 for a two-sided 0.05 α level and four interim analyses plus a final analysis. These spending functions correspond to interim analyses at information fractions at 0.2, 0.4, 0.6, 0.8, and 1.0. However, in practice the information fractions need not be equally spaced. We chose those information fractions to indicate the connection between the earlier discussion of group sequential boundaries and the alpha-spending function. The Pocock-type spending function allocates the alpha more rapidly than the O'Brien-Fleming–type spending function. For the O'Brien-Fleming–type spending function at $t^* = 0.2$, the $\alpha(0.2)$ is less than 0.0001, which corresponds approximately to the very large critical value or boundary value 4.56 in Fig. 15-4. At $t^* = 0.4$, the amount of alpha that can be spent is $\alpha(0.4) - \alpha(0.2)$, which is approximately 0.0006, corresponding to the boundary value 3.23 in Fig. 15-4. That is, the difference in $\alpha(t^*)$ at two consecutive information fractions, t_1^* and t_2^* where $t_1^* < t_2^*$, $\alpha(t_2^*) - \alpha(t_1^*)$, determines the boundary or critical value at t_2^*. Obtaining these critical values consecutively requires numerical calculations similar to that for Pocock and is described elsewhere in detail.[115] Because these spending functions are only approximately equivalent to the Pocock or O'Brien-Fleming boundaries, the actual boundary values will be similar but not exactly the same. However, the practical differences are not important. Programs are available for these calculations.[160]

Many different spending functions can be specified. The O'Brien-Fleming $\alpha_1(t^*)$ and Pocock $\alpha_2(t^*)$ spending functions are specified as follows:

$$\alpha_1(t^*) = 2 - 2\,\Phi(Z_{\alpha/2}/t^*) \qquad \sim \text{O'Brien-Fleming}$$

$$\alpha_2(t^*) = \alpha \bullet ln[1 + (e-1)t^*] \qquad \sim \text{Pocock}$$

$$\alpha_3(t^*) = \alpha \bullet (t^*)^{\theta} \qquad \text{for } \theta > 0$$

The spending function $\alpha_3(t^*)$ spends alpha uniformly during the trial for $\theta = 1$, at a rate somewhat between $\alpha_1(t^*)$ and $\alpha_2(t^*)$. Other spending functions have also been defined.[95,96]

The advantage of the alpha-spending function is that neither the number nor the time of the interim analyses need to be specified in advance. Once the particular spending function is selected, the information fractions t_1^*, t_2^*, ... determine the critical or boundary values exactly. In addition, the frequency of the interim analyses can be changed during the trial and still preserve the prespecified α level. Even if the rationale for changing the frequency depends on the emerging trends, the impact on the overall type-I error rate is almost neglibible.[116,159] These advantages give the spending function approach to group sequential monitoring the flexibility in analysis times that is often required in actual clinical trial settings.[129] However, it must be emphasized that no change of the spending function itself is permitted during the trial.

Applications of group sequential boundaries

As indicated in the Beta-Blocker Heart Attack Trial[46] example, the standardized log rank test can be compared with the standardized boundaries provided by the O'Brien-Fleming, Pocock, or α-spending function approach. However, these group sequential methods are quite widely applicable for statistical tests that can be standardized with a normal distribution and independent increments of information between interim analyses. Besides log rank and other survival tests,[119] comparisons of means, comparison of proportions,[109,152] and comparison of linear regression slopes* can be monitored using this approach. For means and proportions, the information fraction can be approximated by the ratio of the number of participants observed to the total expected. For regression slopes, the information fraction is best determined from the ratio of the inverse of the variance of the regression slope

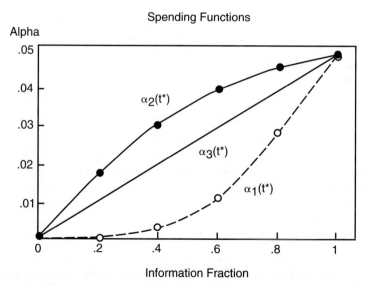

Fig. 15-6 Alpha-spending functions for $K = 5$, two-sided $\alpha = 0.05$ at information fractions 0.2, 0.4, 0.6, 0.8, and 1.0. $\alpha_1(t^*) \sim$ O'Brien-Fleming; $\alpha_2(t^*) \sim$ Pocock; $\alpha_3(t^*) \sim$ uniform.

---

*References 76, 120, 126–128, 161, 176, 181, 189, 195, 205.

differences computed for the current and expected final estimate.[127,205] Considerable work has extended the group sequential methodology to more general linear and nonlinear random effects models for continuous data and to repeated measure' methods for categorical data.[76] Thus for most of the statistical tests that would be applied to common primary outcome measures, the flexible group sequential methods can be used directly.

If the trial continues to the scheduled termination point, p value is often computed to indicate the extremeness of the result. If the standardized statistical test exceeds the critical value, the p value would be less than the corresponding significance level. If a trial is terminated early or continues to the end with the standardized test exceeding or crossing the boundary value, a p value can also be computed.[59] These p values cannot be the nominal p value corresponding to the standardized test statistic. They must be adjusted to account for the repeated statistical testing of the outcome measure and for the particular monitoring boundary employed.[59] Calculation of the p value is relatively straightforward with existing software packages.[160]

Statistical tests of hypotheses are but one of the methods used to evaluate the results of a clinical trial. Once trials are terminated, either on schedule or earlier, confidence intervals are often used to give some sense of the uncertainty in the estimated treatment or intervention effect. For a fixed-sample study, confidence intervals are typically constructed as:

$$\text{(effectiveness estimate)} \pm Z(\alpha) \text{ (standard error of the estimate)}.$$

In the group sequential monitoring setting, this confidence interval will be referred to as the naive estimate since it does not consider the sequential aspects. In general, construction of confidence intervals after the termination of a clinical trial is not as straightforward,* but software exists to aid in the computations.[160] The major problem with naive confidence intervals is that they may not give proper coverage of the unknown but estimated treatment effect. That is, the confidence intervals constructed in this way may not include the true effect size the proper number of times (e.g., 95%). For example, the width of the confidence interval may be too narrow. Several methods have been proposed for constructing a more proper confidence interval,[58,189,199] typically ordering the possible outcomes in different ways. That is, a method is needed to determine if an intervention effect at one time is either more or less extreme than a difference at another time. None of the methods proposed appear to be universally superior, but the ordering originally suggested by Siegmund[171] and adopted by Tsiatis et al.[189] appears to be quite adequate. In this ordering, any treatment comparison statistic that exceeds the group sequential boundary at one time is considered to be more extreme than any result that exceeds

---

*References 21, 58, 94, 105, 107, 157, 167, 171, 189, 199.

the sequential boundary at a later time. While construction of confidence intervals using this ordering of possible outcomes can break down, the cases or circumstances are almost always quite unusual and not likely to occur in practice.[199] It is also interesting that for conservative monitoring boundaries such as the O'Brien-Fleming method, the naive confidence interval does not perform that poorly, due primarily to the extreme early conservatism of the boundary.[167] While more exact confidence intervals can be computed for this case, the naive estimate may still prove useful as a quick estimate to be recalculated later using the method described.[189] Pocock and Hughes[157] have suggested that the point estimate of the effect of the intervention should also be adjusted, since trials that are terminated early tend to exaggerate the size of the true treatment difference. Others have also pointed out the bias in the point estimate.[58,105,197] Kim[105] suggested that a median estimator is less biased.

Confidence intervals can also be used in another manner in the sequential monitoring of interim data. At each interim analysis, a confidence interval could be constructed for the parameter summarizing the treatment effect, such as differences in means, proportions, or hazard ratios. This is referred to as repeated confidence intervals (RCI).[47,62,63,99,100] If the RCI excludes a null difference, or no treatment effect, then the trial might be stopped, claiming a significant treatment effect. It is also possible to continue the trial unless the confidence interval excluded not only no difference, but minimal or clinically uninteresting differences. On the other hand, if all values of clinically meaningful treatment differences are ruled out or fall outside the confidence interval, then that trial might be stopped, claiming that no useful clinical effect is likely. Here, as for confidence intervals after termination, the naive confidence interval is not appropriate. Jennison and Turnball[99,100] have suggested one method for RCI that basically inverts the group sequential test. That is, the confidence interval has the same form as the naive estimate, but the coefficient is the standardized boundary value as determined by the spending function, for example. The RCI has the form:

$$\text{(treatment difference)} \pm Z(k) \text{ (standard error of difference)}$$

where $Z(k)$ is the sequential boundary value at the kth interim analysis. For example, using the O'Brien-Fleming boundaries shown in Fig. 15-4, we would have a coefficient of 4.56 at $k = 1$, $t_1^* = 0.2$ and 3.23 at $k = 2$, $t_2^* = 0.4$. Used in this manner, the RCI and the sequential test of the null hypothesis will yield the same conclusions.

One particular application of the RCI is for trials whose goal is to demonstrate that two interventions or treatments are essentially "equivalent," that is, have an effect that is considered to be within a specified acceptable range and might be used interchangeably. As indicated in the design discussion, clinicians might select the cheaper, less toxic, or less invasive intervention if the effects were close enough. One suggestion for "close enough" or "equivalence" would be treatments whose effects are within 20%.[62,63] Thus RCIs that are contained within a 20% range would suggest that the results are consistent with this working definition of equivalence. For example, if the relative risk were estimated along with an RCI, the working range of equivalence would be from 0.8 to 1.2, where large values indicate inferiority of the intervention being tested. The trial would continue as long as the upper limit of the RCI exceeded 1.2 since we would not have ruled out a treatment worsening by 20% or more. Depending on the trial and the interventions, the trial might also continue until the lower limit of the RCI was larger than 0.8, indicating no improvement by 20% or greater.

Asymmetric boundaries

In most trials, the main purpose is to test whether the intervention is superior to the control. It is not always ethical to continue a study to prove, at the usual levels of significance, that the intervention is harmful relative to a placebo or standard control. This point has been mentioned by several authors[20,40,49,56,180] who discuss methods for group sequential designs in which the hypothesis to be tested is one-sided; that is, to test whether the intervention is superior to the control. They proposed retaining the group sequential upper boundaries of Pocock or O'Brien-Fleming for rejection of H_0 while suggesting various forms of a lower boundary that would imply "acceptance" of H_0. One simple approach is to set the lower boundary at an arbitrary value of Z_i, such as -1.5 or -2.0. If the test statistic goes below that value, the data may be sufficiently suggestive of a harmful effect to justify terminating the trial. This asymmetric boundary attempts to reflect the behavior or attitude of members of many monitoring committees, which recommend stopping a study once the intervention shows a strong, but nonsignificant, trend in an adverse direction. Work by Gould and Pecore[83] suggests ways for early acceptance of the null hypothesis while incorporating costs as well.

An example of asymmetric group sequential boundaries is provided by the CAST. Two interventions (encainide and flecainide) were terminated early using a symmetric two-sided boundary, although the lower boundary for harm was described as advisory by the authors.[17,71] The third drug (moricizine vs. placebo) continued. However, because of the experience with the encainide and flecainide arms, the lower boundary for harm was revised to be less extreme than before.[18]

Curtailed sampling procedures

During the course of monitoring accumulating data, one question often posed is whether the current trend in the data is so impressive that acceptance or rejection of H_0 is already determined, or at least close to being determined. If the results of the trial are such that the conclusions are "known for certain," no matter what the future outcomes might be, then consideration of early termination is in order. A helpful sports analogy is a baseball team "clinching the pennant" after winning a specific game. At that time it is known for certain who has won and who has not won, regardless of the outcome of the remaining games. Playing the remaining games is done for reasons (e.g., fiscal) other than deciding the winner. This idea has been developed for clinical trials and is often referred to as deterministic curtailed sampling. It should be noted that group sequential methods focus on existing data while curtailed sampling in addition considers the data that have not yet been observed.

Alling[1,2] may have introduced this concept when he considered the early stopping question and compared the survival experience in two groups. He used the Wilcoxon test for two samples, a frequently used nonparametric test that ranks survival times and is the basis for one of the primary survival analysis techniques.[77] Alling's method allows stopping decisions to be based on data available during the trial. The trial would be terminated if future data could not change the final conclusion about the null hypothesis. The method is applicable whether all participants are entered at the same time or recruitment occurs over a longer period. However, when the average time to the event is short relative to the time needed to enroll participants, the method is of limited value. The repeated testing problem is irrelevant, because any decision is based on what the significance test will be at the end of the study. Therefore frequent use of this procedure causes no problem with regard to significance level and power.

Many clinical trials with survival time as a response variable have observations that are censored; that is, participants are followed for some length of time and then at some point, no further information about the participant is known or collected. Halperin and Ware[88] extended the method of Alling to the case of censored data, using the Wilcoxon rank statistic. With this method, early termination is particularly likely when the null hypothesis is true or when the expected difference between groups is large. The method is shown to be more effective for small sample sizes than for large studies. The Alling approach to early stopping has also been applied to another commonly used test, the Mantel-Haenszel statistic. However, the Wilcoxon statistic appears to have better early stopping properties than the Mantel-Haenszel statistic.

A deterministic curtailed procedure has been developed[45] for comparing the means of two bounded random variables using the two-sample t-test. It assumes that the response must be between two values, A and B ($A < B$). An approximate solution is an extreme case approach. First, all the estimated remaining responses in one group are given the maximum favorable outcome (i.e., B) and all the remaining responses in the other take on the worst response (i.e., A). The statistic is then computed. Next, the responses are assigned in the opposite way and a second statistic is computed. If neither of these two extreme results alters the conclusion, no additional data are necessary for testing the hypothesis. While this deterministic curtailed approach provides an answer to an interesting question, the requirement for absolute certainly results in a very conservative test and allows little opportunity for early termination.

In some clinical trials, the final outcome may not be absolutely certain, but almost so. To use the baseball analogy again, a first-place team may not have clinched the pennant but is so many games in front of the second place team that it is highly unlikely that it will not, in fact, end up the winner. Another team may be so far behind that it realistically cannot catch up. In clinical trials, the idea is often referred to as stochastic curtailed sampling. It is identical to the concept of conditional power, discussed in the section on extending a trial.

Lan, Simon, and Halperin[122] considered the effect of stochastic curtailed procedures on type-I and type-II error rates. If the null hypothesis, H_0, is tested at time t using the statistic $S(t)$, then at the scheduled end of a trial at time T, the statistic would be $S(T)$. Two cases are considered. First, suppose a trend in favor of rejecting H_0 is observed at time $t < T$, with intervention doing better than control. One then computes the conditional probability, γ_0 of rejecting H_0 at time T; that is, $S(T) > Z_\alpha$, assuming H_0 to be true and given the current data, $S(t)$. If this probability is sufficiently large, one might argue that the favorable trend is not going to disappear. Second, suppose a negative trend, or data consistent with the null hypothesis of no differences, at some pont t. Then, one computes the conditional probability, γ_1, of rejecting H_0 at the end of the trial, time T, given that some alternative H_1 is true, for a sample of reasonable alternatives. This essentially asks how large the true effect must be before the current "negative" trend is likely to be reversed. If the probability of a trend reversal is highly unlikely for a realistic range of alternative hypotheses, trial termination might be considered.

Because there is a small probability that the results will change, a slightly greater risk of a type-I or type-II error rate will exist than would be if the trial continued to the scheduled end.[87] However, it has been shown that the type-I error is bounded very conservatively by α/γ_0 and the type-II error by β/γ_1. For example, if the probability of rejecting the null hypothesis, given the existing data, were 0.85, then the actual type-I error would be no more than 0.05/0.85 or 0.059, instead of 0.05. The actual upper limit is considerably closer to 0.05, but that calculation requires computer simulation. Calculation of these probabilities is relatively straightforward, and Lan and Wittes have described the details.[123]

The Beta-Blocker Heart Attack Trial[46] made considerable use of this approach. As discussed, the interim results were impressive with 1 year of follow-up still remaining. One question posed was whether the strong favorable trend ($Z = 2.82$) could be lost during that year. The probability of rejecting H_0 at the scheduled end of the trial, given the existing trend (γ_0), was approximately 0.90. This meant that the false-positive or type-I error was not more than $\alpha/\gamma_0 = 0.05/0.90$ or 0.056.

Other approaches

Other techniques for interim analysis of accumulating data have also received attention. These include binomial sampling strategies,[174] decision theoretic models,[25] and likelihood or Bayesian methods.* The literature on these methods is extensive, but the methods appear to be used infrequently. Cornfield,[26-28] for example, proposed the use of Bayesian methods in clinical trials. These require specifying a prior probability on the possible values of the unknown parameter. The experiment is performed and based on the data obtained, and the prior probability is adjusted. If the adjustment is large enough, the investigator may change his opinion (i.e., his prior belief). Spiegelhalter et al.[179] and Freedman et al.[69] have implemented Bayesian methods that have frequentist properties similar to boundaries of either the Pocock or O'Brien-Fleming type. It is somewhat reassuring that two methodologies, even from a different theoretical framework, can provide similar monitoring procedures. While the Bayesian view is critical of the hypothesis-testing methods because of the arbitrariness involved, the Bayesian approach is perhaps hampered mostly by the requirement that the investigator formally specify a prior probability on the effect of the intervention. However, if a person in the decision-making process uses all of the factors and methods discussed in this chapter, a Bayesian approach is involved, although in a very informal way.

An ad hoc model has been developed[110] for stopping accrual of participants into a clinical trial while follow-up continues for the occurrence of the event of interest. This approach is only applicable if the intervention is given once upon entry into the trial (e.g., surgery or vaccination).

We have stated that the data monitoring committee should be aware of all the relevant information in the use of the intervention that existed before the trial started or that emerges during the course of a trial. Some have argued that all of this information should be pooled or incorporated and updated sequentially in a formal statistical manner.[125] This is referred to as sequential meta-analysis. We describe meta-analysis in the chapter on analysis issues (Chapter 16). We do not support sequential meta-analysis as a primary approach for monitoring a trial. We believe that the results of the ongoing trial should be first presented alone in the detail described earlier. As supportive evidence for continuation or termination, other analysis may be used, including a pooled analysis of all available external data.

REFERENCES

1. Alling DW: Early decision in the Wilcoxon two sample test, *J Am Stat Assoc* 58:713-720, 1963.
2. Alling DW: Closed sequential tests for binomial probabilities, *Biometrika* 53:73-84, 1966.
3. Anscombe FJ: Sequential medical trials, *J Am Stat Assoc* 58:365-383, 1963.
4. Armitage P: Restricted sequential procedures, *Biometrika* 44:9-26, 1957.

*References 23, 26, 28, 69, 82, 86, 131, 132, 178, 179.

5. Armitage P: *Sequential medical trials,* ed 2, New York, 1975, John Wiley & Sons.

6. Armitage P, McPherson CK, Rowe BC: Repeated significance tests on accumulating data, *J R Stat Soc* 132 A:235-244, 1969.

7. Aspirin Myocardial Infarction Study Research Group: A randomized controlled trial of aspirin in persons recovered from myocardial infarction, *JAMA* 243:661-669, 1980.

8. Baum M, Houghton J, Abrams K: Early stopping rules—clinical perspectives and ethical considerations, *Stats Med* 13:1459-1470, 1994.

9. Beta-Blocker Heart Attack Trial Research Group: A randomized trial of propranolol in participants with acute myocardial infarction. I. Mortality results, *JAMA* 247:1707-1714, 1982.

10. Breslow N, Haug C: Sequential comparison of exponential survival curves, *J Am Stat Assoc* 67:691-697, 1972.

11. Bross I: Sequential medical plans, *Biometrics* 8:188-205, 1952.

12. Burke G: Discussion of Early stopping rules—clinical perspectives and ethical considerations, *Stat Med* 13:1471-1472, 1994.

13. Buyse M: Interim analyses, stopping roles and data monitoring in clinical trials in Europe, *Stat Med* 12:509-520, 1993.

14. Canner PL: Monitoring treatment differences in long-term clinical trials, *Biometrics* 33:603-615, 1977.

15. Canner PL: Monitoring clinical trial data for evidence of adverse or beneficial treatment effects. In Boissel JP, Klimt CR, eds: *Multicenter controlled trials: principles and problems,* Paris, 1979, INSERM.

16. Canner PL: Monitoring of the data for evidence of adverse or beneficial treatment effects, *Controlled Clin Trials* 4:467-483, 1983.

17. Cardiac Arrhythmia Suppression Trial (CAST) Investigators: Preliminary report: Effect of encainide and flecainide on mortality in a randomized trial of arrhythmia suppression after myocardial infarction, *N Engl J Med* 321:406-412, 1989.

18. Cardiac Arrhythmia Suppression Trial - II Investigators: Effect of the antiarrhythmic agent moricizine on survival after myocardial infarction, *N Engl J Med* 327:227-233, 1992.

19. CASS Principal Investigators and Their Associates: Coronary Artery Surgery Study (CASS): a randomized trial of coronary artery bypass surgery, survival data, *Circulation* 68:939-950, 1983.

20. Chalmers TC: Invited remarks, *Clin Pharmacol Ther* 25:649-650, 1979.

21. Chang MN, O'Brien PC: Confidence intervals following group sequential tests, *Controlled Clin Trials* 7:18-26, 1986.

22. Chatterjee SK, Sen PK: Nonparametric testing under progressive censoring, *Calcutta Stat Assoc Bull* 22:13-50, 1973.

23. Choi SC, Pepple PA: Monitoring clinical trials based on predictive probability of significance, *Biometrics* 45:317-323, 1989.

24. Collaborative Group on Antenatal Steroid Therapy: Effect of antenatal dexamethasone administration on the prevention of respiratory distress syndrome, *Am J Obstet Gynecol* 141:276-287, 1981.

25. Colton T: A model for selecting one of two medical treatments, *J Am Stat Assoc* 58:388-400, 1963.

26. Cornfield J: A Bayesian test of some classical hypotheses—with applications to sequential clinical trials, *J Am Stat Assoc* 61:577-594, 1966.

27. Cornfield J: Sequential trials, sequential analysis and the likelihood principle, *Am Stat* 20:18-23, 1966.

28. Cornfield J: Recent methodological contributions to clinical trials, *Am J Epidemiol* 104:408-421, 1976.

29. Coronary Drug Project Research Group: The coronary drug project: initial findings leading to modifications of its research protocol, *JAMA* 214:1303-1313, 1970.

30. Coronary Drug Project Research Group: The coronary drug project: findings leading to further modifications of its protocol with respect to dextrothyroxine, *JAMA* 220:996-1008, 1972.

31. Coronary Drug Project Research Group: The coronary drug project: design, methods, and baseline results, *Circulation* 47(suppl 1):I-1–I-79, 1973.

32. Coronary Drug Project Research Group: The coronary drug project: findings leading to discontinuation of the 2.5-mg/day estrogen group, *JAMA* 226:652-657, 1973.

33. Coronary Drug Project Research Group: Clofibrate and niacin in coronary heart disease, *JAMA* 231:360-381, 1975.

34. Coronary Drug Project Research Group: Practical aspects of decision making in clinical trials: the coronary drug project as a case study, *Controlled Clin Trials* 1:363-376, 1981.
35. Crowley J, Green S, Liu PY, Wolf M: Data monitoring committees and the early stopping guidelines: the Southwest Oncology Group experience, *Stat Med* 13:1391-1400, 1994.
36. Dambrosia JM, Greenhouse SW: Early stopping for sequential restricted tests of binomial distributions, *Biometrics* 39:695-710, 1983.
37. Davis CE: A two sample Wilcoxon test for progressively censored data, *Commun Statist-Theor Meth A* 7:389-398, 1978.
38. DeMets D: Stopping guidelines vs. stopping rules: a practitioners's point of view, *Commun Statist-Theor Meth A* 13:2395-2417, 1984.
39. DeMets D, Lan G: An overview of sequential methods and their application in clinical trials, *Commun Stat Theory Methods* 13:2315-2338, 1984.
40. DeMets D, Ware J: Group sequential methods in clinical trials with a one-sided hypothesis, *Biometrika* 67:651-660, 1980.
41. DeMets DL: Practical aspects in data monitoring: a brief review, *Stat Med* 6:753-760, 1987.
42. DeMets DL: Data monitoring and sequential analysis—an academic perspective, *J AIDS* 3 (suppl 2): S124-S133, 1990.
43. DeMets DL, Ellenberg SS, Fleming TR, Childress JF et al: Data and safety monitoring board and acquired immune deficiency syndrome (AIDS) clinical trials, *Controlled Clin Trials,* in press.
44. DeMets DL, Gail MH: Use of logrank tests and group sequential methods at fixed calendar times, *Biometrics* 41:1039-1044, 1985.
45. DeMets DL, Halperin M: Early stopping in the two-sample problem for bounded random variables, *Controlled Clin Trials* 3:1-11, 1982.
46. DeMets DL, Hardy R, Friedman LM, Lan KKG: Statistical aspects of early termination in the Beta-Blocker Heart Attack Trial, *Controlled Clin Trials* 5:362-372, 1984.
47. DeMets DL, Lan KKG: Discussion of interim analyses: the repeated confidence interval approach by C Jennison and BW Turnbull, *J R Stat Soc* 51B:344, 1989.
48. DeMets DL, Lan KKG: Interim analyses: the alpha spending function approach, *Stat Med* 13: 1341-1352, 1994.
49. DeMets DL, Ware JH: Asymmetric group sequential boundaries for monitoring clinical trials, *Biometrika* 69:661-663, 1982.
50. DeMets DL, Williams GW, Brown BW Jr, and the NOTT Research Group: A case report of data monitoring experience: the nocturnal oxygen therapy trial, *Controlled Clin Trials* 3:113-124, 1982.
51. The Diabetic Retinopathy Study Research Group: Preliminary report on effects of photocoagulation therapy, *Am J Ophthalmol* 81:383-396, 1976.
52. The Diabetic Retinopathy Study Research Group: Photocoagulation treatment of proliferative diabetic retinopathy: the second report of Diabetic Retinopathy Study findings, *Ophthalmology* 85:82-106, 1978.
53. Diabetic Retinopathy Study Research Group: Diabetic retinopathy study: Report No 6. Design, methods, and baseline results, *Invest Ophthalmol Vis Sci* 21:149-209, 1981.
54. Ederer F, Podgor MJ, the Diabetic Retinopathy Study Research Group: Assessing possible late treatment effects in stopping a clinical trial early: diabetic retinopathy study report no 9, *Controlled Clin Trials* 5:373-381, 1984.
55. Ellenberg SS, Myers MW, Blackwelder WC, Hoth DF: The use of external monitoring committees in clinical trials of the National Institute of Allergy and Infectious Diseases, *Stat Med* 13:461-468, 1993.
56. Emerson SS, Fleming TR: Symmetric group sequential test designs, *Biometrics* 45:905-932, 1989.
57. Emerson SS, Fleming TR: Interim analyses in clinical trials, *Oncology* 4:126-133, 1990.
58. Emerson SS, Fleming TR: Parameter estimation following group sequential hypothesis testing, *Biometrika* 77:875-892, 1990.
59. Fairbanks K, Madsen R: P values for tests using a repeated significance test design, *Biometrika* 69:69-74, 1982.
60. Falissard B, Lellouch J: A new procedure for group sequential analysis in clinical trials, *Biometrics* 48:373-388, 1992.

61. Fleming T, DeMets DL: Monitoring of clinical trials: issues and recommendations, *Controlled Clin Trials* 14:183-197, 1993.
62. Fleming TR: Treatment evaluation in active control studies, *Cancer Treat Rep* 17:1061-1065, 1987.
63. Fleming TR: Evaluation of active control trials in AIDS, *J AIDS* 3(suppl):S82-S87, 1990.
64. Fleming TR: Data monitoring committees and capturing relevant information of high quality, *Stat Med* 12:565-570, 1993.
65. Fleming TR, Green SJ, Harrington DP: Considerations for monitoring and evaluating treatment effects in clinical trials, *Controlled Clin Trials* 5:55-66, 1984.
66. Fleming TR, Watelet LF: Approaches to monitoring clinical trials, *JNCI* 81:188-193, 1989.
67. Freedman B: Equipoise and the ethics of clinical research, *N Engl J Med* 317:141-145, 1987.
68. Freedman LS, Lowe D, Macaskill P: Stopping rules for clinical trials, *Stat Med* 2:167-174, 1983.
69. Freedman LS, Spiegelhalter DJ, Parmar MKB: The what, why, and how of Bayesian clinical trials monitoring, *Stat Med* 13:1371-1384, 1994.
70. Friedman L: The NHLBI model: a 25 year history, *Stats Med* 12:425-432, 1993.
71. Friedman L, Bristow JD, Hallstrom A et al: Data monitoring in the cardiac arrhythmia suppression trial, *Online J Curr Clin Trials* Doc 79, July 31, 1993.
72. Furberg C, Campbell R, Pitt B: Letter to the editor (on consensus II). *N Engl J Med* 328:967-968, 1993.
73. Gail M: Monitoring and stopping clinical trials. In Mike V, Stanley K, eds: *Statistics in medical research: methods and issues, with applications in cancer research,* New York, 1982, John Wiley & Sons.
74. Gail M: Nonparametric frequentist methods for monitoring comparative survival studies. In Krishnaiah PR, Sen PK, eds: *Handbook of statistics: parametric methods,* vol 4, Amsterdam, 1984, North Holland Publishing.
75. Gail MH, DeMets DL, Slud EV: Simulation studies on increments of the two-sample log rank score test for survival data, with application to group sequential boundaries. In Johnson R, Crowley J, eds: *Survival analysis. Monograph Ser 2*, Hayward, Calif, 1982, IMS Lecture Notes.
76. Gange SJ, DeMets DL: Sequential monitoring of clinical trials with correlated categorical responses, UW Department of Biostatistics, Tech Rep No 86, July, 1994.
77. Gehan E: A generalized Wilcoxon test for comparing arbitrarily singly censored samples, *Biometrika* 52:203-224, 1965.
78. Geller ND: Discussion of "Interim analysis: The alpha spending approach," *Stat Med* 13:1353-1356, 1994.
79. Geller NL, Stylianou M: Practical issues in the data monitoring of clinical trials: summary of responses to a questionnaire at NIH, *Stat Med* 12:543-552, 1993.
80. George SL: A survey of monitoring practices in cancer clinical trials, *Stat Med* 12:435-450, 1993.
81. George SL: Discussion of "Sequential methods based on the boundaries approach for the clinical comparison of survival times," *Stat Med* 13(13/14):1369-1370, 1994.
82. George SL, Clenchang L, Berry DA, Green MR: Stopping a clinical trial early: frequentist and Bayesian approaches applied to a CALGB trial of non-small-cell lung cancer, *Stats Med* 13(13/14):1313-1328, 1994.
83. Gould AL, Pecore VJ: Group sequential methods for clinical trials allowing early acceptance of Ho and incorporating costs, *Biometrika* 69:75-80, 1982.
84. Green S, Crowley J: Data monitoring committees for Southwest Oncology Group Clinical Trials, *Stat Med* 12(5/6):451-456, 1993.
85. Green SB, Freedman LS: Early stopping of prevention trials when multiple outcomes are of interest: a discussion, *Stats Med* 13(13/14):1479-1484, 1994.
86. Grieve AP: Predictive probability in clinical trials, *Biometrics* 47:323-330, 1991.
87. Halperin M, Lan KKG, Ware JH et al: An aid to data monitoring in long-term clinical trials, *Controlled Clin Trials* 3:311-323, 1982.
88. Halperin M, Ware J: Early decision in a censored Wilcoxon two-sample test for accumulating survival data, *J Am Stat Assoc* 69:414-422, 1974.
89. Harrington D, Crowley J, George SL, Pajak T, Redmond C, Wieand HS: The case against independent monitoring committees, *Stat Med* 13:1411-1414, 1994.

90. Harrington DP, Fleming TR, Green SJ: Procedures for serial testing in censored survival data. In Johnson R, Crowley J, eds: *Survival analysis. Monograph ser 2,* Hayward, Calif, 1982, IMS Lecture Notes.

91. Haybittle JL: Repeated assessment of results in clinical trials of cancer treatment, *Br J Radiol* 44:793-797, 1971.

92. Heart Special Project Committee: Organization, review and administration of cooperative studies (Greenberg Report): A report from the heart special project committee to the National Advisory Council, May, 1967, *Controlled Clin Trials* 9:137-148, 1988.

93. Herson J: Data monitoring boards in the pharmaceutical industry, *Stat Med* 12(5/6):555-562, 1993.

94. Hughes MD, Pocock SJ: Stopping rules and estimation problems in clinical trials, *Stat Med* 7:1231-1241, 1988.

95. Hwang I, Tsiatis A: Approximately optimal one-parameter boundaries for group sequential trials, *Biometrics* 43:193-199, 1987.

96. Hwang IK, Shih WJ: Group sequential designs using a family of type I error probability spending function, *Stat Med* 9:1439-1445, 1990.

97. Hypertension Detection and Follow-up Program Cooperative Group: Five-year findings of the hypertension detection and follow-up program. Reduction in mortality with high blood pressure, including mild hypertension, *JAMA* 242:2562-2571, 1979.

98. ISIS-2 (Second International Study of Infarct Survival) Collaborative Group: Randomized trial of intravenous streptokinase, oral aspirin, both or neither among 17187 cases of suspected acute myocardial infarction: ISIS-2, *Lancet* ii:349-360, 1988.

99. Jennison C, Turnbull BW: Repeated confidence intervals for group sequential clinic trials, *Controlled Clin Trials* 5:33-45, 1984.

100. Jennison C, Turnbull BW: Interim analyses: the repeated confidence interval approach, *J R Stat Soc* 51B:305-361, 1989.

101. Jennison C, Turnbull BW: Statistical approaches to interim monitoring of medical trials: a review and commentary, *Stat Sci* 5:299-317, 1990.

102. Joe H, Koziol JA, Petkau JA: Comparison of procedures for testing the equality of survival distributions, *Biometrics* 37:327-340, 1981.

103. Jones D, Whitehead J: Sequential forms of the log rank and modified Wilcoxon tests for censored data, *Biometrika* 66:105-113, 1979.

104. Jones, DR, Whitehead J: Applications of large-sample sequential tests to the analysis of survival data. In Tagnon HJ, Staquet MJ, eds: *Controversies in cancer—design of trials and treatment,* New York, 1979, Masson.

105. Kim K: Point estimation following group sequential tests, *Biometrics* 45:613-617, 1989.

106. Kim K: Study duration for group sequential clinical trials with censored survival data adjusting for stratification, *Stat Med* 11:1477-1488, 1992.

107. Kim K, De Mets DL: Confidence intervals following group sequential tests in clinical trials, *Biometrics* 4:857-864, 1987.

108. Kim K, DeMets DL: Design and analysis of group sequential tests based on the type I error spending rate function, *Biometrika* 74:149-154, 1987.

109. Kim K, DeMets DL: Sample size determination for group sequential clinical trials with immediate response, *Stat Med* 11:1391-1399, 1992.

110. Kim K, Tsiatis AA: Study duration for clinical trials with survival response and early stopping rule, *Biometrics* 46:81-92, 1990.

111. Klimt CR, Canner PL: Terminating a long-term clinical trial, *Clin Pharmacol Ther* 25:641-646, 1979.

112. Kolata GB: Controversy over study of diabetes drugs continues for nearly a decade, *Science* 203:986-990, 1979.

113. Koziol J, Petkau J: Sequential testing of equality of two survival distributions using the modified Savage statistic, *Biometrika* 65:615-623, 1978.

114. Lachin JM: Sequential clinical trials for normal variates using interval composite hypotheses, *Biometrics* 37:87-101, 1981.

115. Lan KKG, DeMets DL: Discrete sequential boundaries for clinical trials, *Biometrika* 70:659-663, 1983.

116. Lan KKG, DeMets DL: Changing frequency of interim analyses in sequential monitoring, *Biometrics* 45:1017-1020, 1989.

117. Lan KKG, DeMets DL: Group sequential procedures: calendar versus information time, *Stat Med* 8:1191-1198, 1989.

118. Lan KKG, DeMets DL, Halperin M: More flexible sequential and non-sequential designs in long-term clinical trials, *Commun Stat Theory Method* 13:2339-2354, 1984.

119. Lan KKG, Lachin J: Implementation of group sequential logrank tests in a maximum duration trial, *Biometrics* 46:759-770, 1990.

120. Lan KKG, Reboussin DM, DeMets DL: Information and information fractions for design and sequential monitoring of clinical trials, *Commun Stat Theory Methods* 23:403-420, 1994.

121. Lan KKG, Rosenberger WF, Lachin JM: Use of spending functions for occasional or continuous monitoring of data in clinical trials, *Stat Med* 12:2214-2231, 1993.

122. Lan KKG, Simon R, Halperin M: Stochastically curtailed tests in long-term clinical trials, *Commun Stat, Sequent Anal* 1:207-219, 1982.

123. Lan KKG, Wittes J: The B-value: a tool for monitoring data, *Biometrics* 44:579-585, 1988.

124. Lan KKG, Zucker D: Sequential monitoring of clinical trials: the role of information in Brownian motion, *Stat Med* 12:753-765, 1993.

125. Lau J, Antman EM, Jimenez-Silva J, Kupelnick B, Mosteller F, Chalmers TC: Cumulative meta-analysis of therapeutic trials for myocardial infarction, *N Engl J Med* 327:248-254, 1992.

126. Lee JW: Group sequential testing in clinical trials with multivariate observations: a review, *Stat Med* 13:101-111, 1994.

127. Lee JW, DeMets DL: Sequential comparison of change with repeated measurement data, *J Am Stat Assoc* 86:757-762, 1991.

128. Lee JW, DeMets DL: Sequential rank tests with repeated measurements in clinical trials, *J Am Stat Assoc* 87:136-142, 1992.

129. Li Z, Geller NL: On the choice of times for data analysis in group sequential trials, *Biometrics* 47: 745-750, 1991.

130. Liberati A: Conclusions. 1: The relationship between clinical trials and clinical practice: the risks of underestimating its complexity, *Stat Med* 13(13/14):1485-1492, 1994.

131. Louis TA, Carlin BP: Robust Bayesian approaches for monitoring clinical trials, submitted for publication.

132. Machin D: Discussion of "The what, why and how of Bayesian clinical trials monitoring," *Stat Med* 13:1385-1390, 1994.

133. Mantel N: Evaluation of survival data and two new rank order statistics arising in its consideration, *Cancer Chemother Rep* 50:163-170, 1966.

134. McPherson CK, Armitage P: Repeated significance tests on accumulating data when the null hypothesis is not true, *J R Stat Soc* 134 A:15-25, 1971.

135. Meier P: Terminating a trial—the ethical problem, *Clin Pharmacol Ther* 25:633-640, 1979.

136. The MIAMI Trial Research Group: Metoprolol in acute myocardial infarction (MIAMI): a randomized placebo-controlled trial, *Eur Heart J* 6:199-214, 1985.

137. Muenz L, Green S, Byar D: Applications of the Mantel Haenszel statistic to the comparison of survival distributions, *Biometrics* 33:617-626, 1977.

138. Multiple Risk Factor Intervention Trial Research Group: Multiple Risk Factor Interventional Trial. Risk factor changes and mortality results, *JAMA* 248:1465-1477, 1982.

139. Nagelkerke NJD, Hart AAM: The sequential comparison of survival curves, *Biometrika* 67:247-249, 1980.

140. Nocturnal Oxygen Therapy Group: Continuous or nocturnal oxygen therapy in hypoxemic chronic obstructive lung disease, *Ann Intern Med* 93:391-398, 1980.

141. O'Brien PC, Fleming TR: A multiple testing procedure for clinical trials, *Biometrics* 35:549-556, 1979.

142. O'Neill RT: Some FDA perspectives on data monitoring in clinical trials in drug development, *Stat Med* 12:601-608, 1993.

143. O'Neill RT: Conclusions. 2: The relationship between clinical trials and clinical practice: The risks of understanding its complexity, *Stat Med* 13:1493-1500, 1994.

144. Packer M, Carver JR, Rodeheffer RJ, Ivanhoe RJ et al, for the PROMISE Study Research Group: Effect of oral milrinone on mortality in severe chronic heart failure, *N Engl J Med* 325:1468-1475, 1991.

145. Packer M, Rouleau J, Swedberg K, et al and the PROFILE Investigators: Effect of Flosequinan on survival in chronic heart failure: preliminary results of the PROFILE study (abstract), *Circulation* 88 (suppl):I-301, 1993.
146. Parmar MKB, Machin D: Monitoring clinical trials: experience of, and proposals under consideration by, the Cancer Therapy Committee of the British Medical Research Council, *Stat Med* 12:497-504, 1993.
147. Pater JL: The use of data monitoring committees in Canadian trial groups, *Stat Med* 12:505-508, 1993.
148. Pater JL: Timing the collaborative analysis of three trials comparing 5-FU plus folinic (FUFA) to surgery alone in the management of resected colorectal cancer: A national Cancer Institute of Canada Trial Group (NCIC-CTG) perspective, *Stat Med* 13:1337-1340, 1994.
149. Pawitan Y, Hallstrom A: Statistical interim monitoring of the cardiac arrhythmia suppression trial, *Stat Med* 9:1081-1090, 1990.
150. Peto R, Peto J: Asymptotically efficient rank invariant test procedures, *J R Stat Soc* 135A:185-206, 1972.
151. Peto R, Pike MC, Armitage P et al: Design and analysis of randomized clinical trials requiring prolonged observatons of each patient. I. Introduction and design, *Br J Cancer* 34:585-612, 1976.
152. Pocock SJ: Group sequential methods in the design and analysis of clinical trials, *Biometrika* 64:191-199, 1977.
153. Pocock SJ: Size of cancer clinical trials and stopping rules, *Br J Cancer* 38:757-766, 1978.
154. Pocock SJ: Interim analyses for randomized clinical trials: the group sequential approach, *Biometrics* 38:153-162, 1982.
155. Pocock SJ: When to stop a clinical trial, *Br Med J* 305:235-240, 1992.
156. Pocock SJ: Statistical and ethical issues in monitoring clinical trials, *Stat Med* 12:1459-1469, 1993.
157. Pocock SJ, Hughes MD: Practical problems in interim analyses, with particular regard to estimation, *Controlled Clin Trials* 10:2094-2215, 1989.
158. Proschan MA, Follman DA, Geller NL: Monitoring multi-armed trials, *Stat Med* 13:1441-1452, 1994.
159. Proschan MA, Follman DA, Waclawiw MA: Effects of assumption violations on type I error rate in group sequential monitoring, *Biometrics* 48:1131-1143, 1992.
160. Reboussin DM, DeMets DL, Kim K, Lan KKG: Programs for computing group sequential bounds using the Lan-DeMets method, UW Department of Biostatistics, Tech Rep No 60, June, 1992.
161. Reboussin D, Lan KKG, DeMets DL: Group sequential testing of longitudinal data, Tech Report No 72, UW, Department of Biostatistics, August, 1992.
162. Report of the Committee for the Assessment of Biometric Aspects of Controlled Trials of Hypoglycemic Agents, *JAMA* 231:583-608, 1975.
163. Robbins H: Some aspects of sequential design of experiments, *Bull Am Math Soc* 58:527-535, 1952.
164. Robbins H: Statistical methods related to the law or iterated logarithm, *Ann Math Stat* 41:1397-1409, 1970.
165. Robinson J: A lay person's perspective on starting and stopping clinical trials, *Stat Med* 13:1473-1478, 1994.
166. Rockhold FW, Enas GG: Data monitoring and interim analyses in the pharmaceutical industry: ethical and logistical considerations, *Stat Med* 12:471-480, 1993.
167. Rosner GL, Tsiatis AA: Exact confidence intervals following a group sequential trial: a comparison of methods, *Biometrika* 75:723-729, 1988.
168. Seiget D, Milton RC: Further results on a multiple-testing procedure for clinical trials, *Biometrics* 39:921-928, 1983.
169. Sellke T, Siegmund D: Sequential analysis of the proportional hazards model, *Biometrika* 70:315-326, 1983.
170. Shaw LW, Chalmers TC: Ethics in cooperative clinical trials, *Am NY Acad Sci* 169:487-495, 1970.
171. Siegmund D: Estimation following sequential tests, *Biometrika* 65:341-349, 1978.
172. Silverman WA, Agate FJ Jr, Fertig JW: A sequential trial of the nonthermal effect of atmospheric humidity on survival of newborn infants of low birth weight, *Pediatrics* 31:719-724, 1963.
173. Simon R: Some practical aspects of the interim monitoring of clinical trials, *Stat Med* 13:1401-1410, 1994.
174. Simon R, Weiss GH, Hoel DG: Sequential analysis of binomial clinical trials, *Biometrika* 62:195-200, 1975.

175. Slud E, Wei LJ: Two-sample repeated significance tests based on the modified Wilcoxon statistic, *J Am Stat Assoc* 77:862-868, 1982.
176. Smith E, Sempos CT, Smith PE, Gilligan C: Calcium supplementation and bone loss in middle-aged women, *Am J Clin* 50:833-842, 1989.
177. Souhami RL: The clinical importance of early stopping of randomized trials in cancer treatments, *Stat Med* 13:1297-1312, 1994.
178. Spiegelhalter DJ: Probabilitistic prediction in patient management and clinical trials, *Stat Med* 5:421-433, 1986.
179. Spiegelhalter DJ, Freedman LS, Blackburn PR: Monitoring clinical trials: conditional or predictive power? *Controlled Clin Trials* 7:8-17, 1986.
180. Stamler J: Invited remarks, *Clin Pharmacol Ther* 25:651-658, 1979.
181. Su JQ, Lachin JU: Group sequential distribution-free methods for the analysis of multivariate observations, *Biometrics* 48:1033-1042, 1992.
182. Swedberg K, Held, P, Kjekhus J, Rasmussen K, Ryden L, Wedel H: Effects of early administration of enalapril on mortality in patients with acute myocardial infarction—results of the Cooperative New Scandinavian Enalapril Survival Study II (Consensus II), *N Engl J Med* 327:678-684, 1992.
183. Sylvester R, Bartelink H, Rubens R: A reversal of fortune: practical problems in the monitoring and interpretation of an EORTC breast cancer trial, *Stat Med* 13:1329-1336.
184. Task Force of the Working Group on Arrhythmias of the European Society of Cardiology: The early termination of clinical trials: causes, consequences, and control—with special reference to trials in the field of arrhythmias and sudden death, *Circulation* 89:2892-2907, 1994.
185. Truelove SC, Watkinson G, Draper G: Comparison of corticosteroid and sulphasalazine therapy in ulcerative colitis, *Br Med J* 2:1708-1711, 1962.
186. Tsiatis AA: The asymptotic joint distribution of the efficient scores tests for the proportional hazards model calculated over time, *Biometrika* 68:311-315, 1981.
187. Tsiatis AA: Group sequential methods for survival analysis with staggered entry. In Johnson R, Crowley J, eds: *Survival analysis, Monograph Ser 2,* Hayward, Calif, 1982, IMS Lecture Notes.
188. Tsiatis AA: Repeated significance testing for a general class of statistics used in censored survival analysis, *J Am Stat Assoc* 77:855-861, 1982.
189. Tsiatis AA, Rosnar GL, Mehta CR: Exact confidence intervals following a group sequential test, *Biometrics* 40:797-803, 1984.
190. Tukey JW: Some thoughts on clinical trials, especially problems of multiplicity, *Science* 198:679-684, 1977.
191. University Group Diabetes Program: A study of the effects of hypoglycemic agents on vascular complications in patients with adult-onset diabetes. II. Mortality results, *Diabetes* 19(suppl 2):787-830, 1970.
192. University Group Diabetes Program: Effects of hypoglycemic agents on vascular complications in patients with adult-onset diabetes. IV. A preliminary report on phenformin results, *JAMA* 217:777-784, 1971.
193. Wald A: *Sequential analysis,* New York, 1947, John Wiley & Sons.
194. Walters L: Data monitoring committees: the moral case for maximum feasible independence, *Stat Med* 12:575-580, 1993.
195. Wei LJ, Su JQ, Lachin JM: Interim analyses with repeated measurements in a sequential clinical trial, *Biometrika* 77:359-364, 1990.
196. Whitehead J: *The design and analysis of sequential clinical trials,* New York, 1983, Haisted Press.
197. Whitehead J: On the bias of maximum likelihood estimation following a sequential test, *Biometrika* 73:573-581, 1986.
198. Whitehead J: Sequential methods based on the boundaries approach for the clinical comparison of survival times, *Stat Med* 13:1357-1368, 1994.
199. Whitehead J, Facey KM: Analysis after a sequential trial: a comparison of orderings of the sample space. Presented at the Joint Society for Clinical Trials/International Society for Clinical Biostatistics, Brussels, 1991.
200. Whitehead J, Jones D: The analysis of sequential clinical trials, *Biometrika* 66:443-452, 1979.

201. Whitehead J, Jones DR, Ellis SH: The analysis of a sequential clinical trial for the comparison of two lung cancer treatments, *Stat Med* 2:183-190, 1983.
202. Whitehead J, Stratton I: Group sequential clinical trials with triangular continuation regions, *Biometrics* 39:227-236, 1983.
203. Williams GW, Davis RL, Getson AJ, Gould AL, et al: Monitoring of clinical trials and interim analyses from a drug sponsor's point of view, *Stat Med* 12:481-492, 1993.
204. Wittes J: Behind closed doors: the data monitoring board in randomized clinical trials, *Stat Med* 12, 1993.
205. Wu MC, Lan KKG: Sequential monitoring for comparison of changes in a response variable in clinical trials, *Biometrics* 48:765-779, 1992.

CHAPTER 16

Issues in Data Analysis

The analysis of data obtained from a clinical trial represents the outcome of the planning and implementation already described. Primary and secondary questions addressed by the clinical trial can be tested and new hypotheses generated. Data analysis is sometimes viewed as simple and straightforward, requiring little time, effort, or expense. However, careful analysis usually requires a major investment in all three. It must be done with as much care and concern as any of the design or data-gathering aspects. Furthermore, inappropriate statistical analyses can result in misleading conclusions and impair the credibility of the trial.

Several introductory textbooks of statistics* provide excellent descriptions for many basic methods of analysis. Chapter 14 presents essentials for analysis of survival data, since they are frequently of interest in clinical trials and are not covered in most introductory statistics texts. This chapter will focus on some issues in the analysis of data that seem to cause confusion in the medical research community. Some of the proposed solutions are straightforward; others are judgmental. They reflect a viewpoint developed by the authors and colleagues in many collaborative efforts over two decades. Whereas some[7,62,103,109] have taken similar positions, others[121,123] have opposing views on several issues.

FUNDAMENTAL POINT

Excluding randomized participants or observed outcomes from analysis and subgrouping on the basis of outcome or response variables can lead to biased results of unknown magnitude or direction.

WHICH PARTICIPANTS SHOULD BE ANALYZED?

The issue of which participants are to be included in the data analysis often arises in clinical trials. Although a laboratory study may have carefully regulated experimental conditions, even the best designed and managed clinical trial cannot be perfectly implemented. Response variable data may be missing, the protocol may not be completely adhered to, and some participants, in retrospect, will not have

---

*References 8, 19, 20, 39, 61, 79, 114, 144.

met the entrance criteria. Some investigators prefer to remove from the analysis participants who do not fit the inclusion criteria or do not follow the protocol perfectly. Conversely, others believe that once a participant is randomized, that participant should always be followed and included in the analysis. The rationale for each of these positions is considered in the following pages. This chapter has adopted, in part, the terminology used by Peto et al.[109] to classify participants according to the nature and extent of their participation.

Exclusions are people who are screened as potential participants for a randomized trial but who do not meet all of the entry criteria and, therefore, are not randomized. Reasons for exclusion might be related to age, severity of disease, refusal to participate, or any of numerous other determinants evaluated before randomization of a participant to a study group (Chapter 3). Since these potential participants are not randomized, their exclusion does not bias any intervention–control group comparison. Exclusions do, however, influence interpretation of the results of the clinical trial. In some circumstances, follow-up of excluded people can be helpful in determining to what extent the results can be generalized. If the event rate in the control group is considerably lower than anticipated, an investigator may determine whether most high-risk people were excluded or whether the initial assumption was incorrect.

Withdrawals are participants who have been randomized but are deliberately not included in the analysis. As the fundamental point states, omitting participants from analyses can bias the results of the study.[93] If participants are withdrawn, the burden rests with the investigator to convince the scientific community that the analysis has not been biased. However, this can be a difficult task, because no one can be sure that participants were not differentially withdrawn from the study groups. Differential withdrawal can exist even if the number of omitted participants is the same in each group, since the reasons for withdrawal in each group may be different. Consequently, the participants remaining in the trial may not be comparable, undermining one of the reasons for randomization.

Many reasons are given for withdrawing participants from the analysis, such as ineligibility, nonadherence, poor quality data, and occurrence of competing events.

Ineligibility

The most commonly cited reason for withdrawal is that some participants did not meet the entry criteria, a protocol violation unknown at the time of enrollment. Admitting unqualified participants may be the result of a simple clerical error, a laboratory error, a misinterpretation, or a misclassification. Clerical mistakes such as listing wrong sex or age may be obvious. Other errors can arise from differing interpretations of diagnostic studies such as ECGs, x-rays, or biopsies. It is not difficult to find examples in different disease areas.*

---

*References 5, 6, 16, 23, 36, 82, 117, 133.

Withdrawals for ineligibility can involve a relatively large number of participants. In a trial by the Canadian Cooperative Study Group,[23] 64 of the 649 enrolled participants (10%) with stroke were later found to have been ineligible. In this four-armed study, the numbers of ineligible patients in the study groups ranged from 10 to 25. The reasons for the ineligibility of these 64 participants were not reported, nor was their outcome experience. Before cancer cooperative groups implemented phone-in or electronic eligibility checks, 10% to 20% of patients entered into a trial may have been ineligible after further review. By taking more care at the time of randomization, the number of ineligible participants was reduced to less than 5%.

A study design may require enrollment within a defined period after a qualifying episode. Because of this time constraint, data concerning participants' eligibility might not be available or confirmed when the decision is made to enroll them. For example, the Beta-Blocker Heart Attack Trial[16] looked at 2-year mortality in people administered a beta-blocking drug during hospitalization for an acute myocardial infarction. Because of known variability in interpretation, the protocol required that the diagnostic ECGs be read by a central unit. However, this verification took several weeks to accomplish. Local institutions, therefore, interpreted the ECGs and decided whether the patient met the necessary criteria for inclusion. Almost 9% of the enrolled participants did not have their myocardial infarction confirmed and were "incorrectly" randomized. The question then arises: Should the participants be kept in the trial and included in the analysis of the response variable data? The Beta-Blocker Heart Attack Trial protocol required follow-up and analysis of all randomized participants. In this case, it made no important difference. The observed benefits from the intervention were similar in those eligible and in those ineligible.

A more complicated situation occurs when the data needed for enrollment cannot be obtained until hours or days have passed, yet the study design requires initiation of intervention before then. For instance, in the Multicenter Investigation for the Limitation of Infarct Size (MILIS),[117] propranolol, hyaluronidase, or placebo was administered shortly after participants were admitted to the hospital with possible acute myocardial infarctions. In some, the diagnosis of myocardial infarction was not confirmed until after electrocardiographic and serum enzyme changes had been monitored for several days. Such participants were, therefore, randomized on the basis of a preliminary diagnosis of infarction. Subsequent testing may not have supported the initial diagnosis. Another example of this problem involves a study of pregnant women who were likely to deliver prematurely and, therefore, would have children who were at a higher-than-usual risk of being born with respiratory distress syndrome.[36] Corticosteroids administered to the mother prior to delivery were hypothesized to protect the premature child from developing respiratory distress syndrome. Although at the time of the mother's randomization to either intervention or control groups the investigators could not be sure that the delivery would be premature, they needed to decide whether to enroll the mother into the study.

To complicate matters still further, the intervention given to a participant can affect or change the entry diagnosis. For example, in the previously mentioned study to limit infarct size, some patients without a myocardial infarction were randomized because of the need to begin intervention before the diagnosis was confirmed. Moreover, if the interventions succeeded in limiting infarct size, they could have affected the ECG and serum enzyme levels. Participants in the intervention groups with a small myocardial infarction may have shown reduced serum enzyme values and appeared not to have had an infarction. Thus they would not seem to have met the entry criteria. However, this situation could not exist in the placebo group. If the investigators had withdrawn participants who did not meet the study criteria for a myocardial infarction, they would have withdrawn more participants from the intervention groups (those with no infarction plus those with small infarction) than from the control group (those with no infarction). This could have produced a bias in later comparisons. On the other hand, it could be assumed that a similar number of truly ineligible participants were randomized to the intervention groups and to the control group. To maintain comparability, the investigators might have decided to withdraw the same number of participants from each group. The ineligible participants in the control group could have been readily identified. However, the participants in the intervention groups who were truly ineligible had to be distinguished from those made to appear ineligible by the effects of the interventions. This would have been difficult, if not impossible. In the MILIS, all randomized participants were retained in the analysis.[117]

An example of possible bias because of withdrawal of ineligible participants is found in the Anturane Reinfarction Trial, which compared sulfinpyrazone with placebo in participants who had recently suffered a myocardial infarction.[5,6,133] As seen in Table 16-1, of 1629 randomized participants (813 to sulfinpyrazone and 816 to placebo), 71 were subsequently found to be ineligible. Thirty-eight had been assigned to sulfinpyrazone and 33 to placebo. Despite relatively clear definitions of eligibility and comparable numbers of participants withdrawn, mortality among these ineligible participants was 26.3% in the sulfinpyrazone group (10 of 38) and 12.1% in the placebo group (4 of 33).[133] The eligible placebo-group participants had a mortality of 10.9%, similar to the 12.1% seen among the ineligible placebo participants. In contrast, the eligible participants on sulfinpyrazone had a mortality of 8.3%, less than one third that of the ineligible sulfinpyrazone participants. Including

Table 16-1   Mortality by study group and eligibility status in the Anturane Reinfarction Trial

	Randomized	Percentage mortality	Ineligible	Percentage mortality	Eligible	Percentage mortality
Sulfinpyrazone	813	9.1	38	26.3	775	8.3
Placebo	816	10.9	33	12.1	783	10.9

all 1629 participants in the analysis gave 9.1% mortality in the sulfinpyrazone group, and 10.9% mortality in the placebo group ($p = 0.20$). Withdrawing the 71 ineligible participants (and 14 deaths, 10 vs. 4) gave an almost significant $p = 0.07$.

Stimulated by criticisms of the study, the investigators initiated a reevaluation of the Anturane Reinfarction Trial results. An independent group of reviewers examined all reports of deaths in the trial.[5] Instead of 14 deceased participants who were ineligible, it found 19; 12 in the sulfinpyrazone group and 7 in the placebo group. Thus supposedly clear criteria for ineligibility can be judged differently.

Three trial design policies that relate to withdrawals because of entry criteria violations have been discussed by Peto et al.[109] The first policy is not to enroll participants until all the diagnostic tests have been confirmed and all the entry criteria have been carefully checked. Once enrollment occurs, no withdrawals are allowed. For some studies, such as the one on limiting infarct size, this policy cannot be applied because firm diagnoses cannot be ascertained before the time when intervention has to be initiated.

The second policy is to enroll marginal or unconfirmed cases and later withdraw those participants who are proven to have been misdiagnosed. This would be allowed, however, only if the decision to withdraw is based on data collected before enrollment. The process of deciding on withdrawal of a participant from a study group should be done blinded with respect to the participant's outcome and group assignment and as soon as possible after randomization.

A third policy is to enroll some participants with unconfirmed diagnoses and to allow no withdrawals. This procedure is always valid in that investigators compare two randomized groups that are comparable at baseline. However, this policy is conservative because each group contains some participants who might not be able to benefit from intervention. Thus the overall trial may have less power to detect differences of interest.

A modification to these three policies is recommended. Every effort should be made to establish the eligibility of participants prior to any randomization. No withdrawals should be allowed, and the analyses should include all participants enrolled. Subgroup analyses based on eligibility criteria may be performed. If the analyses of data from all enrolled participants and from subgroups agree, the interpretation of the results, at least with respect to participant eligibility, is clear. If the results differ, however, investigators must be very cautious in their interpretation. In general, they should emphasize the analysis with all the enrolled participants because that analysis is always valid.

Any policy on withdrawals should be stated in the study protocol before the start of the study. The actual decision to withdraw specific participants should be done without knowledge of the study group, ideally by someone not directly involved in the trial. Of special concern is withdrawal based on review of selected cases, particularly if the decision rests on a subjective interpretation. Even in double-blind trials, blinding may not be perfect, and investigators may supply information for the eligibility review differentially depending on study group and health status. Therefore withdrawal should be done early in the course of follow-up, before a response variable has occurred, and with a minimum of data exchange between the investigator and the person making the decision to withdraw the participant. This withdrawal approach does not preclude a later challenge by readers of the report, on the basis of potential bias. It should, however, remove the concern that the withdrawal policy depended on the outcome of the trial. The withdrawal rules should not be based on knowledge of study results. Even when these guidelines are followed, if the number of entry criteria violations are substantially different in the study groups, or if the event rates in the withdrawn participants are different between the groups, the question will certainly be raised whether bias played a role in the decision to withdraw a participant.

Nonadherence

Another common reason that participants are withdrawn from the analysis is nonadherence to the prescribed intervention or control regimen.* Nonadherence refers to drop-outs and drop-ins (Chapter 13). Drop-outs are participants in intervention groups who do not continue to adhere to the regimen. Drop-ins are participants in the control arm who start to follow the treatment strategy. The decision not to adhere to the protocol intervention may be made by the participant, his primary care physician, or the trial investigator. Nonadherence may be because of adverse effects of the intervention or control, loss of participant interest, changes in the underlying condition of a participant, or a variety of other reasons.

Withdrawal from analysis of participants who do not adhere to the intervention regimens specified in the study design is often proposed. The motivation for withdrawal of nonadherent participants is that the trial is not a fair test of the ideal intervention with these participants included. For example, there may be a few participants in the intervention group who took little or no therapy. If participants do not take their medication, they certainly cannot benefit from it. There could also be participants in the control group who frequently receive the study medication. The intervention and control groups are thus "contaminated." Proponents of withdrawal of nonadhering participants argue that removal of these participants keeps the trial close to what was intended; that is, a comparison of optimal intervention vs. control. The impact of nonadherence on the trial is that any observed benefits of the intervention, as compared with the control, will be reduced, making the trial less powerful than was planned. Newcombe,[103] for example, discussed the implication of adherence for the analysis as well as design and sample size. We discussed this at length in Chapter 7.

---

*References 24, 40, 41, 49, 50, 52, 55, 78, 81, 87, 90, 99, 104, 110, 111, 113, 116, 128, 130, 137, 142.

A policy of withdrawal from analysis because of participant nonadherence can lead to bias. The overwhelming reason is that participant adherence to a protocol may be related to the intervention. In other words, there may be an interaction between adherence and intervention. Certainty, if nonadherence is greater in one group than another, then withdrawal of nonadherent participants could lead to bias. Even if the frequency of nonadherence is the same for the intervention and control groups, the reasons for nonadherence in each group may differ and involve different types of participants. The concern would always be whether the same type of participant had been withdrawn in the same proportion from each group or whether an imbalance had been created. Of course, an investigator could probably neither confirm nor refute the possibility of bias.

The Coronary Drug Project evaluated several lipid-lowering drugs in people several years after a myocardial infarction. In participants on one of the drugs, clofibrate, total 5-year mortality was 18.2%, as compared with 19.4% in control participants.[40] Among the clofibrate participants, those who had at least 80% adherence to therapy had a mortality of 15%, whereas the poor adherers had a mortality of 24.6% (Table 16-2). This seeming benefit from taking clofibrate was, unfortunately, mirrored in the group taking placebo, 15.1% vs. 28.2%. A similar pattern (Table 16-3) was noted in the Aspirin Myocardial Infarction Study.[137] Overall, no difference in mortality was seen between the aspirin-treated group (10.9%) and the placebo-treated group (9.7%). Good adherers to aspirin had a mortality of 6.1%; poor adherers had a mortality of 21.9%. In the placebo group, the rates were 5.1% and 22%.

A trial of antibiotic prophylaxis in cancer patients also demonstrated a relationship between adherence and benefit in both the intervention and placebo groups.[55] Among the participants assigned to intervention, efficacy in reducing fever or infection was 82% in excellent adherers, 64% in good adherers, and 31% in poor

Table 16-2   Percentage mortality by study group and level of adherence in the Coronary Drug Project

	Overall	Drug adherence	
		≥80%	< 80%
Clofibrate	18.2	15.0	24.6
Placebo	19.4	15.1	28.2

Table 16-3   Percentage mortality by study group and degree of adherence in the Aspirin Myocardial Infarction Study

	Overall	Good adherence	Poor adherence
Aspirin	10.9	6.1	21.9
Placebo	9.7	5.1	22.0

adherers. Among the placebo participants, the corresponding figures were 68%, 56%, and 0%.

One of the interventions in the CDP, high-dose estrogen, produced a somewhat different pattern. As Canner[24] discussed, the mortality of the participants in the placebo group who adhered to the therapy, that is, who took 80% or more of the protocol dose, was 4.8%. The mortality of the placebo participants who did not adhere was 9.9%. Both adherers and nonadherers to estrogen had similar mortality: 6.3% and 6.1%. The finding that nonadherers to placebo had a different outcome from nonadherers to active intervention (9.9% vs. 6.1%) could theoretically lead one to conclude that "it is beneficial to be randomized to the estrogen group and not take the drug."[24]

A third pattern is noted in a three-arm trial comparing two beta-blocking drugs, propranolol and atenolol, with placebo.[142] Approximately equal numbers of participants in each group stopped taking their medication. In the placebo group, adherers and nonadherers had similar mortality: 11.2% and 12.5%, respectively. Nonadherers to the interventions, however, had death rates several times greater than did the adherers: 15.9% to 3.4% in those on propranolol and 17.6% to 2.6% in those on atenolol. Thus, even though the numbers of nonadherers were similar, their characteristics were obviously different.

Pledger[111] provides an analogous example for a schizophrenia trial. Participants were randomized to chlorpromazine or placebo, and 1-year relapse rates were measured. The overall comparison was a 27.8% relapse rate on treatment to 52.8% for placebo-treated patients. Participants were categorized into low or high adherence subgroups. Among the treated participants, the relapse rate was 61.2% for low adherence and 16.8% for high adherence. However, the relapse rate was 74.7% and 28.0% for the corresponding adherence groups on placebo.

Another example of placebo adherence vs. nonadherence is provided by Oakes et al.[104] A trial of 2466 heart attack patients compared diltiazem with placebo over a period of 4 years with time to first cardiac event as the primary outcome. Cardiac death or all-cause mortality were additional outcome measures. The trial was initially analyzed according to intention-to-treat with no significant effect of treatment. Qualitative interaction effects were found with the presence or absence of pulmonary congestion that favored diltiazem for participants without pulmonary congestion and placebo in participants with pulmonary congestion. Interestingly, for participants without pulmonary congestion, the hazard ratio or relative risk for time to first cardiac event was 0.92 for those off placebo compared with those on placebo. For participants with pulmonary congestion, the hazard ratio was 2.86 for participants off placebo compared with those on placebo. For time to first cardiac death and to all-cause mortality, hazard ratios exceeded 1.68 in both pulmonary congestion subgroups. This again suggests that placebo adherence is a powerful prognostic indicator and argues for placebo controls and intention-to-treat analysis.

The definition of nonadherence can also have a major impact on the analysis. This is demonstrated by reanalysis of breast cancer patients by Redmond et al.[113] This trial compared a complex chemotherapy with placebo as adjuvant therapy following surgery with disease-free survival as the primary outcome. One analysis divided patients into good adherers (>85% of therapy), moderate adherers (65% to 84% of therapy), and poor adherers (<65% of therapy). Adherence was defined as the fraction of chemotherapy taken while on the study to what was defined by the protocol as a full course. For this definition, placebo adherers had a superior disease-free survival than moderate adherers who did better than poor adherers. (See Fig. 16-1.) This pattern of outcome in the placebo group is similar to the CDP clofibrate example. The authors[113] did a second analysis, changing the definition of adherence slightly. In this case, adherence was defined as the fraction of chemotherapy taken while on study to what should have been taken while still on study. Note that the previous definition compared chemotherapy taken with what would have been taken had the patient survived to the end and adhered perfectly. This subtle difference scrambled the order of outcome in the placebo group. Here, the poor placebo adherers had the best disease-free survival, and the best placebo adherers had a disease-free survival between the moderate and worst adherers.

Detre and Peduzzi have argued that, although as a general rule nonadherent participants should be analyzed according to the study group to which they were assigned, there can be exceptions. They present an example from the VA Coronary Bypass Surgery Trial.[49] In that trial, several participants assigned to medical intervention crossed over to surgery. Contrary to expectation, these participants were at a

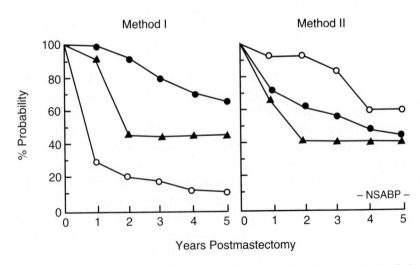

Fig. 16-1 Percentage (%) probability of disease-free survival related to dose level of placebo: methods I and II in National Surgical Adjuvant Breast Program (NSABP).

risk of having an event, after adjusting for a variety of baseline factors, similar to those who did not crossover. Therefore the authors argued that the nonadherers should be kept in their original groups but can be censored at the time of crossover. This may be true, but, as seen in the CDP,[40] adjustment for known variables does not always account for the observed response. The differences in mortality between adherers and nonadherers remained even after adjustment. Thus other unknown or unmeasured variables were of critical importance. The same may hold true for the VA trial.

It has been claimed[121] that if rules for withdrawing participants are specified in advance, withdrawals for nonadherence are legitimate. However, the potential for bias cannot be avoided simply because the investigator states, ahead of time, the intention to withdraw participants. This is true even if the investigator is blinded to the group assignment of a participant at the time of withdrawal. Participants were not withdrawn from the analyses in the above examples. However, had a rule allowing withdrawal of participants with poor adherence been specified in advance, the type of participants withdrawn would have been different in the groups. This could have resulted in the analysis of noncomparable groups of adherers. Unfortunately, as noted, the patterns of possible bias can vary and depend on the precise definition of adherence. Neither the magnitude nor direction of that bias is easily assessed or compensated for in analysis.

Adherence is also a response to the intervention. If the adherence by participants to an intervention is poor compared with that of participants in the control group, widespread use of this therapy in the study population may not be feasible. An intervention may be effective but may be of little value if it cannot be tolerated by a large portion of the participants.

It is therefore recommended that no participants be withdrawn from analysis for lack of adherence. The price an investigator must pay for this policy is possibly to reduce the power of the study because some participants who are included may not be on optimal intervention. For limited or moderate nonadherence, one can compensate for this reduced power by increasing the sample size, as discussed in Chapter 7. Increasing the sample size is costly and undesirable, but the alternative action may bias the comparison of the intervention and control in unpredictable ways.

Poor quality or missing data

Participants may be withdrawn from a trial because their data are found to be of poor quality, the extreme being missing data.*

In long-term trials, participants may be lost to follow-up. In this situation, the status of the participant with regard to many response variables cannot be determined. If mortality is the primary response variable, and if the participant fails to return to

---

*References 29, 30, 46, 53, 54, 56, 60, 72, 73, 85, 86, 88, 91, 117, 139.

the clinic, his survival status may still be obtained. If a death has occurred, the date of death can be ascertained. In the CDP,[41] where survival experience over the course of 60 months was the primary response variable, 4 of 5011 participants were lost to follow-up (one in a placebo group, three in one treatment group, and none in another treatment group). The Lipid Research Clinics Coronary Primary Prevention Trial[90] followed more than 3800 participants for an average of 7.4 years and was able to assess vital status on all. The Physicians' Health Study of more than 20,000 U.S. male physicians had complete follow-up for survival status.[132] Many other large trials, such as GUSTO,[74] have similar, nearly complete follow-up experience. Obtaining such low loss to follow-up rates, however, required special effort.

An investigator may not be able to obtain information on other response variables. This may be a problem for longitudinal studies with repeated measurements. For example, if a participant is to have blood pressure measured at the last follow-up visit 12 months after randomization and the participant does not appear, that 12-month blood pressure can never be retrieved. Even if the participant is contacted later, the later measurement may not truly represent the 12-month blood pressure. In some situations, substitutions may be permitted, but, in general, this will not be a satisfactory solution. An investigator needs to make every effort to have participants come in for their scheduled visits to keep losses to follow-up at a minimum. In the Intermittent Positive Pressure Trial (IPPB), repeated pulmonary function measurements were required for participants with chronic obstructive lung disease.[85] However, some patients who had deteriorated could not perform the required test. A similar problem existed for the MILIS study, where infarct size could not be obtained in many of the sickest patients.[117]

If the number of patients lost to follow-up is different in each of two study groups, there could be a problem in the analysis of the data. A bias could be introduced if the loss is related to the intervention. For example, participants who are taking a particular new drug that has some adverse effects may not be doing well and consequently, miss scheduled clinic visits. Events may occur and be unobserved. These losses to follow-up would probably not be the same in the control group. In this situation, there is a bias favoring the new drug. In reality, it is uncertain whether or not such a bias exists. Even if the number lost to follow-up is the same in each study group, there is still the possibility of bias. The argument that different mechanisms may be involved also applies. The participants who are lost in each group may have been quite different in their prognosis and eventual outcome.

Survival analysis methods, which are discussed in Chapter 14, consider time from initiation of intervention to response. These methods can use the experience of participants up to the time of loss to follow-up if certain conditions are met. For continuous variables, the analytical methods are not as carefully worked out. For example, an investigator may be measuring change in a variable over time. If a participant is lost to follow-up, the observed rate of change may be used to estimate the missing data. In other situations, an investigator might elect to rank the observed response variables and assign a rank to those participants with missing data. He could assign the highest rank to all such participants in the intervention group, while assigning the lowest ranks to those in the control group. Then he could analyze the ranked response variable data. Next, the way in which the investigator assigned highest and lowest ranks could be reversed and the analysis repeated. If the results are consistent, there would be some assurance that the lost information did not have any effect on the overall study conclusions. If the results are inconsistent, the investigator would have to be more cautious in his interpretation. Since losses to follow-up can lead to bias and can complicate the analyses, every effort should be made to keep them to a minimum.

If participants do not adhere to therapy and also do not return for follow-up visits, the primary outcome measured may not be obtained unless the outcome is survival or some easily ascertained event. In this situation, a true "intent-to-treat" analysis is not feasible. Pledger[111] recommends a "last observation carried forward" analysis, also known as an "endpoint" analysis. In these situations, no analysis is fully satisfactory. The best that can be offered is a series of analyses, each exploring different approaches to the problem. If all, or most, are in general agreement qualitatively, then the results are more persuasive. All analyses should be presented, not just the one with the preferred results.

Various other methods for imputation of missing values have been described.* Examples of some of these methods are given by Espeland et al.[60] for a trial measuring carotid artery thickness at multiple anatomical sites using ultrasonography. In trials of this type, typically not all measurements can be made. Several imputation methods are based on a mixed effects linear model where the regression coefficient and a covariance (i.e., variances and correlations) structure are estimated. Once these are known, this regression equation is the basis for the imputation. Several imputation strategies were used based on different methods of estimating the parameters and whether intervention differences were assumed or not. Most of the imputation strategies gave similar results when the trial data were analyzed. The results indicated up to a 20% increase in efficiency compared with just using averages from data that are available.

Techniques such as this are useful if the data are missing at random; that is, the probability of missing data is not dependent on the measurement that would have been observed.[88] Missing completely at random means that the probability of missing data also does not depend on the preceding measurement. If data are missing at the end of an observation period and are not missing at random, the censoring of the data may in fact be informative. This idea is discussed in a later section.

An outlier is an extreme value significantly different from the remaining values. The concern is whether extreme values in the sample should be excluded from the

---

*References 46, 56, 60, 72, 85, 88, 91, 139.

analysis. This question may apply to a laboratory result, to the data from one of several wards in a hospital, or from a clinic in a multicenter trial. Removing outliers is not recommended unless the data can be clearly shown to be erroneous. Even though a value may be an outlier, it could be correct, indicating that on occasion an extreme result is possible. This fact could be important and should not be ignored by eliminating the outlier. Kruskall[86] suggests carrying out an analysis with and without the "wild observation." If the conclusions vary depending on whether the outlier values are included or excluded, one should view any conclusions cautiously. Procedures for detecting extreme observations have been discussed,[29,30,53,54,73] and the publications cited can be consulted for further details.

An interesting example given by Canner et al.[29] concerns the CDP. The authors plotted the distributions of four response variables for each of the 53 clinics in that multicenter trial. Using total mortality as the response variable, no clinics were outlying. When nonfatal myocardial infarction was the outcome, only one clinic was an outlier. With congestive heart failure and angina pectoris, response variables that are probably less well defined, there were nine and eight outlying clinics, respectively.

As indicated previously, data may be missing in a longitudinal study, but the missing information may not have occurred in a random manner. Individuals with chronic obstructive lung disease typically decline in their pulmonary function, and this decline may lead to death. Some participants in the IPPB trial with substantial or rapid decline were not able to have their lung function determined since they were unable to perform the necessary tests.[85] Some patients died because of the decline. In this case, the missing data are not missing at random, and this censoring of the data is said to be informative. One simple method for such cases as the IPPB study is to define a performance level considered to be a clinical event. Then the analysis can be based on time to the clinical event or death, incorporating both pieces of information. Survival analysis, for example, assumes that loss of follow-up is random and independent of risk of the event. Methods have been proposed for the analysis of such data[145,146] but require strong assumptions, and the details are beyond the scope of this text.

Competing events

Competing events may preclude the assessment of the primary response variable. They can reduce the power of the trial by decreasing the number of participants available for follow-up. If the intervention can affect the competing event, there is also the risk of bias. In some clinical trials, the primary response variable may be cause-specific mortality, such as death because of myocardial infarction or sudden death, rather than total mortality. The reason for using cause-specific death as a response variable is that a therapy often has specific mechanisms of action that are effective against a disease or condition. In this situation, measuring death from all causes, most of which are not likely to be affected by the intervention, can dilute the results. For example, a study drug may be antiarrhythmic, and thus sudden car-diac death might be the selected response variable. Other causes of death would be competing events.

Even if the response variable is not cause-specific mortality, death may be a fac-tor in the analysis. This is particularly a problem in long-term trials in the elderly or high-risk populations. If a participant dies, the measurements that would have been obtained are missing. Analysis of nonfatal response variable data on surviving partici-pants has the potential for bias, especially if the mortality rates are different in the two groups.

In a study with cause-specific death as the primary response variable, deaths from other causes are treated statistically as though the participants were lost to fol-low-up from the time of death (Chapter 14), and these deaths are not counted in the analysis. In this situation, the analysis, however, must go beyond merely examining the primary response variable. An intervention may or may not be effective in treat-ing the condition of interest but could be harmful in other respects. Therefore total mortality should be considered as well as the cause-specific fatal event. Similar considerations need to be made when death occurs in studies using nonfatal pri-mary response variables. This argument is more than theoretical. The Coronary Pri-mary Prevention Trial[90] demonstrated a reduction in coronary heart disease mortality and morbidity in participants with elevated cholesterol who were taking the lipid-lowering drug cholestyramine. Total mortality, however, was almost identical in the intervention and placebo control groups. This was because of a larger number of deaths from violent causes in the intervention group. As there was no good explana-tion for this, the investigators attributed it to chance. This may well be the case. However, the same pattern of increased noncardiac mortality appears in other trials of lipid-lowering regimens, including diet.[98]

No completely satisfactory solution exists for handling competing events. At the very least, the investigator should report all major outcome categories, such as total mortality, cause-specific mortality, and morbid events.

COVARIATE ADJUSTMENT

The goal in a clinical trial is to have groups of participants that are comparable except for the intervention being studied. Even if randomization is used, all of the prog-nostic factors may not be perfectly balanced, especially in smaller studies. Even if no prognostic factors are significantly imbalanced in the statistical sense, an investigator may, nevertheless, observe that one or more factors favor one of the groups. In either case, covariate adjustment can be used in the analysis to minimize the effect of the dif-ferences. Covariance analysis for clinical trials has been covered in numerous articles.*

---

*References 1, 3, 9, 13, 22, 25, 27, 28, 42, 43, 57, 58, 67, 100, 106, 118–120, 124, 134, 140, 147.

Adjustment also reduces the variance in the test statistic. If the covariates are highly correlated with outcome, this can produce a more sensitive analysis. The specific adjustment procedure depends on the type of covariate being adjusted for and the type of response variable being analyzed. If a covariate is discrete, or if a continuous variable is converted into intervals and made discreet, the analysis is sometimes referred to as "stratified." A stratified analysis, in general terms, means that the study participants are subdivided into smaller, more homogenous groups, or strata. A comparison is made within each stratum and then averaged over all strata to achieve a summary result for the response variable. This summary result is adjusted for group imbalances in the discrete covariate. If a response variable is discrete, such as the occurrence of an event, the stratified analysis might take the form of a Mantel-Haenszel statistic,[92] described briefly in the appendix to this chapter. Bishop et al.[17] discuss analysis of discrete data in detail.

If the response variable is continuous, the stratified analysis is referred to as analysis of covariance. This uses a model that, typically, is linear in the covariates. A simple example for a response Y and covariate X would be $Y = \alpha_j + \beta(X - \mu) + error$ where β is a coefficient representing the importance of the covariate X and is assumed to be the same in each group, μ is the mean value of X, and α_j is a parameter for the contribution of the overall response variable in the jth group (e.g., $j = 1$ or 2). The basic idea is to adjust the response variable Y for any differences in the covariate X between the two groups. Under appropriate assumptions, the advantage of this method is that the continuous covariate X does not have to be divided into categories. Further details concerning the use of this methodology can be found in statistics textbooks.* If time to an event is the primary response variable, then survival analysis methods are used (Chapter 14). These methods allow for adjustments of discrete or continuous covariates (e.g., Thall and Lachin[134]). However, whenever models are employed, the investigator must be careful to evaluate the assumptions required and how close the data meet those criteria. Analysis of covariance can be attractive, but also abused if a linearity is assumed when the data are nonlinear, if the response curves in the intervention and control groups are not parallel, or if assumptions of normality are not met.[58] Another issue is that if the measurement error in covariates is substantial, the lack of precision can be increased.[100]

Regardless of adjustment procedure, covariates should be measured at baseline. Except for certain factors such as age, sex, or race, any variables that are evaluated after initiation of intervention should be considered as response variables. Group comparisons of the primary response variable, adjusted for other response variables, are discouraged. Interpretation of such analyses is difficult because group comparability may be lost.

---

*References 8, 19, 20, 39, 61, 79, 114, 144.

Surrogates as a Covariate

As discussed earlier, adherence is also a response variable. Adjusting for adherence can lead to misinterpretation of results. Sometimes, adjustment in analysis for adherence may not be obvious.

In a trial of clofibrate,[115] the authors reported that those participants who had the largest reduction in serum cholesterol had the greatest clinical improvement. However, reduction in cholesterol is probably highly correlated with adherence to the intervention regimen. Because adherers in one group may be different from adherers in another group, analyses that adjust for adherence can be biased. This issue was addressed in the Coronary Drug Project.[40] Adjusted for baseline factors, the five-year mortality was 18.8% in the clofibrate group (N = 997) and 20.2% in the placebo group (N = 2535), an insignificant difference. For participants with baseline serum cholesterol greater than or equal to 250 mg/dl, the mortality was 17.5% and 20.6% in the clofibrate and placebo groups, respectively. No difference in mortality between the groups was noted for participants with baseline cholesterol of less than 250 mg/dl (20.0% vs. 19.9%). Those participants with lower baseline cholesterol in the clofibrate group who had a reduction in cholesterol during the trial had a 16.0% mortality, as opposed to a 25.5% mortality for those with a rise in cholesterol (Table 16-4). This would fit the hypothesis that lowering cholesterol is beneficial. However, in those participants with high baseline cholesterol, the situation was reversed. An 18.1% mortality was seen in those who had a fall in cholesterol, and a 15.5% mortality was noted in those who had a rise in cholesterol. The best outcome, therefore, appeared to be in participants receiving clofibrate whose low baseline cholesterol dropped or whose high baseline cholesterol increased. Lack of knowledge about why some people comply or respond to intervention while others do not makes this sort of analysis vulnerable to misinterpretation and bias.

Modeling the impact of adherence on a risk factor and thus on the response has also received attention.[1,57] Regression models have been proposed that attempt to adjust response variable outcome for the amount of risk factor change that could have been attained with optimum adherence. One example of this is provided by Efron and Feldman[57] for a lipid research study. However, Alberts and DeMets[1] show that these models are very sensitive to assumptions about the independence of adherence and health status or response. If these assumptions using these regression models are violated, uninterpretable results emerge, such as that for the clofibrate serum cholesterol example described earlier.

Clinical trials of cancer treatment commonly analyze results by comparing responders with nonresponders.[99,128] That is, those who go into remission or have a reduction in tumor size are compared with those who do not. One survey indicates that such analyses had been done in at least 20% of published reports.[140] The authors of the survey argue that statistical problems, because of lack of random assignment,

Table 16-4   Percentage 5-year mortality in the clofibrate group, by baseline cholesterol and change in cholesterol in the Coronary Drug Project

	Baseline cholesterol	
	< 250 mg/dL	≥ 250 mg/dL
Total	20.0	17.5
Fall in cholesterol	16.0	18.1
Rise in cholesterol	25.5	15.5

and methodologic problems, caused by both classification of response and inherent differences between responders and nonresponders, can occur. These will often lead to misinterpretation of the study results. Anderson et al.[3] provide an example of the bias that can accompany such analyses. They point out that participants "who eventually become responders must survive long enough to be evaluated as responders." This factor can invalidate some statistical tests that compare responders with nonresponders. The authors present two statistical tests that avoid bias. They note, though, that even if the tests indicate a significant difference in survival between responders and nonresponders, one cannot conclude that increased survival is because of tumor response. Thus aggressive intervention, which may be associated with better response, cannot be assumed to be better than less intensive intervention, which may be associated with poorer response. Anderson et al. state that only a truly randomized comparison can say which intervention method is preferable. What is unsaid, and illustrated by the CDP examples, is that even comparison of good responders in the intervention group with good responders in the control can be misleading, because there may be different reasons for good response.

Morgan[99] provides another related example of comparing duration of response in cancer patients, where duration of response is the time from a favorable response such as tumor regression (partial or total) to remission. This is another form of defining a subgroup of posttreatment outcome, that is, tumor response. In a trial comparing two complex chemotherapy regimens (*A* vs. *B*) in small cell lung cancer, the response rates were 64% and 85% with median duration of 245 and 262 days, respectively. When only responders were analyzed, a slight imbalance in prognostic factors was dramatically increased. Extensive disease was evident at baseline in 48% and 21% of the two treatment responder groups. The author[99] points out that while it may be theoretically possible to adjust for prognostic factors, in practice such adjustment may decrease bias but will not eliminate it. Not all prognostic factors are known.

The Cox proportional hazards regression model for the analysis of survival data (Chapter 14) allows for covariates in the regression to vary with time.[42] This has been suggested as a way to adjust for factors such as adherence and level of response. It should be pointed out that this and simple regression models are vulnerable to the same biases described earlier in this chapter. For example, if cholesterol level and cholesterol reduction in the CDP example were used as time-dependent covariates in the Cox model, the estimator of treatment effect would be biased because of the effects shown in Table 16-4.

Rosenbaum[120] provides a nice overview of adjustment for concomitant variables that have been affected by treatment in both observational and randomized studies. He states that "adjustments for posttreatment concomitant variables should be avoided when estimating treatment effects except in rather special circumstances, since adjustments themselves can introduce a bias where none existed previously."

Several additional methodologic attempts to adjust for nonadherence have also been conducted.[87,118,119,130] Newcombe,[103] for example, suggests adjusting estimates of treatment effect on the extent of nonadherence. Robins[118,119] proposes a causal inference model. Lagakos et al.[87] evaluated censoring survival time, or time to an event, at the time point when intervention is terminated. The rationale is that participants are no longer able to completely benefit from the intervention. However, the hazard ratio estimated by this approach is not the hazard that would have been estimated if participants had not terminated intervention.

Baseline variables as covariates

The issue of stratification was first raised in the discussion of randomization (Chapter 5). For large studies, the recommendation is that stratified randomization is usually unnecessary because overall balance would nearly always be achieved and that stratification would be possible in the analysis. For smaller studies, baseline adaptive methods could be considered, but the analysis should include the covariates used in the randomization. In a strict sense, analysis should always be stratified if stratification was used in the randomization. In such cases, the adjusted analysis should include not only those covariates found to be different between the groups, but also those stratified during randomization. Of course, if no stratification is done at randomization, the final analysis is less complicated because it would involve only those covariates that turn out to be imbalanced or to be of special interest.

As stated in Chapter 5, randomization tends to produce comparable groups for both measured and unmeasured baseline covariates. However, not all baseline covariates will be closely matched. Adjusting treatment effect for these baseline disparities continues to be debated. Canner[28] describes two points of view, one that argues that "if done at all, analyses should probably be limited to covariates for which there is a disparity between the treatment groups and that the unadjusted measure is to be preferred." The other view is "to adjust on only a few factors that were known from previous experience to be predictive." Canner[25,28] and Beach and Meier[13] indicate that even for moderate disparity in baseline comparability, or even if the covariates are moderately predictive, it is possible for covariate adjustment to have a nontrivial impact on the measure of intervention effect. However, Canner[28] also points out that it is "often possible to select specific covariates out of a large set in order to achieve a desired result." In addition, Canner[28] shows that this issue is true for both small and large studies. For this reason, it is critical that the process for selecting covariates to be used in the adjustment be specified in the protocol and adhered to in the primary analyses. Other adjustments may be used in the exploratory analyses.

Another issue is testing for covariate interaction in a clinical trial.[22,27,67,107,124] Intervention-covariate interaction is defined when the response to intervention varies according to the value of the covariate.[22] Peto[107] defines intervention-covariate interactions as quantitative or qualitative. Quantitative interactions indicate that the magnitude of intervention effect varies with the covariate. Qualitative interaction involves a change of direction in treatment effect as the covariate changes in value. This is indicated in Fig. 16-2. A qualitative interaction would exist if the benefit of

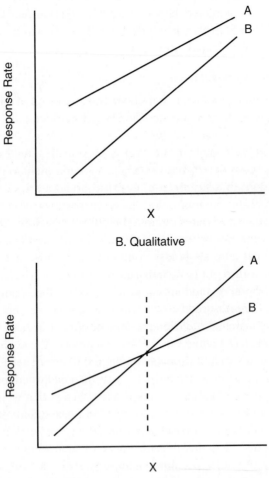

B. Qualitative

Fig. 16-2 Two types of intervention-covariate interactions (see text for explanation).

intervention for blood pressure on mortality varied in degree by the level of baseline blood pressure. Quantitative interaction would exist if lowering blood pressure was beneficial for severe hypertension, but harmful for mild hypertension. Intervention effect will vary by chance across levels of the covariate, even changing direction, so considerable caution must be taken in the interpretation. One can test formally for interaction, but requiring a significant interaction test is much more cautious than reviewing the magnitude of intervention effect within each subgroup. Byar[22] presents a nice example, shown in Table 16-5. Two interventions, A and B, are being compared by the intervention difference in mean response, $Y = \bar{X}_A - \bar{X}_B$, and S is the standard error of Y. In the upper panel, the interaction test is not significant, but examination of the subgroups is highly suggestive of interaction. The lower panel is more convincing for interaction, but we still need to examine each subgroup to understand what is going on.

Methods have been proposed for testing for overall interactions. However, Byar's[22] concluding remarks are noteworthy:

"one should look for treatment-covariate interactions, but, because of the play of chance in multiple comparisons, one should look very cautiously in the spirit of exploratory data analysis rather than that of formal hypothesis testing. Although the newer statistical methods may help decide whether the data suffice to support a claim of qualitative interactions and permit a more precise determination of reasonable p values, it seems to me unlikely that these methods will ever be as reliable a guide to sensible interpretation of data as will medical plausibility and replication of the findings in other studies. We are often warned to specify the interactions we want to test in advance in order to minimize the multiple comparisons problem, but this is often impossible in practice and in any case would be of no help in evaluating unexpected new findings. The best advice remains to look for treatment-covariate interactions but to report them sceptically as hypotheses to be investigated in other studies."

Table 16-5   Examples of apparent treatment-covariate interactions.[22] (Let $Y = \bar{X}_A - \bar{X}_B$.)

	Statistic	SE of Y	p value (2 tail)
Unconvincing			
Overall test	$Y = 2S$	S	0.045
Subsets	$Y_1 = 3S$	$S\sqrt{2}$	0.034
	$Y_2 = 1S$	$S\sqrt{2}$	0.480
Interaction	$Y_1 - Y_2 = 2S$	$2S$	0.317
More convincing			
Overall test	$Y = 2S$	S	0.045
Subsets	$Y_1 = 4S$	$S\sqrt{2}$	0.005
	$Y_2 = 0$	$S\sqrt{2}$	1.000
Interaction	$Y_1 - Y_2 = 4S$	$2S$	0.045

As indicated in Chapter 5, the randomization in multicenter trials should be stratified by clinic. The analysis of such a study should, strictly speaking, incorporate the clinic as a stratification variable. Furthermore, the randomization should be blocked to achieve balance over time in the number of participants randomized to each group. These "blocks" are also strata and, ideally, should be included in the analysis as a covariate. However, there could be a large number of strata, since there may be many clinics and the blocking factor within any clinic is usually anywhere from four to eight participants. Use of these blocking covariates is probably not necessary in the analysis. Some efficiency will be lost for the sake of simplicity, but the sacrifice should be small.

As Fleiss[62] describes, clinics differ in their demography of participants, medical practice, and adherence to all aspects of the protocol. These factors are likely to lead to variation in intervention response from clinic to clinic. In the Beta-Blocker Heart Attack Trial (BHAT),[16] most, but not all, of the 30 clinics showed a mortality benefit from propranolol. A few indicated a negative trend. In the Aspirin Myocardial Infarction Study,[9] a few clinics indicated a benefit to aspirin usage in preventing heart attacks, although most clinics indicated little or no benefit. Most analyses reported probably do not stratify by clinic, but simply lump together all the clinic's results. However, at least one of the primary analyses should average within-clinic differences, an analysis that is always valid, even in the presence of clinic-intervention interaction.[124]

SUBGROUP ANALYSES

While covariance or stratified analysis adjusts the overall comparison of main outcomes for baseline variables, another common analysis technique is to subdivide or subgroup the enrolled participants.* Here the investigator looks specifically at the intervention-control comparison within one or more particular subgroups rather than the overall comparison. One of the most frequently asked questions during the design of a trial or at the time of analysis is, "Among which group of participants is the intervention most beneficial or harmful?" It is important that subgroups be examined. Clinical trials require considerable time and effort to conduct, and the resulting data deserve maximum evaluation. The hope is to refine the primary hypothesis and specify to whom, if anyone, the intervention should be recommended. Nevertheless, care must be exercised in the interpretation of subgroup findings. As discussed earlier in this chapter, categorization of participants by any outcome variable, such as adherence, can lead to biased conclusions. Only baseline factors are appropriate for use in defining subgroups.

Subgroups may be identified in several ways that affect the strength of their results.[83] First, subgroup hypotheses may be specified in the study protocol. Because these are defined in advance, they have the greatest credibility. There is likely to be,

---

*References 4, 64, 65, 83, 84, 89, 102, 126.

however, low power for detecting differences in these subgroups. Therefore investigators should not pay as much attention to statistical significance for subgroup questions as they do for the primary question. Recognizing the low chance of seeing significant differences, descriptions of subgroup effects are often qualitative. On the other hand, testing several questions can increase the chance of a type-I error. Therefore, if one were to perform tests of significance on a large number of subgroup analyses, there will be an increased probability of false-positive results unless adjustments are made.

Some subgroups may be implied but may not be explicitly stated in the protocol. For example, if randomization is stratified by age, sex, or stage of disease, it might be reasonable to infer that subgroup hypotheses related to those factors were in fact considered in advance. Of course, the same problems in interpretation apply here as with prespecified subgroups.

A third type of analysis concerns subgroups identified by other, similar trials. If one study reports that the observed difference between intervention and control appears to be concentrated in a particular subgroup of participants, it is appropriate to see if the same findings occur in another trial, even though that subgroup was not specified in advance. Problems here include comparability of definition. It is unusual for different trials to have baseline information sufficiently similar to allow for characterization of identical subgroups.

On occasion, during the monitoring of a trial, particular subgroup findings may emerge and be of special interest. If additional participants remain to be enrolled into the trial, one approach is to test the new subgroup hypothesis in the later participants. With small numbers of participants, it is unlikely that significant differences will be noted. If, however, the same pattern emerges in the newly created subgroup, the hypothesis is considerably strengthened.

The weakest type of subgrouping involves post hoc analysis, sometimes referred to as "data-dredging" or "fishing." Such analysis is suggested by the data themselves.[51,75,85] Because many comparisons are theoretically possible, tests of significance become difficult to interpret and should be challenged. Such analyses should serve primarily to generate hypotheses for evaluation in other studies. An example of subgrouping that was challenged is in a study of diabetes in Iceland. In this study, male children under the age of 14 and born in October were claimed to be at highest risk. Gouldic[71] challenged whether the month of October was victimized by poststudy analyses biased by knowledge of the results. Peto et al.[85] point out a spurious significant subgroup, suggesting the treatment benefit was primarily in patients born in a specific time period or astrologic sign. Another similar example[51] suggests twice as many patients with bronchial carcinoma were born in March ($p < 0.01$), although this observation could not be reproduced in other studies.[11,44]

Several trials of beta-blocking drugs have been conducted in people with myocardial infarction. One found that the observed benefit was restricted to participants with anterior infarctions.[102] Another claimed improvement only in participants

65 years or younger.[4] In the Beta-Blocker Heart Attack Trial, it was observed that the greatest relative benefit of the intervention was in participants with complications during the infarction.[65] These subgroup findings, however, have not been consistently confirmed in other studies.

Regardless of how subgroups are selected, several factors can provide supporting evidence for the validity of the findings. As mentioned, similar results obtained in several studies strengthen interpretation. Internal consistency within a study is also a factor. If the same subgroup results are observed at most of the sites of a multicenter trial, they are more likely to be true. Plausible, post hoc biologic explanations for the findings, while necessary, are not sufficient. Given almost any outcome, reasonable-sounding explanations can be put forward.

Often, attention is focused on subgroups with the largest intervention-control differences. However, even with only a few subgroups, the likelihood of large but spurious differences in effects of intervention between the most extreme subgroup outcomes can be considerable.[64,83,101,126] Because large, random differences can occur, subgroup findings may easily be overinterpreted. Peto has argued that observed quantitative differences in outcome between various subgroups are to be expected, and they do not imply that the effect of intervention is truly dissimilar.[107]

It has also been suggested that, unless the main overall comparison for the trial is significant, investigators should be particularly conservative in evaluating significant subgroup findings.[109,126] Lee et al. conducted a simulated randomized trial in which participants were randomly allocated to two groups, although no intervention was initiated.[89] Despite the expected lack of overall difference, a subgroup was found that showed a significant difference.

In summary, subgroup analyses are important. However, they must be done and interpreted cautiously.

NOT COUNTING SOME OUTCOME EVENTS

In some prevention trials, the temptation is not to count outcome events that are observed in the early follow-up period. The rationale given for this practice is that these events must have occurred before entry into the trial, but were not detected. For example, if a cancer-prevention trial randomized participants into a vitamin vs. placebo trial, any immediate postrandomization cancer events could not have been prevented since the cancer had to have already been present at entry. Since the intervention could not have prevented these events, their inclusion in the analysis only dilutes the results and decreases power. While such an argument has some appeal, it must be viewed with caution. Rarely are mechanisms of action of therapies or interventions fully understood. More important, any early negative impact of an intervention might be missed if early-outcome events are not counted.

An extreme case of dropping early events might be in a surgical or procedure trial. Participants might be at higher risk of a fatal or irreversible event during the procedure. For example, in a coronary bypass trial, death or nonfatal myocardial infarction during or shortly after surgery should not be eliminated from the analysis. These risks to the patient are part of the overall intervention effect.

Some trials have defined various counting rules for events once participants have dropped out of the study or reached some level of nonadherence. For example, the Anturane Reinfarction Trial[6] suggested that no events after 7 days off intervention should be counted. It is not clear what length of time, if any, is appropriate to eliminate events to avoid bias. For example, if a participant with an acute disease continues to decline and is removed from therapy, bias could be introduced if the therapy itself is contributing to the decline because of adverse effects and toxicity.

In general, just as all participants are included in the analyses, it is greatly preferable to include all events. If the approach of not counting some outcome events is used at all, it should be used rarely, and the data should be presented in both ways.

COMPARISON OF MULTIPLE VARIABLES

If many significance tests are done, some of them may be significant by chance alone. This issue of multiple comparisons includes repeated looks at the same response variable (Chapter 15) and comparisons of multiple variables. Many clinical trials have more than one response variable, and certainly several baseline variables are measured. Thus several statistical comparisons are likely to be made. These would include testing for differences in entry characteristics to establish baseline comparability and subgroup analyses. For example, if an investigator has 100 independent comparisons, five of them, on the average, will be significantly different by chance alone if the 0.05 level of significance is used. The implication of this is that the investigator should be cautious in the interpretation of results if making multiple comparisons. The alternative is to require a more conservative significance level. As noted before, lowering the significance level will reduce the power of a trial. The issue of multiple comparisons has been discussed by Miller,[97] who reviewed many proposed approaches, and Tukey.[136]

One way to counter the problem is to increase the sample size so that a smaller significance level can be used while maintaining the power of the trial. However, in practice, most investigators could probably not afford to enroll the number of participants required to compensate for all the possible comparisons that might be made. As an approximation, if investigators are making k comparisons, each comparison should be made at the significance level α/k. Thus, for $k = 10$ and $\alpha = 0.05$, each test would need to be significant at the 0.005 level. Sample size calculations involving a significance level of 0.005 will dramatically increase the required number of participants. Therefore it is more reasonable to calculate sample size based on one primary response variable comparison and be cautious in claiming significant results for other comparisons.

It is important to evaluate the consistency of the results qualitatively and not stretch formal statistical analysis too far. Most formal comparisons should be stated in advance. Beyond that, one engages in exploratory data analysis to generate ideas for subsequent testing.

USE OF CUTPOINTS

Splitting continuous variables into two categories, for example, by using an arbitrary "cutpoint," is often done in data analysis. This can be misleading, especially if the cutpoint is suggested by the data. As an example, consider the constructed data set the Table 16-6. Heart rate, in beats per minute, was measured before intervention in two groups of 25 participants each. After therapies A and B were administered, the heart rate was again measured. The average changes between groups A and B are not sufficiently different from each other ($p = 0.75$) using a standard t-test. However, if these same data are analyzed by splitting the participants into responders and nonresponders, according to the magnitude of heart-rate reduction, the results can be made to vary. Table 16-7 shows three such possibilities, using reductions of seven, five, and three beats per minute as definitions of response. As indicated, the significance levels, using a chi-square test or Fisher's exact test, change from not significant to significant and back to not significant. This created example suggests that by manipulating the cutpoint, one can observe a significance level less than 0.05 when there does not really seem to be a difference.

In an attempt to understand the mechanisms of action of an intervention, investigators frequently want to compare participants from two groups who experience the same event. Sometimes this retrospective look can suggest factors or variables by which the participants could be subgrouped. If some subgroup is suggested, the investigator should create that subgroup in each study group and make the appropriate comparison. For example, participants in the intervention group who died may be older than those in the control group who died. This retrospective observation might suggest that age is a factor to consider. The appropriate way to test this hypothesis would be to subgroup all participants by age and compare intervention vs. control for each age subgroup.

META-ANALYSIS OF MULTIPLE STUDIES

Often in an area of clinical research, several independent trials are conducted over a period of years. Some of these trials may be large multicenter trials. Other trials may be small, too small to be conclusive on their own, but may have served as a pilot for a larger subsequent study. Regardless of the origins, investigators from a

Table 16-6   Differences in pretherapy and posttherapy heart rate, in beats per minute (HR), for groups *A* and *B*, with 25 participants each

Observation number	A				B		
	Pre-HR	Post-HR	Change in HR		Pre-HR	Post-HR	Change in HR
1	72	72	0		72	70	2
2	74	73	1		71	68	-3
3	77	71	6		75	74	1
4	73	78	-5		74	71	3
5	70	66	4		71	73	-2
6	72	76	-4		73	78	-5
7	72	72	0		71	69	2
8	78	76	2		70	74	-4
9	72	80	-8		79	78	1
10	78	71	7		71	72	-1
11	76	70	6		78	79	-1
12	73	77	-4		72	75	-3
13	77	75	2		73	72	1
14	73	79	-6		72	69	3
15	76	76	0		77	74	3
16	74	76	-2		79	75	4
17	71	69	2		77	75	2
18	72	71	1		75	75	0
19	68	72	-4		71	70	1
20	78	75	3		78	74	4
21	76	76	0		75	80	-5
22	70	63	7		71	72	-1
23	76	70	6		77	77	0
24	78	73	5		79	76	3
25	73	73	0		79	79	0
Mean	73.96	73.2	0.76		74.40	73.96	0.44
Standard deviation	2.88	3.96	4.24		3.18	3.38	2.66

Table 16-7   Comparison of change in heart rate in group *A* vs. *B* by three choices of cutpoints

Beats/min	< 7	≥ 7		< 5	≥ 5		< 3	≥3
Group *A*	25	2		19	6		17	8
Group *B*	25	0		25	0		18	7
Chi-square	$p = 0.15$			$p = 0.009$			$p = 0.76$	
Fisher's exact	$p = 0.49$			$p = 0.022$			$p = 0.99$	

variety of medical disciplines often feel compelled to review the cumulative data from studies involving similar participants and similar intervention strategies to reach a consensus on the overall results.* If this overview is performed by a formal process and with statistical methods for combining all the data in a single analysis, the analysis, it is usually referred to as meta-analysis. While this has been called a new technique,[2] the methods often used are not new.[45] In fact, they were essentially described in 1954 by Cochran[35] and later by Mantel and Haenszel.[92]

Rationale and issues

There are several reasons for conducting an overview or meta-analysis.[†] Probably the most common reason is to obtain more precise estimates of intervention effect and to strengthen the power to observe small, but clinically important, intervention effects. A closely related reason is to evaluate the generalizability of the results across trials, populations, and specific interventions. Subgroup analyses within a trial are often based on too few participants to be definitive or identify qualitative differences in intervention effect. Many are also post hoc and thus unreliable because of both multiplicity of testing and data exploration. However, meta-analysis offers the opportunity to test a limited number of prespecified hypotheses often of interest in planning subsequent trials. If a major clinical trial is being designed, a sensible approach is to base many aspects of the design on the summary of all existing data. This would include definition of population and intervention, control group response rates, expected size of intervention effect, and length of follow-up. Use of meta-analysis is a systematic process to provide this critical information. If a new intervention gains widespread popularity early in its use, a meta-analysis of small trials may provide a balanced perspective, perhaps suggesting the need for a single large properly designed clinical trial to provide a more definitive result. Alternatively, overviews or meta-analyses are of critical importance if the opportunity to conduct a new study no longer exists because of a loss of equipoise, even if this loss is not well justified. In this case, a meta-analysis may be the only solution to try to salvage the most reliable consensus. Another goal of meta-analysis of subgroups is to guide clinicians in their practice in selecting suitable participants for the intervention. Many submissions to the FDA now include a meta-analysis as part of the analysis report.

As indicated, a meta-analysis is the combination of results from similar participants evaluated by similar protocols and receiving similar interventions. The ideal meta-analysis is the standard analysis of a large multicenter trial, stratified by clinical center. Each center plays the role of a small study. Protocols and intervention strategies are identical, and participants are more similar compared with a typical collection of trials. Meta-analysis should never be an excuse for medical research to con-

*References 2, 12, 21, 26, 34, 38, 48, 59, 69, 80, 94-96, 105, 108, 122, 131, 138, 149, 150.
†References 33, 35, 37, 45, 66, 76, 108, 143, 148.

duct numerous small studies, loosely connected, with the expectation that meta-analysis will rescue the definitive result from chaos.

The ideal meta-analysis is the large multicenter trial because this concept focuses on some of the limitations of the typical meta-analysis.[66] While differences exist in the implementation of a clinical protocol across centers, these differences are less than for a collection of independently conducted large or small trials. Typically in meta-analysis, nontrival differences exist in actual intervention, study population, length of follow-up, measures of response, and quality of data.[33] With these and other potential differences, the decision as to which studies are similar enough to justify combining their data represents a challenge.

Many support the concept that the most valid overview or meta-analysis requires all studies conducted be available for inclusion or at least for consideration.[37,108] Furberg[63] provides a review of seven meta-analyses of lipid-lowering trials. Each article presents different inclusion criteria, such as the minimum number of participants or the degree of cholesterol reduction. The results among these metanalyses vary depending on the criteria used. As in a clinical trial protocol, the questions and the criteria should be stated in advance.[33] While it is difficult to decide what similar might mean, a further serious complication is that all trials conducted may not be readily accessible in the literature because of publication bias.[14,125] Not all trials that are started are completed and published. The problem is that trials published are more likely to be positive ($p < 0.05$) or favorable. Trials that are indifferent are not as likely to be published. One unpublished example described by Furberg and Morgan[66] even shows the intervention to be harmful. A study[129] of users of propranolol in patients after a heart attack reported 7 of 45 patients died in the hospital compared with 17 of 46 patients in a matched group of non-users. Controversy over design limitations caused the investigator to conduct two randomized trials, but neither were ever publisheddue to disappointing results. As a further complication, Chalmers et al.[32] point out that a MEDLINE literature search may find only 30% to 60% of published trials. This is due in part to the way results are presented and the way key words are listed.

Investigator bias may determine what response variables get reported in the literature. If protocols were adhered to strictly, investigator bias may not be a problem. However, repeated testing, multiple subgroups, and multiple response variables may not be easy to detect from the published report.[66] Early promising results may draw major attention, but if later results show diminished intervention effects, they may go unnoticed or be harder to find. Much time and persistence are required to get access to all known conducted trials and accurately extract the relevant data. Not all meta-analyses are conducted with the same degree of thoroughness.* Furthermore, authors of overviews are also subject to investigator bias. That is, unless the goals of the meta-analysis are clearly stated a priori, a positive result can be found in this

---

*References 10, 14, 32, 33, 37, 63, 66, 76, 77, 125, 127, 129, 143, 148.

analysis by undertaking numerous attempts. In fact, data dredging for large studies is more likely to find at least one positive result than for a single small study.

The medical literature is filled with meta-analysis of trials covering a wide range of disciplines. Chalmers et al.[34] reviewed the use of anticoagulants in heart attack patients to reduce mortality in six small studies. While only one of the six was individually significant, the combined overall results suggested a statistically significant absolute 4.2% reduction in mortality. The authors suggested no further trials were necessary. However, due to issues raised, this analysis drew serious criticism.[69] Several years later, Yusuf et al.[149] reviewed a much larger number (33) of fibrinolytic trials, focusing largely on the use of streptokinase. This overview had trials with many dissimilarities about dose, route of administration, and setting. Although the meta-analysis for intravenous use of fibrinolytic drugs was impressive, and the authors thought that results were not due to reporting biases, they nevertheless discussed the need for future large-scale, simple trials before widespread use should be recommended. Canner[26] conducted an overview of six randomized clinical trials testing aspirin use in heart attack patients to reduce mortality. His overall meta-analysis suggested a 10% reduction, although not significant ($p = 0.11$). However, there was an apparent heterogeneity of results, and the largest trial had a slightly negative mortality result. The Canner overview was repeated by Hennekens[77] after several more trials had been conducted and the favorable results confirmed.

May et al.[94] conducted an early overview of several modes of therapy for secondary prevention of mortality after a heart attack. Their overview covered antiarrhythmic drugs, lipid-lowering drugs, anticoagulant drugs, beta-blocker drugs, and physical exercise. Although statistical methods were available to combine studies within each treatment class, they chose not to combine results, but simply provide relative risks and confidence interval results graphically for each study. A visual inspection of the trends and variation in trial results provides a summary analysis. Yusuf et al.[150] later provided a more detailed overview of beta blockade studies. While using a similar graphical presentation, they provided a summary odds ratio and its confidence interval. The details of the method are described later. Several meta-analyses of cancer trials have also been conducted,[127] including the use of adjuvant therapy for breast cancer.[80,105] While using multiple chemotherapeutic agents indicated improved relapse-free survival after 3 and 5 years of follow-up, as well as for survival, the dissimilarity among the trials led the authors to call for more trials and better data.

Thompson[135] points out the need to investigate thoroughly sources of heterogeneity, such as clinical differences across studies. These differences may be in populations studied, intervention strategies, outcomes measured, or other logistical aspects. Given such differences, incompatible results among individual studies might be expected. Statistical tests for nonheterogeneity often have low power even in the presence of a moderate heterogeneity. Thompson[135] argues that we should investigate the influence of apparent clinical differences between studies and not rely on formal statistical tests to give us assurance of no heterogeneity. In the presence of apparent heterogeneity, overall summary results should be interpreted cautiously. Thompson describes an example of a meta-analysis of 28 studies evaluating cholesterol lowering and the impact on risk of coronary heart disease. Much heterogeneity is present, and so a simple overall estimate of risk reduction may be misleading. He shows that factors such as age of the cohort, duration of intervention, and size of study are contributing factors. Taking these factors into account made the heterogeneity less extreme and results more interpretable. One analysis showed that the percentage reduction in risk decreased with the age of the participant at the time of the outcome event, a point not seen in the overall meta-analysis. However, Thompson also cautions that such analyses of heterogeneity must also be interpreted cautiously, just as for subgroup analyses in any single trial.

Meta-analysis, as opposed to typical literature reviews, usually puts a p value on the conclusion. The statistical procedure may allow for calculation of a p value, but it implies a precision that may be inappropriate.[112] The possibility that studies may be missed and the issue of study selection may make the interpretation of the p value tenuous. As indicated, quality of data may vary from study to study. Data from some trials may be incomplete, and perhaps not even recognized as such. Thus only very simple and unambiguous outcome variables, such as all-cause mortality, ought to be used for meta-analyses.

Statistical methods

Since meta-analysis became a popular approach to summarizing a collection of studies, numerous publications have addressed several statistical aspects.* Most of this is beyond the scope of this text. However, we will summarize one popular meta-analysis method. This approach combines information on success and failure by intervention group across separate studies; that is, the combination of two tables.

A standard approach, as in the overview paper by May et al.,[94] is to summarize each study with an odds ratio, or a relative risk, along with a 95% confidence interval (CI). That is, suppose each trial can be summarized by a 2-by-2 table where S represents success and F represents failure:

---

*References 15, 18, 26, 31, 45, 47, 68, 70, 141, 150.

Group	Result S	F	TOTAL
Intervention	a	b	
Control	c	d	
Total			m

The number of individuals in each category is indicated by a, b, c, and d, and m is the total. Each study compares the success rate in intervention (P_I) and control (P_C) intervention. The relative risk, $RR = P_I/P_C$, is one summary statistic. Another summary statistic, the odds ratio (OR) that approximates the RR, may also be used. An estimate of the OR is ad/bc, and the 95% CI is:

$$\left(\frac{ad}{bc}\right)\exp\left[\pm 1.96\sqrt{1/a + 1/b + 1/c + 1/d}\right]$$

Typically, the OR estimate and 95% CI is plotted in a single graph for each trial to provide a visual summary. This may be seen in May et al.[94] or in Yusuf et al.[150] Figure 16-3 is taken from Yusuf et al.[149] to indicate the method. This graph summarizes the effects on mortality of 24 trials of fibrinolytic treatment for patients with an acute heart attack. The vertical mark represents the estimated OR, and the horizontal line represents the 95% confidence interval. May et al.[94] went no further in their overview. Yusuf et al.,[150] however, recommended that a single estimation of the OR be obtained, combining all studies.

Two technical approaches are used,[135] both suggested by Cochran[35] in 1954. If all trials included in the meta-analysis are estimating the same true (but unknown) fixed effect of an intervention, the Mantel-Haenszel method[92] is used with a slight variation[150] (summarized in the Appendix). This is similar to the log rank or Mantel-Haenszel method in the chapter on survival analysis. This method is referred to here as the Peto-Yusuf method. If the trials are assumed to have dissimilar or heterogeneous true treatment effects, the intervention effects are described by a random effects model, suggested by Der Simonian and Laird.[47]

The Peto-Yusuf[150] method follows the Cochran-Mantel-Haenszel procedure.[35,92] Let $O_i = a_i$, E_i be the expected value of O_i, and V_i be the variance. Then,

$$O_i = a_i$$

$$E_i = \frac{(a_i + c_i)(a_i + b_i)}{m_i}$$

$$V_i = \frac{(a_i + c_i)(b_i + d_i)(a_i + b_i)(c_i + d_i)}{m_i^2(m_i - 1)}$$

Methods for Combining Randomized Clinical Trials

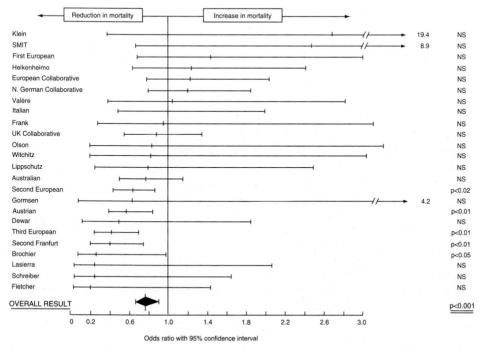

Fig. 16-3 Apparent effects of fibronolytic treatment on mortality in the randomized trials of IV treatment of acute myocardial infarction. Reproduced with permission of the editor, *European Heart Journal* and Dr. S. Yusuf.

and let $O = \Sigma_i \, O_i$, $E = \Sigma_i \, E_i$, and $V_i = \Sigma V_i$, where $i = 1, 2, 3, \dots N$. As shown in Chapter 15, the statistic $Z_{MH} = (O-E)/\sqrt{V}$ has a standard normal distribution. The Peto-Yusuf[150] method estimates the pooled odds ratio, OR_p, as:

$$OR_p = \exp\left[(O - E)/V\right]$$

and the 95% CI as:

$$\exp\left\{\frac{O - E}{V} \pm 1.96/\sqrt{V}\right\}$$

Using this method, the summary pooled odds ratio and 95% CI, shown in Fig. 16-3, can be computed for the 24 fibrinolytic studies.

The method of Der Simonian and Laird[47] compares rate differences within each study and obtains a pooled estimate of the overall rate difference and its standard error. The pooled estimate of the rate difference is a weighted average of the individual study rate differences. The weights are the inverse of the sum of the between and within study variance components of intervention effect. If the studies are relatively similar or homogeneous in intervention effect, the two methods provide very similar results.[15] However, if studies vary in intervention effect, these two methods can produce different results, as illustrated by Berlin et al.[15] and Pocock and Hughes.[112]

In the presence of serious heterogeneity of intervention effect, the appropriateness of obtaining a single point estimate must be questioned. This was part of the reason May et al.[94] did not combine studies. If the heterogeneity is qualitative; that is, some estimates of the *OR* are larger than unity and others less than unity, then a combined single estimate is perhaps not wise. This would be especially true if these estimates indicated a time trend that could occur if dose and participant selection changed with experience with the new intervention.

Despite these problems, many see meta-analysis as an alternative to the extraordinary effort and cost often required to conduct an adequate individual trial. Rather than providing a solution, it perhaps ought to be viewed as a way to present existing data; a way that has strengths and weaknesses, and that must be as critically evaluated as any other information. It would clearly be preferable to combine resources prospectively and collaborate in a single large study. Pooled studies cannot replace individual, well-conducted multicenter trials.

APPENDIX
Mantel-Haenszel statistic

Suppose an investigator is comparing response rates and divides the data into several strata using baseline characteristics. For each stratum i, a 2-by-2 table is constructed.

2-by-2 table for ith stratum

	Response		
	Yes	No	
Intervention	a_i	b_i	$a_i + b_i$
Control	c_i	d_i	$c_i + d_i$
Total	$a_i + c_i$	$b_i + d_i$	n_i

The entries a_i, b_i, c_i, and d_i represent the counts in the four cells, and n_i is the number of participants in the ith stratum. The marginals represent totals in the various categories. The value $(a_i + c_i)/n_i$ represents the overall response rate for the ith stratum. Within the ith stratum, the rates $a_i/(a_i + b_i)$ with $c_i/(c_i + d_i)$ are compared.

The standard chi-square test for 2-by-2 tables could be used to compare group differences in this stratum. However, the investigator is interested in "averaging" the comparison over all the strata. The method for combining several 2-by-2 tables over all tables or strata was described by Cochran[35] and Mantel and Haenszel.[92] The summary statistic, denoted MH, is given by:

$$MH = \frac{\left\{ \sum_{i=1}^{K} \left[a_i - (a+c_i)(a_i+b_i)/n_i \right] \right\}^2}{\sum_{i=1}^{K} (a_i+c_i)(b_i+d_i)(a_i+b_i)(c_i+d_i)/n_i^2(n_i-1)}$$

The MH statistic has a chi-square distribution with one degree of freedom. Tables for this distribution are available in standard statistical textbooks. Any value for MH greater than 3.84 is significant at the 0.05 level, and any value greater than 6.63 is significant at the 0.01 level. This method is particularly appropriate for covariates that are discrete or continuous covariates that have been classified into intervals.

REFERENCES

1. Albert JM, DeMets D: On a model-based approach to estimating efficacy in clinical trials, *Stat Med* 13:2323-2335, 1994.
2. Altman L: New method of analyzing health data stirs debate, *New York Times* Aug 21, 1990.
3. Anderson JR, Cain KC, Gelber RD: Analysis of survival by tumor response, *J Clin Oncol* 1:710-719, 1983.
4. Anderson MP, Bechsgaard P, Frederiksen J et al: Effect of alprenolol on mortality among patients with definite or suspected acute myocardial infarction, *Lancet* ii:865-868, 1979.
5. Anturane Reinfarction Trial Policy Committee: The Anturane Reinfarction Trial: reevaluation of outcome, *N Engl J Med* 306:1005-1008, 1982.
6. The Anturane Reinfarction Trial Research Group: Sulfinpyrazone in the prevention of sudden death after myocardial infarction, *N Engl J Med* 302:250-256, 1980.
7. Armitage P: The analysis of data from clinical trials, *The Statistician* 28:171-183, 1980.
8. Armitage P: *Statistical methods in medical research*, New York, 1977, John Wiley & Sons.
9. Aspirin Myocardial Infarction Study (AMIS), Research Group: AMIS, a randomized controlled trial of aspirin in persons recovered from myocardial infarction, *JAMA* 243:661-669, 1980.
10. Bailey KR: Inter-study differences: how should they influence the interpretation and analysis of results? *Stat Med* 6:351-358, 1987.
11. Bass C, Strackee J: Lung cancer and month of birth, *Lancet* I:47, 1964.
12. Baum ML, Anish DS, Chalmers TC et al: A survey of clinical trials of antibiotic prophylaxis in colon surgery: evidence against further use of no-treatment controls, *N Engl J Med* 305:795-799, 1981.
13. Beach ML, Meier P: Choosing covariates in the analysis of clinical trials, *Controlled Clin Trials* 10:161S-175S, 1989.
14. Berlin JA, Begg CB, Louis TA: An assessment of publication bias using a sample of published clinical trials, *J Am Stat Assoc* 84:381-392, 1989.
15. Berlin JA, Laird NM, Sacks HS, Chalmers TC: A comparison of statistical methods for combining event rates from clinical trials, *Stat Med* 8:141-151, 1989.
16. Beta-blocker Heart Attack Trial Research Group: A randomized trial of propranolol in patients with acute myocardial infarction. 1. Mortality results, *JAMA* 247:1707-1714, 1982.
17. Bishop YM, Fienberg SE, Holland PW: *Discrete multivariate analysis: theory and practice*, Cambridge, 1975, MIT Press.
18. Brand R, Kragt H: Importance of trends in the interpretation of an overall odds ratio in the meta-analysis of clinical trials, *Stat Med* 11:2077-2082, 1992.

19. Brown BW, Hollander M: *Statistics: a biomedical introduction*, New York, 1977, John Wiley & Sons.
20. Brownlee KA: *Statistical theory and methodology in science and engineering*, New York, 1965, John Wiley & Sons.
21. Budetti PP, McManus P: Assessing the effectiveness of neonatal intensive care, *Med Care* 20:1027-1039, 1982.
22. Byar DB: Assessing apparent treatment—covariate interactions in randomized clinical trials, *Stat Med* 4:255-263, 1985.
23. The Canadian Cooperative Study Group: A randomized trial of aspirin and sulfinpyrazone in threatened stroke, *N Engl J Med* 299:53-59, 1978.
24. Canner PL: Monitoring clinical trial data for evidence of adverse or beneficial treatment effects. In Boissel JP, Klimt CR, eds: *Multicenter controlled trials: principles and problems*, Paris, 1979, INSERM.
25. Canner PL: Choice of covariates in the adjustment of treatment effects. Presented at the Society for Clinical Trials Annual Scientific Sessions, San Francisco, 1981.
26. Canner PL: Aspirin in coronary heart disease: comparison of six clinical trials, *Isr J Med Sci* 19:413-423, 1983.
27. Canner PL: Further aspects of data analysis, *Controlled Clin Trials* 4:485-503, 1983.
28. Canner PL: Covariate adjustment of treatment effects in clinical trials, *Controlled Clin Trials* 12:359-366, 1991.
29. Canner PL, Huang YB, Meinert CL: On the detection of outlier clinics in medical and surgical trials: I. Practical considerations, *Controlled Clin Trials* 2:231-240, 1981.
30. Canner PL, Huang YB, Meinert CL: On the detection of outlier clinics in medical and surgical trials: II. Theoretical considerations, *Controlled Clin Trials* 2:241-252, 1981.
31. Carroll RJ, Stefanski LA: Measurement error, instrumental variables and corrections for attenuation with applications to meta-analyses, *Stat Med* 13:1265-1282, 1994.
32. Chalmers TC, Frank CS, Reitman D: Minimizing the three stages of publication bias, *JAMA* 263:1392-1395, 1990.
33. Chalmers TC, Levin H, Sacks HS, Reitman D, Berrier J, Nagalingam R: Meta-analysis of clinical trials as a scientific discipline. I: Control of bias and comparison with large co-operative trials, *Stat Med* 6:315-326, 1987.
34. Chalmers TC, Matta RJ, Smith H Jr, Kunzier AM: Evidence favoring the use of anticoagulants in the hospital phase of acute myocardial infarction, *N Engl J Med* 297:1091-1096, 1977.
35. Cochran WG: Some methods for strengthening the common chi-square tests, *Biometrics* 10:417-451, 1954.
36. Collaborative Group on Antenatal Steroid Therapy: Effect of antenatal dexamethasone administration on the prevention of respiratory distress syndrome, *Am J Obstet Gynecol* 141:276-287, 1981.
37. Collins R, Gray R, Godwin J, Peto R: Avoidance of large biases and large random errors in the assessment of moderate treatment effects: the need for systematic overviews, *Stat Med* 6:245-250, 1987.
38. Collins R, Yusuf S, Peto R: Overview of randomized trials of diuretics in pregnancy, *Br Med J* 290:17-23, 1985.
39. Colton T: *Statistics in medicine,* Boston, 1974, Little Brown.
40. Coronary Drug Project Research Group: Influence of adherence to treatment and response of cholesterol on mortality in the Coronary Drug Project, *N Engl J Med* 303:1038-1041, 1980.
41. Coronary Drug Project Research Group: Clofibrate and niacin in coronary heart disease, *JAMA* 231:360-381, 1975.
42. Cox DR: Regression models and lifetables, *J R Stat Soc* Ser 34 B:187-202, 1972.
43. Crager MR: Analysis of covariance in parallel-group clinical trials with pretreatment baselines, *Biometrics* 43:895-901, 1987.
44. Davies JM: Cancer and date of birth, *Br Med J* 2:1535, 1963.
45. DeMets DL: Methods for combining randomized clinical trials: strengths and limitations, *Stat Med* 6:341-348, 1987.
46. Dempster AP, Laird NM, Rubin DB: Maximum likelihood from incomplete data via the EM algorithm, *J Royal Stat Soc* 39B:1-38, 1977.
47. DerSimonian R, Laird N: Meta-analysis in clinical trials, *Controlled Clin Trials* 7:177-188, 1986.
48. DeSilva RA, Hennekens CH, Lown B, Casscells W: Lignocaine prophylaxis in acute myocardial infarction: an evaluation of randomized trials, *Lancet* ii:855-858, 1981.

49. Detre K, Peduzzi P: The problems of attributing deaths of nonadherers: the VA coronary bypass experience, *Controlled Clin Trials* 3:355-364, 1982.
50. Diggle PJ: Testing for random dropouts in repeated measurement data, *Biometrics* 45:1255-1258, 1989.
51. Dijkstra BKS: Origin of carcinoma bronchus, *J Natl Cancer Inst* 31:511-519, 1963.
52. Dillman RO, Seagren SL, Propert KJ, Guerra J, et al: A randomized trial of induction chemotherapy plus high-dose radiation versus radiation alone in stage III non-small-cell lung cancer, *N Engl J Med* 323:940-945, 1990.
53. Dixon WJ: Processing data for outliers, *Biometrics* 9:74-89, 1953.
54. Dixon WJ: Rejection of observations. In Sarhan AE, Greenberg BG, eds: *Contributions to order statistics,* New York, 1962, John Wiley & Sons.
55. Dolin R, Reichman R, Madore H, et al: A controlled trial of amantadine and rimantadine in the prophylaxis of influenza A infection, *N Engl J Med* 307:580-583, 1982.
56. Efron B: Missing data and the bootstrap, *J Am Stat Assoc* 89:463-474, 1994.
57. Efron B, Feldman D: Adherence as an explanatory variable in clinical trials, *J Am Stat Assoc* 86: 9-17, 1991.
58. Egger MJ, Coleman ML, Ward JR, Reading JC, et al: Uses and abuses of analysis of covariance in clinical trials, *Controlled Clin Trials* 6:12-24, 1985.
59. Elashoff JD: Combining results of clinical trials, *Gastroenterology* 75:1170-1174, 1978 (editorial).
60. Espeland MA, Byington RP, Hire D, Davis VG, et al: Analysis strategies for serial multivariate ultrasonographic data that are incomplete, *Stat Med* 11:1041-1056, 1992.
61. Fisher L, Van Belle G: *Biostatistics—A methodology for the health sciences,* New York, 1993, John Wiley & Sons.
62. Fleiss JL: Analysis of data from multiclinic trials, *Controlled Clin Trials* 7:267-275, 1986.
63. Furberg C: Lipid-lowering trials—Results and limitations, *Am Heart J,* 128:1304-1308, 1994.
64. Furberg CD, Byington RP: What do subgroup analyses reveal about differential response to beta-blocker therapy? The Beta-Blocker Heart Attack Trial Experience, *Circulation* 67(suppl 1):I-98–I-101, 1983.
65. Furberg CD, Hawkins CM, Lichstein E: Effect of propranolol in postinfarction patients with mechanical or electrical complications, *Circulation* 69:761-765, 1984.
66. Furberg CD, Morgan TM: Lessons from overviews of cardiovascular trials, *Stat Med* 6:295-299, 1987.
67. Gail M, Simon R: Testing for qualitative interactions between treatment effects and patient subsets, *Biometrics* 41:361-372, 1985.
68. Galbraith RG: A note on graphical presentation of estimated odds ratios from several clinical trials, *Stat Med* 7:889-894, 1988.
69. Goldman L, Feinstein AR: Anticoagulants and myocardial infarction: the problems of pooling, drowning, and floating, *Ann Intern Med* 90:92-94, 1979.
70. Goodman SN: Meta-analysis and evidence, *Controlled Clin Trials* 10:188-204, 1989.
71. Goudie RB: The birthday fallacy and statistics of Icelandic diabetes, *Lancet* ii:1173, 1981.
72. Greenless JS, Reece WS, Zieschang KD: Imputation of missing values when the probability of response depends on the variable being imputed, *J Am Stat Assoc* 77:251-261, 1982.
73. Grubbs FE: Procedures for detecting outlying observations in samples, *Technometrics* 11:1-21, 1969.
74. GUSTO Investigators: An international randomized trial comparing four thrombolytic strategies for acute myocardial infarction, *N Engl J Med* 329(10):673-682, 1993.
75. Helgason T, Jonasson MR: Evidence for a food additive as a cause of ketosis-prone diabetes, *Lancet* 2:716-720, 1981.
76. Hennekens CH, Buring JE, Hebert PR: Implications of overviews of randomized trials, *Stat Med* 6:397-402, 1987.
77. Hennekens C, Buring JE, Sandercock P, Collins R, et al: Aspirin and other antiplatelet agents in the secondary and primary prevention of cardiovascular disease, *Circulation* 880:749-756, 1989.
78. Heyting A, Tolboom JT, Essers JG: Statistical handling of dropouts in longitudinal clinical trials, *Stat Med* 11:2043-2061, 1992.
79. Hill AB: *Principles of medical statistics,* ed 9, New York, 1971, Oxford University Press.
80. Himel HN, Liberati A, Gelber RD, Chalmers TC: Adjuvant chemotherapy for breast cancer— A pooled estimate based on published randomized control trials, *J Am Med Assoc* 256:1148-1159, 1986.

81. Hoover DR, Munoz A, Carey V, Taylor JMG et al, and the Multicenter AIDS Cohort Study: Using events from dropouts in nonparametric survival function estimation with application to incubation of AIDS, *J Am Stat Assoc* 88:37-43, 1993.

82. Ingle JN, Ahmann DL, Green SJ, Edmonson JH, et al: Randomized clinical trial of diethylstibestrol versus tamoxifen in postmenopausal women with advanced breast cancer, *N Engl J Med* 304: 16-21, 1981.

83. Ingelfinger JA, Mosteller F, Thibodeau LA, Ware JH: *Biostatistics in clinical medicine*, New York, 1983, MacMillan.

84. The Intermittent Positive Pressure Breathing Trial Group: Intermittent positive pressure breathing therapy of chronic obstructive pulmonary disease—A clinical trial, *Ann Intern Med* 99:612-620, 1983.

85. ISIS-2 (Second International Study of Infarct Survival) Collaborative Group: Randomized trial of intravenous streptokinase, oral aspirin, both or neither, among 17187 cases of suspected acute myocardial infarction: ISIS-2, *Lancet* ii:349-360, 1988.

86. Kruskal WH: Some remarks on wild observations, *Technometrics* 2:1-3, 1960.

87. Lagakos SW, Lim LL-Y, Robins JM: Adjusting for early treatment termination in comparative clinical trials, *Stat Med* 9:1417-1424, 1990.

88. Laird NM: Missing data in longitudinal studies, *Stat Med* 7:305-315, 1988.

89. Lee KL, McNeer JF, Starmer CF et al: Clinical judgment and statistics: lessons from a simulated randomized trial in coronary artery disease, *Circulation* 61:508-515, 1980.

90. Lipid Research Clinics Program: The Lipid Research Clinics Coronary Primary Prevention Trial results. 1. Reduction in incidence of coronary heart disease, *JAMA* 251:351-364, 1984.

91. Little RJA, Rubin DB: *Statistical analysis with missing data*, New York, 1987, John Wiley & Sons.

92. Mantel N, Haenszel W: Statistical aspects of the analysis of data from retrospective studies of disease, *J Natl Cancer Inst* 22:719-748, 1959.

93. May GS, DeMets DL, Friedman LM et al: The randomized clinical trial: bias in analysis, *Circulation* 64:669-673, 1981.

94. May GS, Furberg CD, Eberlein KA, Geraci BJ: Secondary prevention after myocardial infarction: a review of short-term acute phase trials, *Prog Cardiovasc Dis* 25:335-359, 1983.

95. Meinert CL: Meta-analysis: science or religion? *Controlled Clin Trials* 10:257S-263S, 1989.

96. Messer J, Reitman D, Sacks HS et al: Association of adrenocorticosteroid therapy and peptic ulcer-disease, *N Engl J Med* 309:21-24, 1983.

97. Miller RG Jr: *Simultaneous statistical inference*, New York, 1966, McGraw-Hill.

98. Mitchell RJ: What constitutes evidence on the dietary prevention of coronary heart disease? Cozy beliefs or harsh facts? *Int J Cardiol* 5:287-298, 1984.

99. Morgan TM: Analysis of duration of response: a problem of oncology trials, *Controlled Clin Trials* 9:11-18, 1988.

100. Morgan TM, Elashoff RM: Effect of covariate measurement error in randomized clinical trials, *Stat Med* 6:31-41, 1987.

101. Moses LE: The series of consecutive cases as a device for assessing outcomes of intervention, *N Engl J Med* 311:705-710, 1984.

102. Multicentre International Study: Improvement in prognosis of myocardial infarction by long-term beta-adrenoreceptor blockade using practolol, *Br Med J* 3:735-740, 1975.

103. Newcombe RG: Explanatory and pragmatic estimates of the treatment effect when deviations from allocated treatment occur, *Stat Med* 7:1179-1186, 1988.

104. Oakes D, Moss AJ, Fleiss JL, Bigger JR et al, and the Multicenter Diltiazem Post-Infarction Trial Research Group: Use of adherence measures in an analysis of the effect of diltiazem on mortality and reinfarction after myocardial infarction, *J Am Stat Assoc* 88:44-49, 1993.

105. Office of Medical Applications of Research, National Institutes of Health: Adjuvant chemotherapy for breast cancer, *JAMA* 254:3461, 1985.

106. Oye RK, Shapiro MF: Reporting results from chemotherapy trials, *JAMA* 252:2722-2725, 1984.

107. Peto R: Statistical aspects of cancer trials, In Halnan KE, ed: *Treatment of Cancer*, London, 1982, Chapman & Hall.

108. Peto R: Why do we need systematic overviews of randomized trials? (Modified transcript of an oral presentation). *Stat Med* 6:233-240, 1987.

109. Peto R, Pike MC, Armitage P et al: Design and analysis of randomized clinical trials requiring pro-longed observation of each patient. 1. Introduction and design, *Br J Cancer* 34:585-612, 1976.
110. Pizzo PA, Robichaud KJ, Edwards BK et al: Oral antibiotic prophylaxis in patients with cancer: a double-blind randomized placebo-controlled trial, *J Pediatr* 102:125-133, 1983.
111. Pledger GW: Basic statistics: importance of adherence, *J Clin Res Pharmacoepidemiol* 6:77-81, 1992.
112. Pocock SJ, Hughes MD: Estimation issues in clinical trials and overviews, *Stat Med* 9:657-671, 1990.
113. Redmond C, Fisher B, Wieand HS: The methodologic dilemma in retrospectively correlating the amount of chemotherapy received in adjuvant therapy protocols with disease-free survival, *Cancer Treat Rep* 67:519-526, 1983.
114. Remington RD, Schork MA: *Statistics with applications to the biological and health sciences,* Englewood Cliffs, NJ, 1970, Prentice-Hall.
115. Report from the Committee of Principal Investigators: A cooperative trial in the primary prevention of ischaemic heart disease using clofibrate, *Br Heart J* 40:1069-1118, 1978.
116. Ridout MS: Testing for random dropouts in repeated measurement data, *Biometrics* 47:1617-1621, 1991.
117. Roberts R, Croft C, Gold HK et al: Effect of propranolol on myocardial infarct size in a randomized blinded multicenter trial, *N Engl J Med* 311:218-225, 1984.
118. Robins JM: The analysis of randomized and non-randomized AIDs treatment trials using a new approach to causal inference in longitudinal studies. In Sechrest L, Freeman H, Mulley A, eds: *Health service research methodology: a focus on AIDS,* US Public Health Service, 1989.
119. Robins JM, Tsiatis AA: Correcting for non-adherence in randomized trials using rank preserving structural failure time models, *Commun Stat-Theory Methods* 20:2609-2631, 1991.
120. Rosenbaum PR: The consequences of adjustment for a concomitant variable that has been affected by the treatment, *J R Stat Soc* 147A(Pt 5):656-666, 1984.
121. Sackett DL, Gent M: Controversy in counting and attributing events in clinical trials, *N Engl J Med* 301:1410-1412, 1979.
122. Sacks HS, Berrier J, Reitman D, Ancona-Berk, VA et al: Meta-analyses of randomized controlled trials, *N Engl J Med* 316:450-455, 1987.
123. Schwartz D, Lellouch J: Explanatory and pragmatic attitudes in therapeutic trials, *J Chronic Dis* 20:637-648, 1967.
124. Shuster J, van Eys J: Interaction between prognostic factors and treatment, *Controlled Clin Trials* 4:209-214, 1983.
125. Simes RJ: Confronting publication bias: a cohort design for meta-analysis, *Stat Med* 6:11-29, 1987.
126. Simon R: Patient subsets and variation in therapeutic efficacy, *Br J Clin Pharmacol* 14:473-482, 1982.
127. Simon R: The role of overviews in cancer therapeutics, *Stat Med* 6:389-394, 1987.
128. Simon R, Makuch RW: A non-parametric graphical representation of the relationship between survival and the occurrence of an event: application to responder versus non-responder bias, *Stat Med* 3:35-44, 1984.
129. Snow PJD: Effect of propranolol in myocardial infaction, *Lancet* 2:551-553, 1965.
130. Sommer A, Zeger SL: On estimating efficacy from clinical trials, *Stat Med* 10:45-52, 1991.
131. Stampfer MJ, Goldhaber SZ, Yusuf S et al: Effect of intravenous streptokinase on acute myocardial infarction. Pooled results from randomized trials, *N Engl J Med* 307:1180-1182, 1982.
132. Steering Committee of the Physicians' Health Study Research Group: Final report on the aspirin component of the ongoing Physicians' Health Study, *N Engl J Med* 321:129-135, 1989.
133. Temple R, Pledger GW: The FDA's critique of the Anturane Reinfarction Trial, *N Engl J Med* 303:1488-1492, 1980.
134. Thall PF, Lachin JM: Assessment of stratum-covariate interaction in Cox's proportional hazards regression model, *Stat Med* 5:73-83, 1986.
135. Thompson S: Why sources of heterogeneity in meta-analysis should be investigated, *Br Med J* 309: 1351-1355, 1994.
136. Tukey JW: Some thoughts on clinical trials, especially problems of multiplicity, *Science* 198:679-684, 1977.

137. Verter J, Friedman L: Adherence measures in the Aspirin Myocardial Infarction Study (AMIS), *Controlled Clin Trials* 5:306, 1984 (abstract).

138. Wang PH, Lau J, Chalmers TC: Meta-analysis of effects of intensive blood-glucose control on late complications of type I diabetes, *Lancet* 341:1306-1309, 1993.

139. Wei CGC, Tanner MA: A Monte Carlo implementation of the EM algorithm and the poor man's data augmentation algorithms, *J Am Stat Assoc* 85:699-704, 1990.

140. Weiss GB, Bunce H, Hokanson JA: Comparing survival of responders and nonresponders after treatment: a potential source of confusion interpreting cancer clinical trials, *Controlled Clin Trials* 4:43-52, 1983.

141. Whitehead A, Whitehead J: A general parametric approach to the meta-analysis of randomized clinical trials, *Stat Med* 10:1665-1677, 1991.

142. Wilcox RG, Roland JM, Banks DC et al: Randomised trial comparing propranolol with atenolol in immediate treatment of suspected myocardial infarction, *Br Med J* 1:885-888, 1980.

143. Wilcox RE: Problems in the medical interpretation of overviews, *Stat Med* 6:269-276, 1987.

144. Woolson R: *Statistical methods for the analysis of biomedical data*, New York, 1987, John Wiley & Sons.

145. Wu M, Bailey K: Estimation and comparison of changes in the presence of informative right censoring: conditional linear model, *Biometrics* 44:939-955, 1989.

146. Wu M, Carrell R: Estimation and comparison of changes in the presence of informative right censoring by modeling the censoring process, *Biometrics* 44:175-188, 1988.

147. Yates F: The analysis of multiple classifications with unequal numbers in the different classes, *J Am Stat Assoc* 29:51-66, 1934.

148. Yusuf S: Obtaining medically meaningful answers from an overview of randomized clinical trials, *Stat Med* 6:281-286, 1987.

149. Yusuf S, Collins R, Peto R, Furberg C, et al: Intravenous and intracoronary fibrinolytic therapy in acute myocardial infarction: overview of results on mortality, reinfarction and side-effects from 33 randomized controlled trials, *Eur Heart J* 6:556-585, 1985.

150. Yusuf S, Peto R, Lewis J, Collins R, et al: Beta blockade during and after myocardial infarction: an overview of the randomized trials, *Prog Cardiovasc Dis* 27:335-371, 1985.

Closeout

In any clinical trial, appropriate plans for the closeout phase must be developed. This phase starts with the final follow-up visit of the first participant enrolled and lasts until all analyses have been completed. It is evident that well before the scheduled end of the trial, a fairly detailed plan is needed for this phase if the study is to terminate in an orderly manner. One must be prepared to implement or modify this plan since unexpected results, either beneficial or harmful, may require that the trial be stopped early.

The literature on the topic of closeout is very scant. Bell et al.[2] contrast the closeout procedures and problems in a study requiring early termination with those from a study stopping on schedule. Krol[19] describes the closeout of the Coronary Drug Project (CDP), a large-scale, multi-armed trial. It is possible that certain subgroups of participants will be taken off intervention earlier than scheduled.*

This chapter will address several closeout topics. Although many of them relate to large single-center or multicenter trials, they may also apply to smaller studies. Topics discussed include technical procedures for the termination of the trial, post-study follow-up, clean-up and storage of data, and dissemination of trial results. Obviously, the details of the closeout plan have to be tailored to the particular trial.

FUNDAMENTAL POINT

The closeout of a clinical trial is usually a fairly complex process that requires careful planning if it is to be accomplished in an orderly fashion.

TERMINATION PROCEDURES

If each participant in a clinical trial is to be followed for a fixed period, the closeout phase will be of at least the same duration as the enrollment phase. In many cases, this means several months to years. Since terminating the follow-up of some participants while others are still being actively followed can create problems in long-term trials, this closeout design may not be desirable. An alternative and frequently used plan involves following all participants to a common termination date, or

---

*References 6, 7, 10, 20, 24, 25.

when this is not feasible, to a compressed closeout period. The termination date is determined by two factors: the date that the last participant is enrolled, and the minimum length of follow-up period that the protocol requires. In other words, if the last participant is enrolled March 15, 1993, and the minimum scheduled follow-up is 3 years, the common termination date would be March 15, 1996.

There are several disadvantages to the use of long closeouts. First, in most blinded trials, the code for each participant is broken at the last scheduled follow-up visit. If the unblinding must occur over a span of many months or years, there is the possibility of accidentally breaking the blind of participants still actively followed in the trial. For example, more than one participant in a drug trial may be given study medications with the same bottle code (Chapter 6). This plan is not optimal because breaking the blind for one participant of four who get bottles with the same code may unblind the other three. In addition, the investigator may start associating a certain symptom or constellation of symptoms and signs with particular drug codes.

Second, the investigator's obligation to a participant means that at the final follow-up visit the investigator needs to advise the participant regarding possible continued intervention. If the closeout is extended over a long period, as it would be if each participant were followed for the same duration, any early recommendation to an individual participant would have to be based on incomplete follow-up data that may not reflect the trial conclusion. Moreover, information could "leak" to participants still in the trial, thus affecting the integrity of the trial. Although it is highly desirable to provide each participant with a recommendation regarding continued treatment, doing so may not be possible until the study is completely over. When unblinding occurs over a span of months or years, the investigator is in the uncomfortable position of ending a participant's participation in the trial and asking him or her to wait months before being told the study results and advised what to do. If the incomplete results are clearcut, one can easily arrive at such recommendations. However, in such an instance, the investigator would be confronted with an ethical dilemma. How can he recommend that a participant start, continue, or discontinue a new intervention while keeping other participants in the trial?

An advantage of adopting the common termination design is the added power of the trial, which extends the follow-up period beyond the minimum time for all but the last participant enrolled. In a trial with 2 years of uniform recruitment, the additional follow-up period would increase by an average of almost 1 year. In addition, in terms of participant-years of follow-up, this approach might be more cost efficient when clinic staff is supported solely by the sponsor of the trial. With all participants followed to the end of the study, full support of personnel can be justified until all participants have been seen for the last time. In trials where the participants are phased out after a fixed time of follow-up, an increase in the staff/participant ratio may be unavoidable.

Despite the problem with following all participants for a fixed length of time, this approach may be preferable in certain trials, particularly those with a relatively short follow-up phase. In such studies, there may be no realistic alternative. In addition, it may not be logistically feasible to conduct a large number of closeout visits in a short time. Depending on the content of the last visit, availability of staff, and weekly clinic hours, seeing 100 to 150 participants at a clinic may require several weeks. A decision on the type of follow-up plan should be based on the scientific question and logistics.

After enrollment, the last follow-up visit is the most important visit. It is particularly so in trials where the main response variables are continuous variables such as laboratory data or a performance measure. By necessity, the response variable data must be obtained for each participant at the last follow-up visit because it marks the end of follow-up. If the participant fails to show up for the last visit, the investigator will lack data. When the response variable is the occurrence of a specific event, such as a fatal myocardial infarction, the situation may be different if the information can be obtained without having the participant complete a visit.

Termination of a long-term study can be difficult because of the bonding that often develops between participants and clinic staff.[2] The final visit needs to be carefully planned to deal not only with this issue, but also with the obligation to inform the participants of which medication they were on (in a blinded study), their individual study data, and the overall study findings (typically at a later time). Referral of the participant to a regular source of medical care is another important issue. The final visit is also an opportunity to ask specific questions regarding blinding, adherence, and attitudes and to get feedback on their experience of study participation.

If a participant suffers an event after the last follow-up visit, but before all participants have been seen for the final visit, the investigator must decide whether that response variable should be included in the data analysis. The simplest solution is to let the last follow-up visit denote each participant's termination of the trial. For participants who do not show up for the last visit, the investigator has to decide when to make the final ascertainment. If death is a response variable, vital status is usually determined as of the last day that the participant is eligible to be seen.

It is important in any trial to obtain, to the extent possible, response variable data on every enrolled participant. The uncertainty of the overall results rises as the number of participants for whom response variable data are missing increases. For example, assume that death from any cause is the primary response variable in a trial and the observed mortality is 15% in one group and 10% in the other group. Depending on study size, this group difference might be statistically significant. However, if 10% of the participants in each group were lost to follow-up, the observed outcome of the trial may be in question. One cannot assume that the mortality experience among those lost to follow-up is the same as for those who stayed in the trial, or that those lost to follow-up in one group have a mortality experience identical to those lost to follow-up in the other group. Equally important, there should be no differential assessment in the study groups. Therefore every effort should be made to ensure that the final ascertainment of response variables is as complete as possible.

Several means have been used to track participants and determine their vital status. These means include the use of a person's Social Security number, relatives, or employers. In countries with national registries, which now include the United States, mortality surveillance is simpler and probably more complete than in countries without such registries. Agencies that specialize in locating people have been used in several trials. This area is very sensitive, because a search may be considered an intrusion into the privacy of the participant. The integrity of a trial and its results plus the participant's initial agreement to participate in the trial have to be weighed against a person's right to protect his privacy. Investigators may want to include in the informed consent form a sentence stating that the participants agree to have their vital status determined at the end of the trial even if they have by then stopped participating actively.

POSTSTUDY FOLLOW-UP

Participant follow-up after the termination of a trial may be composed of two activities. One involves short-term follow-up during a "cooling-off" period when participants are off intervention but still being followed. The other is long-term follow-up of possible toxicity or benefit. These activities are separate from the moral obligation of the investigator to facilitate, when necessary, a participant's return to the usual medical care system, to ensure that study recommendations are communicated to his or her private physician, and at times to continue the participant on a beneficial new intervention.

A cooling-off period to find out how soon laboratory values or symptoms return to pretrial level or status ought to be considered in trials where the intervention is being stopped at the last follow-up visit. A cooling-off period is particularly important when the trial results are negative or inconclusive, when the intervention is not available for nonstudy use, or when no recommendations as to continued intervention can be made. The effect of the intervention may last long after a drug has been stopped, and side effects or "toxic" changes revealed by laboratory measurements may not disappear until weeks after intervention has ended. For certain drugs, such as beta-blockers, the intervention should not be stopped abruptly. A tapering of the dosage may require additional clinic visits.

Poststudy follow-up of participants is a rather complex process. First, the investigator must decide what should be monitored. Mortality surveillance can be cumbersome and is worth undertaking only if there is a reasonable expectation of getting an almost complete record of vital status. Usually, the justification for long-term poststudy surveillance is a trend or unexpected finding in the trial or a finding from another source.

Obtaining information on nonfatal events is usually complicated, and, in general, its value is questionable. However, a classical illustration that poststudy follow-up for toxicity can prove valuable is the finding of severe toxic effects attributed to diethylstilbestrol (DES). The purported carcinogenic effect occurred 15 to 20 years after the drug was administered and occurred in female offspring who were exposed in utero.[14] Similarly, use of unopposed estrogen has been reported to be associated with an increased risk of endometrial cancer 15 or more years after therapy was stopped.[16]

In 1975, the results of a trial of clofibrate in people with elevated lipids[23] indicated an excess of cases of cancer in the clofibrate group compared with the control group. The question was raised whether the participants assigned to clofibrate in the CDP[8] also showed an increase in cancer incidence. This was not the case. Only 3% of the deaths during the trial were cancer related. Subsequently, the WHO study of clofibrate reported that all-cause mortality was increased in the intervention group.[5] At the same time, the CDP investigators decided that poststudy follow-up was scientifically and ethically important, and such a study was undertaken. The example brings up a question: should investigators of large-scale clinical trials make arrangements for surveillance in case, at some future time, the need for such a study were to arise? The implementation of any poststudy surveillance plan raises complications. A key complication is to find a way of keeping participants' names and addresses in a central registry without infringement upon the privacy of the individuals. The investigator must also decide, with little evidence, on the optimal duration of surveillance after the termination of a trial (e.g., 2, 5, or 20 years).

A second issue of poststudy surveillance is related to a possible beneficial effect of intervention. In any intervention trial, assumptions must be made with respect to time between initiation of intervention and the occurrence of full beneficial effect. For many drugs, this so-called lag time is assumed to be zero. However, if the intervention is a lipid-lowering drug or a dietary change and the response variable is coronary mortality, the lag time might be a couple of years. The problem with such an intervention is that the maximum practical follow-up may not be long enough for a beneficial effect to appear. Extended surveillance after completion of active treatment may be considered in such studies. In fact, the CDP follow-up study showed unexpected benefit in one of the intervention groups. At the conclusion of the trial, the nicotinic acid participants had significantly fewer nonfatal reinfarctions, but no difference in survival was detected.[8] Total mortality, after an average 6.5 years in the trial on drug, plus an additional 9 years after the trial, however, was significantly less in the group assigned to nicotinic acid than in the placebo group.[4]

There are several possible interpretations of this finding. It is possible that this observation is real, and that the benefit simply took longer than expected to appear.

As one plausible mechanism, the earlier reduction in nonfatal myocardial infarction may have finally affected prognosis. Of course, the results may also be due to chance. A major difficulty in interpreting the data relates to the lack of knowledge about what the participants in the intervention and control groups did with respect to lipid lowering and other regimens in the intervening 9 years. Although there was no reason to expect that there was differential use of any intervention affecting mortality, such could have been the case.

Many of the very large trials have monitored participants (or subsets thereof) after close-out to determine whether behavioral effects of the study intervention have been sustained[9] or participants have adhered to recommendations regarding continued treatment.[9,15,17] In a trial of partial ileal bypass surgery, there was an interest in documenting the duration of the lipid-lowering effect.[3]

As already pointed out, knowledge of the response variable of interest for almost every participant is required if long-term surveillance after completion of regular follow-up is to be worthwhile. The degree of completeness attainable depends on several factors, such as the response itself, the length of surveillance time, the community where the trial was conducted, and the aggressiveness of the investigator.

DATA CLEAN-UP AND VERIFICATION

Despite attempts to collect complete, consistent, and error-free data, perfection is unlikely to be achieved. Monitoring systems are likely to reveal missing forms, unanswered items on forms, and conflicting data.

The importance of continuous monitoring of study forms and data throughout a trial is emphasized elsewhere (Chapter 10). It helps to minimize the job of cleaning up data at the end of the study. Nevertheless, some final data editing will no doubt be necessary. The timing of this process is important. Data editing should be initiated as soon as possible, because it is difficult to get full staff cooperation after a trial and its funding are over, especially difficult in a multicenter trial, where each investigator tends to pursue other interests once the study ends. It is also necessary to be realistic in the clean-up process. This means "freezing" the files at a reasonable time after the termination of participant follow-up and accepting some incomplete data. Obviously, the efforts during clean-up should be directed toward the most important areas; those crucial to answering the primary question.

Any clinical trial may be faced with having its results reviewed, questioned, and even audited. Traditionally, this review has been a scientific one. However, because special interest groups may want to look at the data, the key results should be properly verified, documented, and filed in an easily retrievable manner. The extent of this additional documentation of important data will depend on the design of each trial. Various models have been used. A simple model requires each investigator to send a duplicate of all death or major event forms on an ongoing basis to a member of the data monitoring committee. In one multicenter study, the investigators were asked at the end of follow-up to send a list of all deceased participants along with date of death to an office independent of the data coordinating center. In another trial,[1] an outside group of experts audited the data before the results were published. An extreme example employed in a large multicenter trial was the establishment of a second data coordinating center.[22] Duplicates of the key study forms were submitted to this center, which generated separate data reports. This approach is obviously costly. Common to all models is an attempt to maintain credibility. Most models have been used in large-scale, industry-sponsored trials with the data coordinating center maintained by the sponsor.

Verification of data may be time-consuming; thus it can conflict with the desire of the investigator to publish the findings as early as possible. While publication of important information should not be delayed unnecessarily, results should not be put into print before key data have been verified.

STORAGE OF STUDY MATERIAL

There are three principal reasons for storage of hard copy study material after a trial has been terminated. The first two, dealing with poststudy harm or benefit and with the possibility of an audit, have been mentioned. The third reason is scientific. In planning for a new trial, an investigator may want to obtain unpublished data from other investigators who have conducted trials in a similar population or tested the same intervention. Similarly, in preparation of a review article, a meta-analysis, or a paper on the natural history of a disease, an investigator may want to obtain additional information from published trials. Tables and figures in scientific papers seldom include everything that may be of interest. No uniform mechanism exists today for getting access to such study material from terminated trials. If information is available, it may not be in a reasonable and easily retrievable form. Substantial cooperation is usually required from the investigators originally involved in the data collection and analysis.

The responsibility of an investigator is to ensure that relevant data are accessible in an organized fashion after the termination of a trial. That is not to say data need be made accessible while a study is in progress. The risk is that other investigators might analyze the data and arrive at different interpretations of the results. However, further analysis and discussion of various interpretations of trial data are usually scientifically sound and ought to be encouraged.

In most trials, an excess of study material is collected, and storing everything may not make sense. The investigator has to consider logistics, the duration of the storage period, and cost. He also has to keep in mind that biological material, for example, deteriorates with time, data tapes require regular maintenance, and laboratory methods change.

One set of documents such as trial protocol, manual of procedures, study forms, and the analytic material, such as data tapes, should be kept by the investigator. In addition, a list containing identifying information for all participants who participated in a trial ought to be stored at the institution where the investigation occurred. Local regulations sometimes require that individual participant data such as copies of study forms, laboratory reports, ECGs, and x-rays be filed for a defined period with the participant's medical records. Storage of these data on microfilm may ease the problem of inadequate space. The actual trial results and their interpretation are usually published and can be retrieved through a library search. Exceptions are obviously findings that never reach the scientific literature. It may also be desirable in these cases to file draft manuscripts along with other documentation and analytic material.

DISSEMINATION OF RESULTS

The reporting of findings from a small single-center trial is usually straightforward. The individual participants are often told about the results at the last follow-up visit or shortly afterward, and the medical community is informed through scientific publications. However, there are situations that make the dissemination of findings difficult, especially the order in which the various interested parties are informed. Particularly in multicenter studies where the participants are referred by physicians not involved in the trial, the investigators have an obligation to tell these physicians about the conclusions, preferably before they read about it in the newspaper or are informed by their patients. In trials with clinics geographically scattered, all investigators have to be brought together to learn the results. In certain instances, the sponsoring party has a desire to make the findings known publicly at a press conference. However, although an early press conference followed by an article in a newspaper may be politically important to the sponsor of the trial, it may offend the participants, the referring physicians, and the medical community. They may all feel that they have a right to be informed before the results are reported in the lay press. One sequence has been suggested by Klimt and Canner.[18] First, the study leadership informs the other investigators who, in turn, inform the participants. The private physicians of the participants are also told, in confidence, of the findings. The results are then published in the scientific press, after which they may be more widely disseminated in other forums.

In special situations, when a therapy of public health importance is found to be particularly effective or harmful, physicians and the public need to be alerted in a timely manner. Although guidelines have been issued by the NIH,[13] there is ongoing debate about how to get the word out.[21] The guidelines charge the sponsoring institute with the distribution of significant information "via electronic and other special releases." Efforts are to be targeted to groups of physicians most directly affected.

After early termination of a trial assessing the effect of intravenous injection of immunoglobulin in preventing bacterial infections in children with the AIDS virus, a mass mailing went out to 18,000 pediatricians.[21] Other dissemination channels include notification of relevant professional societies and voluntary organizations. The National Library of Medicine is charged with announcing clinical alerts,[13] places full texts in the MEDLINE system, faxes them to all medical schools in the United States, and mails them to 3800 institutional members of the National Network of Libraries of Medicine. However, alerts are not always well received. A Clinical Alert from the National Cancer Institute on the value of adjuvant chemotherapy for node-negative cancer triggered pointed complaints from practicing oncologists.[21] It appears to be difficult to please everyone. The agreement by major journals to conduct an expedited peer review and to be more flexible in accepting early public release of important findings is a major step forward.[13,21]

If a serious adverse reaction is uncovered, there may be additional requirements to inform the appropriate regulatory agency (in case of a drug or device trial) and the sponsor (if a manufacturer or distributor). A "Dear Doctor" letter may be disseminated widely, or other means of rapidly alerting the medical community and the public may be implemented. The manufacturers of two antiarrhythmic drugs were required by the FDA to send out such a letter describing the findings of the Cardiac Arrhythmia Suppression Trial.[24] In severe cases, the medication may be taken off the market. An added complication of the dissemination process is the new requirement for the sponsor, if a pharmaceutical company, to announce without delay unpublished "price-sensitive" information.[11]

Another concern is the sometimes long delays between the presentation of trial findings at a scientific meeting and the publication of the full trial reports in peer-reviewed journals.[12] Clinicians are placed in difficult positions by having to make treatment decisions if the lay press reports on elements of findings many months prior to the publication of the trial data in full. The messages released by the lay press are typically very simple. To minimize this problem, three recommendations have been made[12]: (1) "congress organizers should insist that published abstracts contain sufficient data to justify the conclusions of the presentation," (2) "investigators should not present results of any study that is likely to influence clinical management until they are in a position to write a full paper,"and (3) "journal editors must be willing ... to expedite the publication of such papers." These recommendations are reasonable, but there may be exceptions.

REFERENCES

1. Anturane Reinfarction Trial Research Group: Sulfinpyrazone in the prevention of cardiac death after myocardial infarction, *N Engl J Med* 298:289-295, 1978.
2. Bell RL, Curb JD, Friedman LM et al: Termination of clinical trials: The Beta-Blocker Heart Attack Trial and the Hypertension Detection and Follow-up Program experience, *Controlled Clin Trials* 6:102-111, 1985.

3. Buchwald H, Varco RL, Matts JP et al: Effect of partial ileal bypass surgery on mortality and morbidity from coronary heart disease in patients with hypercholesterolemia. Report of the Program on the Surgical Control of the Hyperlipidemias (POSCH), *N Engl J Med* 323:946-955, 1990.

4. Canner PL, Berge KG, Wenger NK et al: Fifteen year mortality in Coronary Drug Project patients: long-term benefit with niacin, *JACC* 8:1245-1255, 1986.

5. Committee of Principal Investigators: WHO cooperative trial on primary prevention of ischaemic heart disease using clofibrate to lower serum cholesterol: mortality follow-up, *Lancet* ii:379-385, 1980.

6. Coronary Drug Project Research Group: The Coronary Drug Project: findings leading to further modifications of its protocol with respect to dextrothyroxine, *JAMA* 220:996-1008, 1972.

7. Coronary Drug Project Research Group: The Coronary Drug Project: findings leading to discontinuation of the 2.5-mg/day estrogen group, *JAMA* 226:652-657, 1973.

8. Coronary Drug Project Research Group: Clofibrate and niacin in coronary heart disease, *JAMA* 231: 360-381, 1975.

9. Cutler JA, Grandits GA, Grimm RH et al: Risk factor changes after cessation of intervention in the Multiple Risk Factor Intervention Trial, *Prev Med* 20:183-196, 1991.

10. Diabetic Retinopathy Study Research Group: Preliminary report on effects of photocoagulation therapy, *Am J Ophthalmol* 81:383-396, 1976.

11. Editorial. Early announcements, *Lancet* 342:1001-1002, 1993.

12. Editorial. Reporting clinical trials message and medium, *Lancet* 344:347-348, 1994.

13. Healy B: From the National Institutes of Health, *JAMA* 269:3069, 1993.

14. Herbst AL, Ulfelder H, Poskanzer DC: Adenocarcinoma of the vagina: association of maternal stilbestrol therapy with tumor appearance in young women, *N Engl J Med* 284:878-881, 1971.

15. Heinonen OP, Huttunen JK, Manninen V et al: The Helsinki Heart Study: coronary heart disease incidence during an extended follow-up, *J Intern Med* 235:41-49, 1994.

16. Paganini-Hill A, Ross RK, Henderson BE: Endometrial cancer and patterns of use of estrogen replacement therapy: a cohort study, *Br J Cancer* 59:445-557, 1989.

17. Hypertension Detection and Follow-up Program Cooperative Group: Persistence of reduction in blood pressure and mortality of participants in the Hypertension Detection and Follow-up Program, *JAMA* 259:2113-2122, 1988.

18. Klimt CR, Canner PL: Terminating a long-term clinical trial, *Clin Pharmacol Ther* 25:641-646, 1979.

19. Krol WF: Closing down the study, *Controlled Clin Trials* 4:505-512, 1983.

20. Moertel CG, Fleming TR, Haller D-G et al: Levamisole and fluorouracil for adjuvant therapy of resected colon carcinoma, *N Engl J Med* 322:352-358, 1990.

21. Palca J: Conflict over release of clinical research data, *Science* 251:374-375, 1990.

22. Persantine-Aspirin Reinfarction Study Research Group: Persantine and aspirin in coronary heart disease, *Circulation* 62:449-461, 1980.

23. Report from the Committee of Principal Investigators: A cooperative trial in the primary prevention of ischaemic heart disease using clofibrate, *Br Heart J* 40:1069-1118, 1978.

24. The Cardiac Arrhythmia Suppression Trial (CAST) Investigators: Preliminary report: effect of encainide and flecainide on mortality in a randomized trial of arrhythmia suppression after myocardial infarction, *N Engl J Med* 321:406-412, 1989.

25. Volberding PA, Lagakos SW, Koch MA et al: Zidovudine in asymptomatic human immunodeficiency virus infection, *N Engl J Med* 322:941-949, 1990.

CHAPTER 18

Reporting and
Interpreting of Results

The final phase in any experiment is to interpret and report the results. Finding the answer to a challenging question is the goal of any research endeavor. Proper communication of the results to clinicians also provides the basis for advances in medicine.[13] To communicate appropriately, the investigators have to review their results critically and avoid the temptation of overinterpretation. They are in the privileged position of knowing the quality and limitations of the data better than anyone else. Therefore they have the responsibility for presenting the results clearly and concisely, together with any issues that might bear on their interpretation. Investigators should devote adequate care, time, and attention to this critical part of the conduct of clinical trials.

A study may be reported in a scientific journal, but publication is in no way an endorsement of its results or conclusions. Even if the journal uses referees to assess each prospective publication, there is no assurance that they have sufficient experience and knowledge of the issues of design, conduct, and analysis to judge the reported study.[27] As pointed out by the editor of the *New England Journal of Medicine*,[54] "In choosing manuscripts for publication we make every effort to winnow out those that are clearly unsound, but we cannot promise that those we do publish are absolutely true…. Good journals try to facilitate this process [of medical progress] by identifying noteworthy contributions from among the great mass of material that now overloads our scientific communication system. Everyone should understand, however, that this evaluative function is not quite the same thing as endorsement." This point was recently illustrated.[20] The favorable results of a multicenter trial accompanied by a very positive editorial were published in the journal only 2 weeks before an Advisory Committee of the FDA voted unanimously against recommending that the intervention, a respiratory syncytial virus immune globulin, be licensed. In the end, it is up to the reader of a scientific article to assess it critically and to decide how to make best use of the reported findings.

In this chapter, we discuss guidelines for reporting, interpretation of findings, and publication bias, and the answers to three specific questions that should be considered in preparing a report: (1) Did the trial work as planned? (2) How do the findings compare with those from other studies? (3) What are the clinical implications of the findings?

FUNDAMENTAL POINT

The investigators have an obligation to review their study and its findings critically and to present sufficient information so that readers can properly evaluate the trial.

Any report of a clinical trial should include sufficient methodologic information, so the readers can assess the adequacy of the methods employed. The titles of chapters of this text almost serve as a checklist. The quality of a trial is typically judged based on the thoroughness and completeness of the material and methods sections of the report.

GUIDELINES FOR REPORTING

There are many guidelines on how to report a clinical trial. The International Committee of Medical Journal Editors has issued a set of uniform requirements that are endorsed by a vast number of journals.[38] Other guidelines have a special focus, such as the reporting of cancer trials or statistical methods.* Specific journals have adapted their own guidelines.[58] In addition, journals have their *Instructions for Authors* that address issues of format and content.

With the enormous number of scientific articles published annually, more than 2 million,[1] it is impossible for clinicians to keep up with the flow of information. More informative abstracts help clinicians who browse through journals on a regular basis. Valid and informative abstracts are important because clinical decisions are often influenced by abstracts alone.[34] For reporting clinical investigations, many journals have adopted the recommendation[1] for structured abstracts, which include information on objective, design, setting, patients or other participants, intervention(s), measurements and main results, and conclusion(s). The early experience of structured abstracts was reviewed by Haynes et al., and comments were "supportive and appreciative." Those authors recommend some modifications of the guidelines.[35] We strongly endorse the use of the structured abstract.

Decisions of authorship are both sensitive and important.[36,37] It is critical that decisions are made at an early stage. Recent cases of scientific fraud have reminded us that being an author carries certain responsibilities and should not be used as a means to show gratitude. Guidelines regarding qualifications for authorship are now included in general guidelines for manuscripts.[37,61] In a surprising decision, the *New England Journal of Medicine* in 1991 instituted guidelines that prohibit group authorship (common to large multicenter studies), restrict authorship to 12 (with a possibility for waiver), and limit the space devoted to acknowledgment.[40] Meinert[45] came to the defense of group authorship and expressed concern over the possible

---

*References 4, 6, 15, 38, 48, 58, 63.

effect of this policy on multicenter work. We believe that group authorship is an important part of clinical trials research. Fairness and equity require proper crediting to those who have made major contributions to the design, conduct, and analysis, not just the few that served on the writing group.

Presentation of the data analysis is also important.* There is a common misunderstanding of the meaning of p values. Only about one fifth of the respondents to a multiple choice question understood the proper meaning of a p value.[62] The p value tells us the probability that an observed difference may have occurred by chance. It conveys information about the level of doubt, not the magnitude of clinical importance of this difference. A p value of 0.05 in a very large trial may be evidence of a weak effect, while in a small sample it can be of a strong effect.[57] The point estimate (the observed result) with its 95% confidence interval (CI) provides us with the best estimates of the size of a difference. The width of the CI is another measure of uncertainty. The p value and the CI are related arithmetically; thus, if the 95% CI excludes 0, the difference is statistically significant with $p < 0.05$. The CI permits the readers to use their own value for the smallest clinically important difference in making treatment decisions.[8] Some journals have taken the lead and now require more extensive use of CIs. We advocate reporting of p values, point estimates, and CIs for the major results.

INTERPRETATION

Several articles have been written to help clinicians in their appraisal of a clinical study.† Readers should be aware that many publications have deficiencies and can even be misleading. Pocock[51] has given three reasons why readers need to be cautious: (1) some authors produce inadequate trial reports, (2) journal editors and referees allow them to be published, and (3) journals favor positive findings. For example, a review of trials of antibiotic prophylaxis found that 20% of the abstracts omitted important information or implied unjustified conclusions.[21] Pocock et al.[52] examined 45 trials and concluded that the reporting "appears to be biased toward an exaggeration of treatment differences" and that there was an overuse of significance levels. Also in a 1982 report, statistical errors were uncovered in a large proportion of 86 controlled trials in obstetrics and pediatrics journals, and only 10% of the conclusions were considered justified.[2] More recently, "doubtful or invalid statements" were found in 76% of 196 trials of nonsteroidal antiinflammatory drugs in rheumatoid arthritis.[31] Inadequate reporting of the methods of randomization and baseline comparability was found in 30% to 40% of 80 randomized clinical trials in leading medical journals.[3] The criteria for tumor response from articles published in

---

*References 8–11, 23, 26, 29, 57.
†References 14, 25, 32, 33, 46, 49.

three major journals were incompletely reported and variable, and contributed to the wide variations in reported response rates.[60]

Baar and Tannock[5] constructed a hypothetical trial and reported its results in two separate articles; one with errors of reporting and omissions similar to those "extracted from" leading cancer journals and the other with appropriate methods. This exercise illustrates how the same results can be interpreted and reported differently.

The way in which results are presented can affect treatment decisions.[24,42,47] Almost half of a group of surveyed physicians were more impressed and indicated a higher likelihood of treating their patients when the results of a trial were presented as a relative change in outcome rate compared with an absolute change (difference in the incidence of the outcome event).[24] A relative treatment effect is difficult to interpret without a knowledge of the event rate in the comparison group. The use of a "summary measure," such as the number of persons who need to be treated to prevent one event, had the weakest impact on clinicians' views of therapeutic effectiveness.[47] We recommend that authors report both absolute and relative changes in outcome rates.

PUBLICATION BIAS

We believe that the timely preparation and submission of the trial results— whether positive, neutral, or negative—ought to be every investigator's obligation. The written report is the public forum that all the work of a clinical trial finally faces. Regrettably, negative trials are more likely to remain unpublished than positive trials. The first evidence of this publication bias came from a survey of the psychological literature. Sterling[59] noted in 1959 that 97% of 294 articles involving hypothesis testing reported a statistically significant result. The situation is similar for medical journals several decades later; about 85% of articles—clinical trials and observational studies—reported statistically significant results.[18] Simes[56] compared the results of published trials with those from trials from an international cancer registry. A pooled analysis of published therapeutic trials in advanced ovarian cancer demonstrated a significant advantage for a combination therapy. However, the survival ratio was lower and statistically nonsignificant when the pooled analysis was based on the findings of all registered trials. Several surveys of investigators also provide evidence of publication biases. Similarly, it has been shown that many abstracts are never followed by full publications.[28] In a survey, Dickerson et al.[17] found that among 178 unpublished trials with a trend specified, 14% favored the new therapy, compared with 55% among 767 published reports ($p < 0.001$). Analysis of factors associated with this bias are, in addition to neutral and negative findings, small sample size and possibly pharmaceutical source of funding.[16] Rejection of a manuscript by a journal is an infrequent reason.[16,19] However, authors are no doubt aware that it is difficult to publish neutral results, and they may never write these manuscripts that are likely to be rejected. A survey of the reference lists of trials of nonsteroidal antiinflammatory drugs revealed a bias toward references with positive outcomes.[30] Journals ought to select trials for publication according to the quality of their conduct rather than according to whether the *p* value is significant.

DID THE TRIAL WORK AS PLANNED?

The foundation of any clinical trial is the effort to make sure that the study groups are initially comparable, so that differences between the groups over time can be reasonably attributed to the effect of the intervention. Randomization is the preferred method used to obtain baseline comparability. The use of randomization does not necessarily guarantee balance at baseline in the distribution of known or unknown prognostic factors. Baseline imbalance is fairly common in small trials but may also exist in large trials. Therefore both a detailed description of the randomization process and an evaluation of baseline comparability are essential. Should the trial be nonrandomized, the credibility of the findings hinges even more on an adequate documentation of this comparability. For each group, baseline data should include means and standard deviations of known and possible prognostic factors. Note that the absence of a statistically significant difference for any of these factors does not mean that the groups are balanced. In small studies, large differences are required to reach statistical significance. In addition, small trends for individual factors can have an impact if they are in the same direction. A multivariate analysis to evaluate balance may be advantageous. Of course, the fact that major prognostic factors may be unknown will produce some uncertainty with regard to baseline balance. Adjustment of the findings on the basis of observed baseline imbalance should be performed, and any difference between unadjusted and adjusted analyses should be carefully explained.

Double-blindness is a desirable feature of a clinical trial design because, as already discussed, it diminishes bias in the assessment of response variables that require some element of judgment. However, few studies are truly double-blinded to all parties from start to finish. While an individual side effect may be insufficient to unblind the investigator, a constellation of effects often reveals the group assignment. A specific drug effect, such as a marked fall in blood pressure in an antihypertensive drug trial, or the absence of such an effect, might also indicate which is the treatment group. Although the success of blinding may be difficult for the investigator to assess, an evaluation should be done. Readers of a publication ought to be informed about the degree of unblinding. An evaluation such as the one provided by Karlowski et al.[39] is commendable. In a recently completed double-blind, placebo-controlled trial of a lipid-lowering agent, the participants were asked at the close-out visit whether they had their lipids analyzed during the 3-year treatment period. More than half of them admitted that they had. It is possible that information on the lipid values could have led to an increased cross-over rate in the placebo group.

In estimating sample size, investigators often make assumptions regarding the rate of nonadherence. Throughout follow-up, efforts are made to maintain optimal adherence with the intervention under study and to monitor adherence. When interpreting the findings, one can then gauge whether the initial assumptions were borne out by what actually happened. When adherence assumptions have been too optimistic, the ability of the trial to test adequately the primary question may be less than planned. The study results must be reported and discussed with the power of the trial in mind. In trials showing a beneficial effect of a specific intervention, non-adherence is usually a minor concern. Two interpretations of the effect of non-adherence are possible. Of course, it may be argued that the intervention would have been even more beneficial had adherence been higher. On the other hand, if all participants (including those who for various reasons did not adhere entirely to the dosage schedule of a trial) had been on full dose, there could have been further adverse or toxic effects in the intervention group.

Also of interest is the comparability of groups during the follow-up period with respect to concomitant interventions. Drug use other than the study intervention, changes in lifestyle, and general medical care, if they affect the response variable, need to be measured. Of course, as mentioned in Chapter 16, adjustment on post-randomization variables is inappropriate. As a consequence, when imbalances exist, the study results must be interpreted cautiously.

When the results of a trial indicate no statistically significant difference between the study groups, there are several possible explanations. The dose of the studied intervention may have been too low or too high; the technical skills of those providing the intervention (e.g., surgical procedure) may have been inadequate; the sample size may have been too small, giving the trial insufficient power to test the hypothesis (Chapter 7); there may have been major adherence problems; concomitant interventions may have reduced the effect that would otherwise have been seen; or the outcome measurements may not have been sensitive enough or the analyses may have been inadequate. Finally, chance is another obvious explanation. The authors should provide the readers with enough information in the methods and in the results for them to judge for themselves why an intervention may not have worked. In the discussion, the authors should also offer their best understanding of why no difference was found.

What are the limitations of the findings? One needs to know the degree of completeness of data to evaluate a trial. A typical shortcoming, particularly in long-term trials, is that the investigator may lose track of some participants. These participants are usually different from those who remain in the trial, and their event rate may not be the same. Vigorous attempts should be made to limit the number of persons lost to follow-up. The credibility of the findings may be questioned in trials in which the number of participants lost to follow-up is large in relation to the number of events. A conservative approach in this context is to assume the "worst case." The worst-case approach assumes the occurrence of an event in each participant lost to follow-up in the group with lower incidence of the response variable, and it assumes no events in the comparison group. After application of the worst-case approach, if the overall conclusions of the trial remain unchanged, they are strengthened. However, if the worst-case analysis changes the conclusions, the trial may have less credibility. The degree of confidence in the conclusion will depend on the extent to which the outcome could be altered by the missing information.

As addressed in Chapter 16, results may be questionable if participants randomized into a trial are withdrawn from the analysis. Withdrawal after randomization violates the randomization and is a bad practice, one to be avoided. Investigators who support the concept of allowing withdrawals from the analysis should be required to include in their reporting of results analyses both with and without withdrawals. If both analyses give approximately the same result, the findings are confirmed. However, if the results of the two analyses differ, the interpretation of the study may remain unclear, and reasons for the differences need to be explored.

In evaluating possible benefit of an intervention, more than one response variable is often assessed, which raises the issue of multiple comparisons (Chapter 16). In essence, the chance of finding a nominally statistically significant result increases with the number of comparisons. This is true whether there are multiple response variables, repeated comparisons for the same response variable, or subgroup analyses, or whether various combinations of response variables are tested. In the survey of 45 trials in three leading medical journals, the median number of significance tests per trial was 8; more than 20 tests were reported in 6 trials.[52] The potential impact of this multiple testing on the findings and conclusion of a trial ought to be considered. A conservative approach in the interpretation of statistical tests is again recommended. When several comparisons have been made, a more extreme statistic might be required before a statistically significant difference could be claimed. One approach is to require a p value of less than 0.01 for a limited number of secondary outcomes to declare a treatment difference statistically significant. An alternative approach is to consider the subsidiary analyses exploratory and hypothesis-generating.[52] Authors of a report should indicate the total number of comparisons made during a trial and in the analysis phase (not just those selected for reporting). Readers should focus attention on p values for protocol-specified comparisons.

The main objective of any trial is to answer the primary question. Findings related to one of the secondary questions may be interesting, but they should be put in the proper perspective. Are the findings for the related primary and secondary response variables consistent? If not, attempts ought to be made to explain discrepancies. Explaining inconsistencies was particularly important in the Cooperative Trial in the Primary Prevention of Ischaemic Heart Disease.[55] In that trial, the intervention group showed a statistically significant reduction in the incidence of major ischaemic heart disease (primary response variable) but a significant increase in mortality from any cause (secondary response variable). In all studies, evidence for possible serious adverse effects from the intervention needs to be presented. In the final conclusion, the overall benefit should be weighed against the risk of harm. This assessment, however, is too infrequently done (Chapter 11).

HOW DO THE FINDINGS COMPARE WITH RESULTS FROM OTHER STUDIES?

The findings from a clinical trial should be placed in the context of current knowledge. Are they consistent with knowledge of basic science, including presumed mechanisms of action of the intervention? Proof of why an intervention works is seldom available. Nevertheless, when the outcome can be explained in terms of known biological actions, the conclusions are strengthened. Do the findings confirm the results of studies with similar interventions or different interventions in similar populations?

It is important here to keep in mind that a substantial proportion of initiated and even completed trials are never published. Additionally, reviews of the completeness of reference lists suggest that trials with neutral or negative results tend to be omitted.[30] Among published trials, the response to a given drug or drug combination can vary markedly.[5,44,50] The reported response rates to fluorouracil therapy vary between 8% and 85% for metastatic colorectal cancer.[5] Much of this variation may be explained by differences in patient selection, treatment regimen, and concomitant intervention, but major differences may also reflect the way the data were analyzed and reported. In a review of 51 randomized clinical trials in congestive heart failure, the authors attributed conflicting results to lack of uniform diagnostic criteria.[44] In a thoughtful editorial, Packer pointed out that several other factors could explain discordant results. He suggested that the characteristics of the enrolled patients may be more important than the definition of congestive heart failure. Differences in design—sample size, dose, and duration of intervention—may affect the trial findings. Other factors might be differences in criteria of efficacy and publication policy. Results of positive trials tend to be published several times, for example, both in a regular journal report and in a journal supplement funded by the pharmaceutical industry. Bero et al.[7] analyzed the symposium issues of 11 journals and concluded that the number increased steadily between 1966 and 1989, that they often had promotional attributes, that they were less likely to be peer-reviewed, and that they were more likely to have misleading titles.

Generally, credibility of a particular finding increases with the proportion of good independent studies that come to the same conclusion. Inconsistent results are not uncommon in research. In such cases, the problem for both the investigators and the readers is to try to determine the true effect of an intervention. How and why results differ need to be explored. The use of confidence limits has the advantage of allowing the readers to compare findings and assess whether the results of different trials could, in fact, be consistent.

WHAT ARE THE CLINICAL IMPLICATIONS OF THE FINDINGS?

It is appropriate, of course, to generalize the results to the study population, that is, those people who would have been eligible for and participated in the trial. The next step, suggesting that the trial results be applied to a more general population (the majority of which would not even meet the eligibility criteria of the trial) is more tenuous. The readers must judge for themselves whether such an extrapolation is appropriate.

A similar argument applies to the intervention itself. How general are the findings? If the intervention involved a special procedure, such as surgery or counseling, is its application outside the trial setting likely to produce the same response? In a drug trial, the question of dose-effect relationship is often raised. Would a higher dose of the drug have given different results? Can the same claims be made for different drugs that have a similar structure or pharmacological action? Can the results of an intervention be generalized even more broadly? For example, are all lipid-lowering regimens (diet, drug, or partial ileal bypass surgery) equivalent in testing the general hypothesis that lowering of serum cholesterol reduces the incidence of coronary heart disease, or is the answer specific to the mode of intervention? See Chapter 3 for a further discussion of generalization.

The majority of today's therapeutic interventions have not been properly tested in randomized clinical trials[22]; approval may have been granted on the basis of surrogate endpoints, or drugs may have multiple indications, only some of which are proven. Skillful marketing has a major impact on practice patterns. The marked regional differences in drug sales cannot be explained on the basis of science because regions have access to the same scientific information. It is difficult to tease out the impact of clinical trials on medical practice from other factors such as marketing and treatment guidelines. There are several examples of trials that have changed practice patterns.[12,41,53] Similarly, there are examples where practice was predominantly influenced by the other factors.[43]

As with all research, a clinical trial will often raise as many questions as it answers. Suggestions for further research should be discussed. Finally, the investigator might allude to the social, economic, and medical implications of the study findings. How many lives can be saved? How many working days will be gained? Can symptoms be alleviated? Economic implications or cost effectiveness are important. Any benefit has to be weighed against the cost and feasibility of use in routine medical practice rather than in the special setting of a clinical trial.

REFERENCES

1. Ad hoc Working Group for Critical Appraisal of the Medical Literature: A proposal for more informative abstracts of clinical articles, *Ann Intern Med* 106:598-604, 1987.
2. Altman DG: Statistics in medical journals, *Stat Med* 1:59-71, 1982.
3. Altman DG, Doré CJ: Randomization and baseline comparisons in clinical trials, *Lancet* 335:149-153, 1990.
4. Antczak AA, Tank J, Chalmers TC: Quality assessment of randomized clinical trials in dental research. I. Methods, *Periodontal Res* 21:305-314, 1986.
5. Baar J, Tannock I: Analyzing the same data in two ways: a demonstration model to illustrate the reporting and misreporting of clinical trials, *J Clin Oncol* 7:969-978, 1989.
6. Bailar JC, Mosteller I: Guidelines for statistical reporting in articles for medical journals. Amplifications and explanations, *Ann Intern Med* 108:266-273, 1988.
7. Bero LA, Galbraith A, Rennie D: The publication of sponsored symposiums in medical journals, *N Engl J Med* 327:1135-1140, 1992.
8. Berry G: Statistical significance and confidence intervals, *Med J Aust* 144:618-619, 1986.
9. Braitman LE: Confidence intervals extract clinically useful information from data, *Ann Intern Med* 108:296-298, 1988.
10. Braitman LE: Statistical estimates and clinical trials, *J Biopharm Stat* 3:249-256, 1993.
11. Bulpitt CJ: Confidence intervals, *Lancet* i:494-497, 1987.
12. Collins R, Julian D: British Heart Foundation surveys (1987 and 1989) of United Kingdom treatment policies for acute myocardial infarction, *Br Heart J* 66:250-255, 1991.
13. Comroe JH Jr: The road from research to new diagnosis and therapy, *Science* 200:931-937, 1978.
14. Cuddy PG, Elenbaas RM, Elenbaas JK: Evaluating the medical literature, *Ann Emerg Med* 12:549-555, 610-620, 679-686, 1993.
15. DerSimonian R, Charette LJ, McPeek B, Mosteller F: Reporting on the methods in clinical trials, *N Engl J Med* 306:1332-1337, 1982.
16. Dickerson K: The existence of publication bias and risk factors for its occurrence, *JAMA* 263:1385-1389, 1990.
17. Dickerson K, Chan S, Chalmers TC et al: Publication bias and clinical trials, *Controlled Clin Trials* 8:343-353, 1987.
18. Dickerson K, Min YI: Publication bias: the problem that won't go away, *Ann NY Acad Sci* 703:135-146, 1993.
19. Easterbrook PJ, Berlin JA, Gopalan R, Matthews DR: Publication bias in clinical research, *Lancet* 337:867-872, 1991.
20. Ellenberg SS, Epstein JS, Fratantoni JC et al: A trial of RSV immune globulin in infants and young children: the FDA view, *N Engl J Med* 331:203-204, 1994.
21. Evans M, Pollock AV: Trials on trial. A review of trials of antibiotic prophylaxis, *Arch Surg* 119:109-113, 1984.
22. Fineberg HV: Clinical evaluation: how does it influence medical practice? *Bull Cancer* 74:333-346, 1987.
23. Freeman PR: The role of p-values in analyzing trial results, *Stat Med* 12:1443-1452, 1993.
24. Forrow L, Taylor WC, Arnold RM: Absolutely relative: how research results are summarized can affect treatment decisions, *Am J Med* 92:121-124, 1992.
25. Fowkes FGR, Fulton PM: Critical appraisal of published research: introductory guidelines, *Br Med J* 302:1136-1140, 1991.
26. Gardner MJ, Altman DG: Confidence interval rather than *p*-values: estimation rather than hypothesis testing, *Br Med J* 292:746-750, 1986.
27. Glantz SA: Biostatistics: how to detect, correct and prevent errors in the medical literature, *Circulation* 61:1-7, 1980.
28. Goldman L, Loscalzo A: Fate of cardiology research orginally published in abstract form, *N Engl J Med* 303:255-259, 1980.
29. Goodman SN, Berlin JA: The use of predicted confidence intervals when planning experiments and the misuse of power when interpreting results, *Ann Intern Med* 121:200-206, 1994.

30. Gøtzsche PC: Reference bias in reports of drug trials, *Br Med J* 295:652-659, 1987.
31. Gøtzsche PC: Methodology and overt and hidden bias in reports of 196 double-blind trials of non-steroidal anti-inflammatory drugs in rheumatoid arthritis, *Controlled Clin Trials* 10:31-56, 1989.
32. Guyatt GH, Sackett DL, Cook DJ, for the Evidence-Based Medicine Working Group: Users' guide to the medical literature: II. How to use an article about therapy or prevention: A. Are the results of the study valid? *JAMA* 270:2598-2601, 1993.
33. Haynes RB, McKibbon KA, Fitzgerald D et al: How to keep up with the medical literature, *Ann Intern Med* 105:149-153, 309-312, 474-478, 636-640, 810-816, 978-984, 1986.
34. Haynes RB, McKibbon KA, Walker CJ et al: A study on the use and usefulness of online access to MEDLINE in clinical settings, *Ann Intern Med* 112:78-84, 1990.
35. Haynes RB, Muldew CD, Huth EJ et al: More informative abstracts revisited, *Ann Intern Med* 113:69-76, 1990.
36. Huth EJ: Preparing to write. In: *How to write and publish papers in medical sciences,* Philadelphia, 1982, ISI Press.
37. Huth EJ: Guidelines for authorship of medical papers, *Ann Intern Med* 104:269-274, 1986.
38. International Committee of Medical Journal Editors: Uniform requirements for manuscripts submitted to biomedical journals, *Ann Intern Med* 108:258-265, 1988.
39. Karlowski TR, Chalmers TC, Frenkel LD et al: Ascorbic acid for the common cold: a prophylactic and therapeutic trial, *JAMA* 231:1038-1042, 1975.
40. Kassirer JP, Angell M: On authorship and acknowledgments, *N Engl J Med* 325:1510-1512, 1991.
41. Lamas GA, Pfeffer MA, Hamm P et al: Do the results of randomized clinical trials of cardiovascular drugs influence medical practice? *N Engl J Med* 327:241-247, 1992.
42. Laupacis A, Sackett DL, Roberts RS: An assessment of clinically useful measures of the consequences of treatment, *N Engl J Med* 318:1728-1733, 1988.
43. Manolio TM, Cutler JA, Furberg CD et al: Trends in pharmacologic management of hypertension in the United States, *Arch Intern Med* 155:829-837, 1995.
44. Marantz PR, Alderman MH, Tobin JN: Diagnostic heterogeneity in clinical trials for congestive heart failure, *Ann Intern Med* 109:55-61, 1988.
45. Meinert CL: In defense of the corporate author for multicenter trials, *Controlled Clin Trials* 14:255-260, 1993.
46. Moon TE: Interpretation of cancer prevention trials, *Prev Med* 18:721-731, 1989.
47. Naylor CD, Chen E, Strauss B: Measured enthusiasm: does the method of reporting trial results alter perceptions of therapeutic effectiveness? *Ann Intern Med* 117:916-921, 1992.
48. Oxman AD: Checklist for review articles, *Br Med J* 309:648-651, 1994.
49. Oxman AD, Sackett DL, Guyatt GH, for the Evidence-Based Medicine Working Group: Users' guides to the medical literature: I. How to get started, *JAMA* 270:2093-2095, 1993.
50. Packer M: Clinical trials in congestive heart failure: why do studies report conflicting results, *Ann Intern Med* 109:3-5, 1988.
51. Pocock SJ: *Clinical trials. A practical approach,* Chichester, 1983, John Wiley & Sons.
52. Pocock SJ, Hughes MD, Lee RJ: Statistical problems in the reporting of clinical trials. A survey of three medical journals, *N Engl J Med* 317:426-432, 1987.
53. Psaty BM, Koepsell TD, Yanez D et al: Temporal patterns of antihypertensive medication use among older adults, 1989-1992: an effect of the major clinical trials on clinical practice? *JAMA* 273:1436-1438, 1995.
54. Relman AS: What a good medical journal does, *The New York Times* Section IV; p 22, March 19, 1978.
55. Report from the Committee of Principle Investigators: A cooperative trial in the primary prevention of ischaemic heart disease using clofibrate, *Br Heart J* 40:1069-1118, 1978.
56. Simes RJ: Publication bias: the case for an international registry of clinical trials, *J Clin Oncol* 4:1529-1541, 1987.
57. Simon R: Confidence intervals for reporting results of clinical trials, *Ann Intern Med* 105:429-435, 1986.
58. Simon R, Wittes RE: Methodologic guidelines for reports of clinical trials, *Cancer Treat Rep* 69:1-3, 1985.

59. Sterling TD: Publication decisions and their possible effects on inferences drawn from test of significance—or vice versa, *JASA* 54:30-34, 1959.

60. Tonkin K, Tritchler D, Tannock I: Criteria of tumor response used in clinical trials of chemotherapy, *J Clin Oncol* 3:870-875, 1985.

61. Whitehouse S, Mellinger RC: Responsibilities of authorship: justification for the multiauthored scientific paper, *Henry Ford Hosp Med J* 36:67-69, 1988.

62. Wulff HR, Anderson B, Brandenholf P, Guttler F: What do doctors know about statistics? *Stat Med* 6:3-10, 1987.

63. Zelen M: Guidelines for publishing papers on cancer clinical trials: responsibilities of editors and authors, *J Clin Oncol* 1:164-169, 1983.

CHAPTER 19

Multicenter Trials

A multicenter trial is a collaborative effort that involves more than one independent center in the tasks of enrolling and following study participants. Early contributions to the design of these trials were made by Hill.[9] Greenberg[13] provided a general discussion of methods.

There has been a dramatic increase in the number of multicenter trials in the last two decades. Of course, the sizes of these have varied, depending on the requirements of the study. Multicenter studies are more difficult and more expensive to perform than single-center studies, and they bring perhaps less professional reward because of the need to share credit among many investigators. Nevertheless, they are carried out because single sites cannot enroll enough participants.[15] Levin et al.[17] provide many examples of "the importance and the need for well-designed cooperative efforts to achieve clinical investigations of the highest quality." Much of the groundwork for the development, organization, and conduct of a multicenter trial was laid in the Coronary Drug Project (CDP).[7] A detailed description of multicenter trials is given by Meinert.[20] This chapter will discuss the reasons such studies are conducted and briefly review some steps in their planning, design, and conduct.

FUNDAMENTAL POINT

Anyone responsible for organizing and conducting a multicenter study should have a full understanding of the complexity of the undertaking. Problems in conduct of the trial most often originate from inadequate and unclear communication between the participating investigators, all of whom must agree to follow a common study protocol.

REASONS FOR MULTICENTER TRIALS

1. The main rationale for multicenter trials is to recruit the adequate number of participants within a reasonable time. Many clinical trials have been, and still are, performed without a good estimate of the number of participants likely to be required to test adequately the main hypothesis. Yet, if the primary response variable is an event that occurs relatively infrequently, or small group differences are to be detected, sample size requirements will be large (Chapter 7).

Studies requiring hundreds of participants usually cannot be done at one center. For example, in the Aspirin Myocardial Infarction Study,[2] 30 centers enrolled the necessary 4200 patients with a history of a heart attack in 1 year and followed them for an additional 3 years. The largest of these centers enrolled slightly more than 200 participants. Let us assume uniform annual rates of enrollment, uniform annual mortality, and follow-up of all participants to a common termination date. If an investigator were interested only in the experience of the participants over the initial 3 years after enrollment, assuming no further benefit from intervention after that time, then the single largest center would have required 21 years to recruit participants and 24 years to complete the study. Even if the investigator were interested simply in an equivalent number of person–years of intervention, regardless of the number of years a participant received the intervention, this one center would have taken approximately 12 years to complete the study.

A 24-year study and even a 12-year study may be impractical and may develop major problems. New advances in therapy and methodology during the years may make the study obsolete. Mortality from causes other than the one of interest may become more important in the later years of the study and dilute any effect of the intervention. It may not be reasonable to expect an intervention to continue to provide the same relative benefit over the course of many years. In addition, participants and investigators are likely to lose interest in the trial and may elect not to participate further. There is also a good chance that they may move from the area. Finally, answers from the trial that might benefit other people will be delayed for a generation. For these reasons, most investigators prefer to engage in studies of shorter duration.

2. A multicenter study may assure a more representative sample of the study or target population. Geography, race, socioeconomic status, and lifestyle of participants may be more representative of the general population if participants are enrolled by many centers. These factors may be important in the ability to generalize the findings of the trial. Severity and sequelae of hypertension, for example, are seemingly race related. A study of hypertensive patients from either a totally African-American or totally white community are likely to yield findings that may not necessarily apply to a more diverse population. Similarly, a study of pulmonary disease in an air-polluted industrial center might not give the same results as a study in a rural area.

3. A multicenter study enables investigators with similar interests and skills to work together on a common problem. Science and medicine, like many other disciplines, are competitive. Nevertheless, investigators may find that there are times when their own interests and those of science require them to cooperate. Thus many scientists collaborate to solve particularly vexing clinical and public health problems and to advance knowledge in areas of common interest. A multicenter trial also gives capable, clinically oriented persons, who might otherwise not become involved in research activities, an opportunity to contribute to science.

CONDUCT OF MULTICENTER TRIALS

One of the earlier multicenter clinical trials was the Coronary Drug Project (CDP).[7] This study provided an initial model for many of the techniques currently employed. Some techniques have been refined in subsequent trials. As in all active disciplines, concepts are frequently changing. Nonetheless, the following series of steps are one reasonable way to approach the planning and conduct of a multicenter trial. They consist of a distillation of experience from several of these studies.

First, a group should be established to be responsible for organizing and overseeing the various phases of the study (planning, participant recruitment, participant follow-up, phaseout, data analysis, and paper writing) and its various centers and committees. This group often consists of people in government agencies, private research organizations, educational institutions, or private industry, with input from appropriate consultants. Use of consultants who are experts in the field of study, in biostatistics, and in the management of multicenter clinical trials is encouraged. The organizing group needs to have authority to operate effectively and for the study to function efficiently.

Second, to determine the feasibility of a study, the organizing group should make a thorough search of the literature and review of other information. Sample size requirements should be calculated. Reasonable estimates must be made regarding control group event rate, anticipated effect of intervention, and participant adherence to therapy. The organizing group also has to evaluate key issues such as total cost, participant availability, availability of competent cooperating investigators, timeliness of the study, and regulatory requirements. After such an assessment, is the trial worth pursuing? Are there sufficient preliminary indications that the intervention under investigation indeed might work? On the other hand, is there so much suggestive (though inconclusive) evidence in favor of the new intervention that it might be difficult ethically to allocate participants to a control group? Since planning for the study may take a year or more, feasibility must constantly be reevaluated, even up to the time of the actual start of participant recruitment. New or impending evidence may at any time cause cancellation, postponement, or redesign of the trial. In some instances, a pilot or feasibility study is useful in answering specific questions important for the design and conduct of a full-scale trial.

Third, multicenter studies require not only clinical centers to recruit participants, but also a coordinating center to help design and manage the trial and to collect and analyze data from all other centers. Additional centers are often needed to perform specialized activities, such as conducting key laboratory tests, reading angiograms or x-rays, reading pathology slides, and distributing study drugs. While the specialized centers may perform multiple services, it is usually not advisable to permit a clinical center to perform these services. If a specialized center and a clinical center are in the same institution, each should have a separate staff. Otherwise, unblinding and, therefore, bias could result. Even if unblinding or bias is avoided, there might be criticism that such a bias could have occurred, and this could raise unnecessary questions about the entire clinical trial.

As Croke[8] reported, a major consideration when selecting clinical center investigators is availability of appropriate participants. The trial has to go where the participants are. Clearly, experience in clinical trials and scientific expertise are desirable features for investigators, but they are not crucial to overall success. Well-known scientists who add stature to a study are not always successful in collaborative ventures. The chief reason is often their inability to devote sufficient time to the trial. In a comprehensive study of factors associated with enrollment of eligible participants with documented myocardial infarction, Shea et al.[24] found positive correlations with institutions in which patients were cared for by staff other than private attending physicians and with the presence of a committed nurse-coordinator.

The selection of the coordinating center is of utmost importance. In addition to helping design the trial, this center is responsible for implementing the randomization scheme, for carrying out day-to-day trial activities, and for collecting, monitoring, editing, and analyzing data. The coordinating center must be in constant communication with all other centers. Its staff must have expertise in areas such as biostatistics, computer technology, epidemiology, medicine, and management to respond expeditiously to daily problems that arise in a trial. These might range from simple questions, such as how to code a particular item on a questionnaire, to requests for special data analyses that may require modifications of established statistical methods. In all, the staff at the coordinating center must be experienced, capable, responsive, and dedicated to handle its workload in a timely fashion. A trial can succeed despite inadequate performance of one or two clinical centers, but a poorly performing coordinating center can materially affect the success of a multicenter trial.

A key element in any coordinating center is not only the presence of integrity, but the appearance of integrity. Any suspicion of conflict of interest can damage the trial. It is for this reason that pharmaceutical firms who support trials sometimes use outside institutions or organizations as coordinating centers. Since the personnel in the coordinating center control the data and the analyses, they should be seen to have no overriding interest in the outcome of a trial. Meinert[20] has described the functions of the coordinating center in detail.

It is also obvious that the centers selected to perform specialized activities need expertise in their particular fields. Equally important is the capacity to handle the large workloads of a multicenter trial with research-level quality. Even with careful selection of these centers, backlogs of work are a frequent source of frustration during the course of a trial.

Fourth, it is preferable for the organizing group to provide prospective investigators with a fairly detailed outline of the key elements of the study design as early as possible. This results in more efficient initiation of the trial and allows each investigator to plan better his staffing and cost requirements. Rather than presenting a final protocol to the investigators, it is recommended that they be given time to discuss and, if necessary, modify the trial design. This process allows them to contribute their own ideas, to have an opportunity to participate in the design of the trial, and to become familiar with all aspects of the study. It may also improve the design. The investigators need a protocol that is acceptable to them and their colleagues at their local institution. This process usually requires several planning sessions before the start of participant recruitment.

If there are many investigators and several difficult protocol decisions, it is useful during the planning stage to have specific groups of investigators address these issues. Working groups can focus on individual problems and prepare reports for all investigators. Of course, if the initial outline has been well thought out and developed, few major design modifications will be necessary. Any design change must be carefully examined to ensure that the basic objectives and feasibility of the study are not threatened. This caveat applies particularly to modifications of participant eligibility criteria. Investigators are understandably concerned about their ability to enroll a sufficient number of participants. In an effort to make recruitment easier, they may favor less stringent eligibility criteria. Any such decisions need to be examined to ensure that they do not have an adverse impact on the objectives of the trial and on sample size requirements. The benefit of easier recruitment may be outweighed by the need for a larger sample size. Planning meetings serve to make all investigators aware of the wide diversity of opinions. Inevitably, compromises consistent with good science must be reached on difficult issues, and some investigators may not be completely satisfied with all aspects of a trial. However, all are usually able to support the final design. *All investigators in a cooperative trial must agree to follow the common study protocol.*

Fifth, an organizational structure for the trial should be established with clear areas of responsibility and lines of authority. Many have been developed.[3-5,16,19] The following structure has stood the test of time.

Data monitoring committee. The data monitoring committee, which should be independent of the investigators and any sponsor of the trial, is charged with periodically monitoring baseline, toxicity, and response-variable data, and evaluating center performance.[11] In light of recent concerns about clinical-trial integrity,[1,6,10] the independence of this group is especially important. It reports to either the organizing group or the study sponsor (which may be one and the same). In several studies, the functions of the committee have been performed by two separate groups, by one group, or by one group with a subcommittee. The use of two groups, one to review data and another to advise on policy matters, has the theoretical advantage of providing an additional level of review. However, if the policy advisory group also has direct responsibility for data review, it can discharge its duties more effectively. That is because it has a more intimate knowledge of study data and can directly request from the coordinating center any additional data analyses that may assist it during its deliberations. Therefore we recommend that the trial should have either a single committee or a subcommittee of the main group that is responsible for data review and must report to the committee as a whole. The coordinating center should present tabulated and graphic data and appropriate analyses to the data monitoring committee for review. The committee has the responsibility to recommend to the organizers or to the sponsor of the trial early termination in case of unanticipated toxicity, greater-than-expected benefit, or high likelihood of indifferent results. (See Chapter 15.) Members of this committee should be knowledgeable in the field under study, in clinical trials methodology, and in biostatistics. Some people also suggest adding a participant advocate to the group. The qualifications of this person will vary, depending on the nature of the trial. The ethical responsibilities of the data monitoring committee to the participants, and to the integrity of the study, should be clearly established. These responsibilities for participant safety are particularly important in double-blind studies, since the individual investigators are unaware of the group assignments.

Steering committee. In large studies, the steering committee, sometimes called an executive committee, provides scientific direction for the study at the operational level. Its membership is made up of a subset of investigators participating in the trial. Depending on the length of the study, some key investigators may be permanent members of the steering committee to provide continuity. Others may be chosen or elected for shorter terms. Subcommittees are often established to consider on a study-wide level specific issues such as adherence, quality control, classification of response variables, and publication policies and then report to the steering committee.

It may also be important to authorize a small subgroup to make executive decisions between steering committee meetings. Most "housekeeping" tasks and day-to-day decisions can be more easily accomplished in this manner. A large committee, for example, it unable to monitor a trial on a daily basis, write memoranda, or prepare agendas. Since committee meetings can rarely be called on short notice, issues requiring rapid decisions must be addressed by an executive group. It is important, however, that major questions be discussed with the investigators.

Assembly of investigators. The assembly of investigators represents all of the centers participating in the trial. In small studies, this assembly may be the same as the steering committee. In large studies, the steering committee would become too large to perform its duties effectively if it included all investigators. In this model, the principal investigator for each center is a voting member of the assembly. The purposes of assembly meetings, which may be attended by other study personnel, are to allow for votes on major issues, to keep all investigators acquainted with the progress of the trial, and to provide an opportunity for staff training and education. Given the complexity of many trials, this last purpose is often the most important.

The committee structure for the multicenter Beta-Blocker Heart Attack Trial[3] was a fairly typical example. Two subcommittees (mortality classification and non-fatal events) dealt with evaluation of response variables. Such central evaluation, with the participant's identity and intervention group assignment blinded, helped to assure unbiased classification of reported events and to ensure consistent application of criteria for particular events. Other subcommittees, such as adherence and quality control, were responsible for assuring high-quality data by monitoring performance and initiating corrective action if needed. Usually, there are subcommittees that develop and review study publications and presentations (editorial subcommittee and bibliography subcommittee). Finally, there are subcommittees with specialized functions depending on the nature of the trial. In the Beta-Blocker Heart Attack Trial, a subcommittee addressed issues concerning conduct and analysis of ambulatory electrocardiographic recordings. These bodies were purposely called subcommittees to emphasize that they were responsible to the steering committee.

In some other trials, the committee structure has become too complex and leads to inefficiencies. Trials with few centers function best with a simple structure. If committees, subcommittees, and task forces multiply, the process of handling routine problems becomes difficult. Studies that involve multiple disciplines especially need a carefully crafted organizational structure. Investigators from different fields tend to look at issues from various perspectives. Although this variety can be beneficial, under some circumstances it can obstruct the orderly conduct of a trial. Investigators may seek to increase their own areas of responsibility and, in the process, change the scope of the study. What starts out as a moderately complex trial can end up being an almost unmanageable undertaking.

Sixth, despite special problems, multicenter trials should try to maintain standards of quality as high as those attainable in carefully conducted single-center trials. Therefore strong emphasis should be placed on training and standardization. It is obviously extremely important that staff at all centers understand the protocol definitions and how to complete forms and perform tests. Differences in performance among centers and between individuals in a single center are unavoidable. They can, however, be minimized by proper training, certification procedures, retesting, and when necessary, retraining of staff. These efforts need to be implemented before a trial begins. (See Chapter 10 for a discussion of quality control.) Not until the steering committee is satisfied that staff are capable of performing necessary procedures should a clinical center be allowed to begin enrolling participants. Meetings of the assembly of investigators are essential to the successful conduct of the trial because they provide opportunities to discuss common problems and review proper ways to collect data and complete study forms. In one trial, very elaborate and extensive standardization, certification, and periodic retesting were undertaken to ensure that methodology and procedures for laboratory determinations were identical at the various centers.[18] Such standardization was rather costly but essential to the completion of the goals of that study.

The large and simple trials[27] typically involve a large number of participating centers, many of which are nonacademic institutions. Education, training, and standardization may not get the same attention as in other trial models. Clinician-investigators need to understand the basic concepts and intent of clinical trials and how the rules of research—which may sometimes seem arbitrary—differ from the way they practice medicine. The reliance on hard endpoints, such as all-cause mortality, and the limited data collection in this kind of multicenter trial tend to reduce the need for elaborate quality-control procedures.

Certain functions in a multicenter trial are best performed by properly selected special centers.[20] The advantages of centrally performing laboratory tests, reading x-rays, evaluating pathology specimens, or coding electrocardiograms include unbiased assessment, reduced variability, ease of quality control, and high quality of performance. The disadvantages of centralized determinations include the cost and time required for shipping, and the risk of losing study material.

Seventh, there needs to be close monitoring of the performance of all centers. Participant recruitment, quality of data collection and processing, quality of laboratory procedures, and adherence of participants to protocol should be evaluated frequently. The exact frequency is determined by the time span for which investigators are willing to allow errors or nonperformance to go undetected. Of course, cost and personnel considerations may dictate a lower frequency than desired. Tables 19-1 through 19-3 are typical of the kinds of information that investigators have used to compare clinical center performance. Table 19-1 compares the average time required for each clinical center to complete and send forms to the coordinating center. Center B in the present 6 months stands out as doing poorly, and it has become worse when compared with previous performance. Table 19-2 shows that center B also has a large number of unsubmitted forms. As seen in Table 19-3, clinical centers A and B are sub-

Table 19-1 Average processing time for follow-up visit (FV) forms

Clinic	Previous 6 Months		Present 6 Months	
	No. of FV forms received	Days from visit to receipt of forms	No. of FV forms received	Days from visit to receipt of forms
A	292	25.8	290	8.7
B	157	22.9	117	29.0
C	210	16.0	198	16.2
D	174	11.6	173	10.4
E	182	8.3	185	12.7
Total	1015	17.8	963	13.8

Table used in Aspirin Myocardial Infarction Study: Coordinating Center, University of Maryland.

Table 19-2   Number of follow-up visit forms not received at coordinating center more than 1 month past the visit window, by clinic

Clinic	Jan. 13, 1978	July 28, 1978
A	8	0
B	21	65
C	0	1
D	1	0
E	0	0
Total	30	66

Table used in Aspirin Myocardial Infarction Study: Coordinating Center, University of Maryland.

Table 19-3   Percentage of follow-up visit forms with one or more errors, by clinic and month of follow-up

Clinic	Feb.	Mar.	Apr.	May	June	July	Total	Total previous 6 months	Errors per form*	No. of forms processed
A	30.0	29.6	29.6	29.7	35.1	29.3	30.3	33.2	6.11	290
B	25.0	14.3	20.8	28.0	—	28.3	24.2	24.2	6.66	117
C	0.0	14.1	3.4	8.1	27.3	13.8	12.1	16.2	5.21	198
D	22.2	16.7	6.3	20.9	9.7	26.3	16.2	17.8	6.21	173
E	4.8	10.3	19.6	13.6	21.2	20.8	15.7	18.7	4.38	185
Total	17.0	18.5	17.0	20.4	20.9	23.8	20.6	23.1	5.68	963

Table used in Aspirin Myocardial Infarction Study: Coordinating Center, University of Maryland.
*Errors per form are calculated by dividing the number of errors by the number of forms failing edit.

mitting many forms with errors. It is useful to identify those centers that are performing below average. Often specific problems can be identified and corrected. For example, in one study, evidence of left ventricular hypertrophy was identified much more often in the ECGs from one center than from the other centers. Only after looking into the reasons for this was it discovered that the internal standard on that clinical center's electrocardiograph machine was incorrectly calibrated.

In all clinical trials, recruitment of participants is difficult. In a cooperative clinical trial, however, there is an opportunity for some clinical centers to compensate for the inadequate performance of other centers. The clinical centers should understand that, while friendly competition keeps everybody working, the real goal is overall success, and what some centers cannot do, another perhaps can. Therefore, it is important to encourage the good centers to recruit as many participants as possible.

Eighth, publication, presentation, and authorship policies should be determined in advance. Authorship becomes a critical issue when there are multiple investigators, many of whose academic careers depend on publication. Unfortunately, there is no completely satisfactory way to recognize the contribution of each investigator. A common compromise is to put the study name immediately under the paper title and to acknowledge the writers of the paper, either in a footnote or under the title, next to the study name. All key investigators are then listed at the end of the paper. The policy may also vary according to the type of paper (main or subsidiary). The group authorship of manuscripts from multicenter trials has been challenged by some medical journals.[12,14,21]

Involvement of the sponsor as an author of the main manuscripts from a major trial can be contentious, especially if it is a commercial firm that stands to benefit from a favorable presentation of the trial results. Most sponsors accept a hands-off policy and leave it to the investigators to write the scientific papers. Typically, they are given 1 month to preview a manuscript, particularly for patent or regulatory issues. This review should not unnecessarily delay the publication of the trial results. Regrettably, there are multiple examples of interference that conflicts with academic freedom.

In one four-center trial, the investigators at one of the centers reported their own findings before the total group had an opportunity to do so.[25,28] Such an action is not compatible with a collaborative effort. It undermines the goal of a multicenter trial of having enough participants to answer a question and, perhaps more important, the trust among investigators. Many academic institutions have taken a strong stand against this principle of collaboration and in defense of academic freedom for each investigator. However, we believe that those unwilling to abide by the rule for common authorship should not participate in collaborative studies.

Advance planning of authorship policy may eliminate subsequent misunderstandings. However, fair recognition of junior staff will always be difficult.[22] Study leadership often gets credit and recognition for work done largely by people whose contributions may remain unknown to the scientific community. One way to alleviate this problem is to appoint as many capable junior staff members as possible to subcommittees. Such staff members should also be encouraged to develop studies ancillary to the main trial. This approach will enable them to claim authorship for their own work while using the basic structure of the trial to get access to participants and supporting data. Such ancillary studies may be performed on only a subgroup of participants and must not interfere with the main effort through unblinding, by harming the participants, or by causing the participants to leave the trial. Sackett and Naylor[23] discuss the issues for and against allowing publication of ancillary studies before the main trial is completed.

GENERAL COMMENTS

Even if investigators think they have identified all potential difficulties and have taken care to prevent them, new problems will always arise. This is particularly true of multicenter trials because of their size, complexity, and large number of investigators with diverse backgrounds and interests. To forestall and minimize problems, the need for adequate studywide communication must be stressed. If communication among the various components of the study lapses or is vague, the trial can rapidly deteriorate. It is the responsibility of the coordinating center to keep in frequent contact (by telephone, letter, and visit) with all the other centers. This contact must be initiated by both the coordinating center and the other centers. The study leaders also need to maintain contact with the various centers and committees, closely monitoring the conduct of the trial.

The difficulties in getting groups of clinicians to work together using a common protocol was recently reported.[26] A group of experienced Italian scientists tried to engage general practitioners in a drug trial of patients with isolated systolic hypertension. The well-established principles for organizing a collaborative study were followed. The practitioners were informed and trained and were also given the opportunity to comment on the study protocol. Unfortunately, only 88 of the 806 general practitioners who had agreed to participate eventually started recruitment. Sixty-three practitioners enrolled at least one participant. Due to poor cooperation, the study was stopped after completion of its feasibility phase. A major problem was the practitioners' difficulties in withdrawing drug therapy. "The change from the role of confident and reassuring prescriber to an attitude of uncertainty (which attracted consensus in the preparatory meetings) raised instinctive resistance in practice, leading to the withdrawal of the general practitioner rather than the patient's treatment."

Cost is always a concern in multicenter trials. These studies are generally expensive because of their complexity, size, and elaborate committee structure. Expense can be minimized by asking only pertinent questions on forms, by reducing the number of laboratory tests, and by performing only necessary quality monitoring; in essence, by simplifying data collection.[27] Accomplishing these economies demands constant attention, particularly during the planning phase. The investigators in a multicenter trial traditionally represent diverse interests. Given the opportunity, most of them would pursue these interests. Few would like to miss an opportunity to add to the main trial questions or examinations of particular importance to them. These additions are often important scientifically. However, it is easy for a trial to become overbuilt and get out of control. It is usually a good policy to restrict additions to the basic study protocol. Special caution should be taken when the argument for inclusion is, "it would be interesting to know." The purpose of every procedure and item on the study forms should be clearly defined in advance and a test hypothesis formulated, if possible. Certain questions require the whole group. Still others cannot be answered, even if all participants are included. Therefore, in each instance, thought should be given to sample size and power calculations.

REFERENCES

1. Angell M, Kassirer JP: Setting the research straight in the breast-cancer trials, *N Engl J Med* 330: 1448-1450, 1994.
2. Aspirin Myocardial Infarction Study Research Group: A randomized, controlled trial of aspirin in persons recovered from myocardial infarction, *JAMA* 243:661-669, 1980.
3. Byington RP, for the Beta-Blocker Heart Attack Trial Research Group: Beta-Blocker Heart Attack Trial: design, methods, and baseline results, *Controlled Clin Trials* 5:382-437, 1984.

4. Carbone PP: Organization of clinical onocology in the USA: role of cancer centers, cooperative groups and community hospitals, *Eur J Cancer Clin Oncol* 21:119-154, 1985.

5. Carbone PP, Tormey DC: Organizing multicenter trials: lessons from the cooperative oncology groups, *Prev Med* 20:162-169, 1991.

6. Cohen J: Clinical trial monitoring: hit or miss? *Science* 264:1534-1537, 1994.

7. Coronary Drug Project Research Group, Canner PL, ed: The Coronary Drug Project: methods and lessons of a multicenter clinical trial, *Controlled Clin Trials* 4:273-541, 1983.

8. Croke G: Recruitment for the National Cooperative Gallstone Study, *Clin Pharmacol Ther* 25:691-694, 1979.

9. Fleiss JL: Multicentre clinical trials: Bradford Hill's contributions and some subsequent developments, *Stat Med* 1:353-359, 1982.

10. Fleming TR, DeMets DL: Monitoring of clinical trials: issues and recommendations, *Controlled Clin Trials* 14:183-197, 1993.

11. Friedman L, DeMets D: The data monitoring committee: how it operates and why, *IRB* 3:6-8, 1981.

12. Goldberg MF: Changes in the Archives, *Arch Ophthalmol* 111:39-40, 1993.

13. Greenberg BG: Conduct of cooperative field and clinical trials, *Am Stat* 13:13-28, June 1959.

14. Kassirer JP, Angell M: On authorship and acknowledgments, *N Engl J Med* 325:1510-1512, 1991.

15. Klimt CR: Principles of multi-center clinical studies. In Boissel JP, Klimt CR, ed: *Multi-center controlled trials. Principles and problems,* Paris, 1979, INSERM.

16. Lachin JM, Marks JW, Schoenfield LJ et al: Design and methodological considerations in the National Cooperative Gallstone Study: a multicenter clinical trial, *Controlled Clin Trials* 2:177-229, 1981.

17. Levin WC, Fink DJ, Porter S et al: Cooperative clinical investigation: a modality of medical science, *JAMA* 227:1295-1296, 1974.

18. Lipid Research Clinics Program Manual of Laboratory Operations: Lipid and lipoprotein analysis, vol 1, Washington, DC; DHEW Publ No (NIH)75-628, 1975.

19. Meinert CL: Organization of multicenter clinical trials, *Controlled Clin Trials* 1:305-312, 1981.

20. Meinert CL: *Clinical trials. Design, conduct and analysis,* New York, 1986, Oxford University Press.

21. Meinert CL: In defense of the corporate author for multicenter trials, *Controlled Clin Trials* 14:255-260, 1993.

22. Remington RD: Problems of university-based scientists associated with clinical trials, *Clin Pharmacol Ther* 25:662-665, 1979.

23. Sackett DL, Naylor CD: Should there be early publication of ancillary studies prior to the first primary report of an unblinded randomized clinical trial? *J Clin Epidemiol* 46:395-402, 1993.

24. Shea S, Bigger JT, Campion J, et al: Enrollment in clinical trials: institutional factors affecting enrollment in the Cardiac Arrhythmia Suppression Trial (CAST), *Controlled Clin Trials* 13:466-486, 1992.

25. Strauss RG, Connett JE, Gale RP et al: A controlled trial of prophylactic granulocyte transfusions during initial induction chemotherapy for acute myelogenous leukemia, *N Engl J Med* 305:597-603, 1981.

26. Tognoni G, Alli C, Avanzini F et al: Randomised clinical trials in general practice: lessons from a failure, *Br Med J* 303:969-971, 1991.

27. Yusuf S, Collins R, Peto R: Why do we need some large, simple, randomized trials? *Stat Med* 3:409-420, 1984.

28. Winston DJ, Ho WG, Gale RP: Prophylactic granulocyte transfusions during chemotherapy of acute nonlymphocytic leukemia, *Ann Intern Med* 94:616-622, 1981.

INDEX